PHARMACOECONOMICS
From Theory to Practice

Drug Discovery Series

Series Editor

Andrew A. Carmen

illumina, Inc.
San Diego, California

PHARMACOECONOMICS
From Theory to Practice

Edited by
RENÉE J. G. ARNOLD

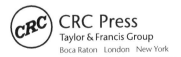

CRC Press
Taylor & Francis Group
Boca Raton London New York

CRC Press is an imprint of the
Taylor & Francis Group, an **informa** business

Chapter 8 is copyright 2010 by Dr. Lieven Annemans.

CRC Press
Taylor & Francis Group
6000 Broken Sound Parkway NW, Suite 300
Boca Raton, FL 33487-2742

© 2010 by Taylor and Francis Group, LLC
CRC Press is an imprint of Taylor & Francis Group, an Informa business

No claim to original U.S. Government works

Printed in the United States of America on acid-free paper
10 9 8 7 6 5 4 3 2 1

International Standard Book Number: 978-1-4200-8422-1 (Hardback)

Library of Congress Cataloging-in-Publication Data

Pharmacoeconomics : from theory to practice / editor, Renee J.G. Arnold.
    p. ; cm. -- (Drug discovery series ; 13)
  Includes bibliographical references and index.
  ISBN 978-1-4200-8422-1 (hardcover : alk. paper)
  1. Drugs--Cost effectiveness. 2. Pharmacy--Economic aspects. 3. Decision making. I.
Arnold, Renee J. G. II. Title. III. Series: Drug discovery
  series ; 13.
  [DNLM: 1. Economics, Pharmaceutical. 2. Costs and Cost Analysis. 3. Decision
Making. 4. Outcome Assessment (Health Care)--economics. QV 736 P5374 2010]
  RS100.P433 2010
  338.4'76151--dc22

                                                        2009032763

Visit the Taylor & Francis Web site at
http://www.taylorandfrancis.com

and the CRC Press Web site at
http://www.crcpress.com

Contents

Preface

The genesis of this book was the pharmacoeconomics research and other outcomes projects my colleagues and I have completed for our pharmaceutical company and government clients over many years. The chapter ideas came specifically from the Introduction to Pharmacoeconomics course I developed and currently teach for the Mount Sinai School of Medicine Master of Public Health program. I have collaborated extensively with many of the colleagues who have written chapters for this book, and I am truly grateful to these extremely busy people, who have contributed their valuable time and collective wisdom to make it useful and practical. Some of the views expressed herein may be controversial but, after all, experts may still disagree and some disagreement is healthy if it leads to useful dialogue and changes in practice that will benefit populations and individual patients.

This book is meant to provide an introduction to the major concepts and principles of pharmacoeconomics, with particular emphasis on modeling, methodologies, and data sources and application to real world dilemmas. Readers will learn about the international use of pharmacoeconomics in drug regulation, drug approval, and pricing. They are also given examples of pharmacoeconomic models used to support these purposes in government, the pharmaceutical industry, and healthcare settings (e.g., pharmacoeconomic analyses of a public health vaccination program). In particular, the example of collaboration among members of the pharmaceutical industry, academia, and government in the development of the recently approved human papillomavirus vaccine is used as a running theme through the majority of the chapters to demonstrate the full range of ethical and moral issues, as well as overall public health and commercial concerns that are often involved in decisions entailing pharmacoeconomic issues. Lest readers think these issues esoteric or untimely, they are referred to a recent Institute of Medicine Report (Institute of Medicine of the National Academies, Roundtable on evidence-based medicine: Learning healthcare system concepts, 2008) that stated that the best value is derived by "applying the evidence we have about the medical care that is most effective" and also by improving our "timely generation of evidence on the relative effectiveness, efficiency, and safety of available and emerging interventions." These principles are being embodied, for example, in the much-discussed potential U.S. Institute for Comparative Effectiveness Research (interestingly, the same acronym as an oft-used concept in pharmacoeconomics, that of the incremental cost-effectiveness ratio, or ICER) and in guidances rendered by the U.K.'s National Institute for Health and Clinical Excellence (NICE). Pharmacogenomics, or the use of personalized medicine, will be combined with cost-effectiveness analyses to inform and improve healthcare decision-making. For example, a recent theoretical Markov model showed pharmacogenomic-guided dosing for anticoagulation with warfarin to not be cost effective in patients with nonvalvular atrial fibrillation. Interestingly, another recently published algorithm using logistic regression from international retrospective databases showed that incorporating pharmacogenetic information was more likely to result in a therapeutic international normalized ratio (INR), the major method of determining anticoagulation, than use of clinical data alone. However, the data used to inform the Markov model were published studies that did not include the latter study, and the algorithm did not indicate the clinical diagnoses, nor the clinical outcomes, of the patients who were more or less likely to be within a therapeutic INR. Thus, improved and cost-effective decisions, using the best available evidence-based medicine, will require that both clinical and economic expertise, as epitomized in this book, be used.

Acknowledgments

I gratefully acknowledge my colleague and friend, Dr. Sean Ekins, who prompted me to write this book and also contributed a chapter. In addition, the expert assistance of Kirsten Groesser, a graduate student in the Mount Sinai School of Medicine Master of Public Health program, was particularly appreciated.

Editor

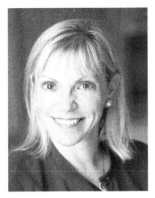

Renée J. Goldberg Arnold completed her undergraduate training at the University of Maryland and received her Doctor of Pharmacy degree from the University of Southern California in Los Angeles. She also completed a one-year post-doctoral residency at University Hospital in San Diego, which is affiliated with the University of California at San Francisco School of Pharmacy. Dr. Arnold was previously President and Co-Founder of Pharmacon International, Inc. Center for Health Outcomes Excellence; Senior Vice President, Medical Director, William J. Bologna International, Inc., a pharmaceutical marketing and advertising agency; and Assistant Professor of Clinical Pharmacy at the Arnold & Marie Schwartz College of Pharmacy and Health Sciences, Long Island University (LIU) in Brooklyn, New York. Her research interests at that time were plasma amino acid concentrations in very low birth weight infants and home-infusion total parenteral nutrition.

Dr. Arnold is currently President and CEO, Arnold Consultancy & Technology LLC, with headquarter offices in New York City, where she develops and oversees outcomes research and affiliated software for the pharmaceutical, biotech, and device industry, and federal government programs. Her special interest in evidence-based health derives from her research that deals with use of technology to collect or model real-world data for use in rational decision-making by healthcare practitioners and policy makers. For example, the company recently developed and published the results of an interactive decision tree model to compare the cost and diagnostic abilities of ultrasound performed with and without the use of an oral contrast material. An interactive program was developed that was used to train 200 representatives nationwide on formulary issues associated with use of the contrast material and was also used in discussions with reimbursement officials (CMS) in the U.S. government.

Dr. Arnold's academic titles include Adjunct Associate Professor, Master of Public Health program, Department of Community and Preventive Medicine at the Mount Sinai School of Medicine, where she has developed the pharmacoeconomics coursework and is a preceptor for MD/MPH students completing their MPH practicums. She is also Full Adjunct Professor, Division of Social Sciences and Administrative Sciences, at LIU. In that capacity, she serves as a preceptor for undergraduate and graduate students completing rotations in health outcomes and pharmacoeconomics research. Dr. Arnold also initiated internship and postdoctoral fellowship programs in pharmacoeconomics at Arnold Consultancy & Technology LLC and is a founding member and former Chair of the Education Committee of the International Society for Pharmacoeconomics and Outcomes Research (ISPOR), as well as current Chair of the Health/Disease Management Special Interest Group. In addition, she is a licensed pharmacist. Dr. Arnold is the author of numerous articles in the areas of pharmacology, pharmacoeconomics, and cost containment strategies and is a co-author of five book chapters, one in cardiovascular therapeutics, another in pharmacoeconomic analyses in cardiovascular disease, the third in computer applications in pharmaceutical research and development, the fourth in quality of life and cost of atopic dermatitis and the fifth in the reliability and validity of claims and medication databases as data sources for health/disease management programs.

Contributors

Lieven Annemans, MSc, MMan, PhD
Professor of Health Economics
Ghent University,
Brussels, Belgium

Renée J.G. Arnold
Arnold Consultancy & Technology
New York, New York
and
Master of Public Health Program
Department of Community and
    Preventive Medicine
Mount Sinai School of Medicine
New York, New York
and
Division of Social and Administrative
    Sciences
Arnold and Marie Schwartz College of
    Pharmacy
Long Island University
Brooklyn, New York

David Atkins, MD, MPH
Quality Enhancement Research
    Initiative (QUERI)
Department of Veterans Affairs
Washington, DC

Sanjeev Balu
Global Health Economics & Outcomes
    Research
Pharmaceutical Products Group Abbott
    Laboratories
Abbott Park, Illinois

J. Robert Beck, MD
Fox Chase Cancer Center
Philadelphia, Pennsylvania

Stuart Birks
Centre for Public Policy Evaluation
Massey University
Palmerston North, New Zealand

Dianne Bryant, MSc, PhD
Faculty of Health Sciences
Elborn College
University of Western Ontario
London, Ontario

J. Jaime Caro, MDCM, FRCPC, FACP
United BioSource Corporation
Lexington, Massachusetts
and
Division of General Internal Medicine
Royal Victoria Hospital
McGill University
Montreal, Quebec

Erik J. Dasbach, PhD
Health Economic Statistics
Merck Research Laboratories
North Wales, Pennsylvania

Michael Drummond, PhD
Centre for Health Economics
University of York
York, United Kingdom

Sean Ekins
Arnold Consultancy & Technology
    LLC
New York, New York

Elamin H. Elbasha
Health Economic Statistics
Merck Research Laboratories
North Wales, Pennsylvania

Rachael L. Fleurence, PhD, MBA
United BioSource Corporation
Bethesda, Maryland

Denis Getsios
United BioSource Corporation
Halifax, Nova Scotia

Gordon Guyatt, MD, MSc
Department of Clinical Epidemiology
    & Biostatistics
Hamilton Health Sciences Centre
McMaster University
Hamilton, Ontario

Alan Haycox, PhD
Health Economics Unit
University of Liverpool Management
    School
Liverpool, United Kingdom

Ralph P. Insinga, PhD
Health Economic Statistics
Merck Research Laboratories
North Wales, Pennsylvania

William F. McGhan, PharmD, PhD
Philadelphia College of Pharmacy
University of the Sciences in
    Philadelphia
Philadelphia, Pennsylvania

Prof. Maarten J. Postma
PharmacoEpidemiology &
    PharmacoEconomics
Department of Pharmacy
University of Groningen
Groningen, Netherlands

Mark S. Roberts, MD, MPP
Decision Sciences and Clinical Systems
    Modeling
General Internal Medicine
Department of Medicine
University of Pittsburgh School of
    Medicine
Pittsburgh, Pennsylvania

Kenneth J. Smith, MD, MS
Decision Sciences and Clinical Systems
    Modeling
General Internal Medicine
Department of Medicine
University of Pittsburgh School of
    Medicine
Pittsburgh, Pennsylvania

Corinna Sorenson, MPH, MHSA
LSE Health
London School of Economics
London, United Kingdom

Ryung Suh, MD
Senior Fellow
National Opinion Research Center
    (NORC)
University of Chicago
Chicago, Illinois

1 Introduction to Pharmacoeconomics

William F. McGhan

CONTENTS

> The desires to consume medicines and use pharmacoeconomics are perhaps the greatest features that distinguish humans from animals.
>
> **—Adapted from William Osler**

1.1 INTRODUCTION

Practitioners, patients, and health agencies face a multitude of conundrums as the development of new therapies seems boundless, while the money to purchase these cures is limited. How does one decide which are the best medicines to use within restricted budgets? The continuing impact of cost-containment is causing administrators and policy makers in all health fields to examine closely the costs and benefits of both proposed and existing interventions. It is increasingly obvious that purchasers and public agencies are demanding that health treatments be evaluated in terms of clinical and humanistic outcomes against the costs incurred.

Pharmacoeconomics is the field of study that evaluates the behavior or welfare of individuals, firms, and markets relevant to the use of pharmaceutical products, services, and programs.[1] The focus is frequently on the cost (inputs) and consequences (outcomes) of that use. Of necessity, it addresses the clinical, economic, and humanistic aspect of health care interventions (often diagrammed as the ECHO Model,

1

ECHO Model:
Economic, Clinical, and Humanistic Outcomes

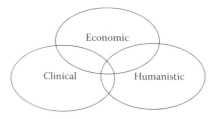

FIGURE 1.1   ECHO Model. (Kozma, CM et al. Economic, clinical, and humanistic outcomes: A planning model for pharmacoeconomic research. *Clin Ther.* 15: (1993): 1121–32.)

Figure 1.1)[2] in the prevention, diagnosis, treatment, and management of disease. Pharmacoeconomics is a collection of descriptive and analytic techniques for evaluating pharmaceutical interventions, spanning individual patients to the health care system as a whole. Pharmacoeconomic techniques include cost-minimization, cost-effectiveness, cost-utility, cost-benefit, cost of illness, cost-consequence, and any other economic analytic technique that provides valuable information to health care decision makers for the allocation of scarce resources. Pharmacoeconomics is often referred to as "health economics" or "health outcomes research," especially when it includes comparison with non-pharmaceutical therapy or preventive strategies such as surgical interventions, medical devices, or screening techniques.

Pharmacoeconomic tools are vitally important in analyzing the potential value for individual patients and the public. These methods supplement the traditional marketplace value as measured by the prices that the patient or patron is willing to pay. With government agencies and third parties' continuing concern about the higher expenditures for prescriptions, pharmaceutical manufacturers and pharmacy managers are highly cognizant that pharmaceutical interventions and services require comparative cost-justification and continual surveillance to assure cost-effective outcomes.[3–6]

From pharmaceutical research, we have seen significant therapeutic advances and breakthroughs. From health care delivery entrepreneurs we have seen numerous expanding roles for pharmacists, nurses, and physician assistants, with services such as home intravenous therapy, drug-level monitoring, parenteral nutrition management, hospice care, self-care counseling, and genetic screening for customizing therapy, among other innovations. The use of valid economic evaluation methods to measure the value and impact of new interventions can increase acceptance and appropriate use of such programs by third-party payers, government agencies, and consumers.[7–9]

There is increasing scrutiny over all aspects of health care as we attempt to balance limited finances and resources against optimal outcomes. Cost-effectiveness evaluations of pharmaceutical options are becoming mandatory for attaining adequate reimbursement and payment for services.[10,11] Pharmacoeconomic methods help document the costs and benefits of therapies and pharmaceutical services, and establish priorities for those options to help in appropriately allocating resources in ever-changing health care landscapes.

1.2 ANALYTICAL PERSPECTIVES

Point of view is a vital consideration in pharmacoeconomics. If a medicine is providing a positive benefit in relation to cost in terms of value to society as a whole, the service may not be valued in the same way by separate segments of society. For example, a drug therapy that reduces the number of admissions or patient days in an acute care institution is positive from society's point of view but not necessarily from that of the institution's administrator, who depends on a high number of patient admissions to meet expenses. Thus, one must determine whose interests are being served when identifying outcome criteria for evaluation. When considering pharmacoeconomic perspectives, one must always consider who pays the costs and who receives the benefits. A favorable economic analysis that showed savings in clinic utilization from the employer perspective would probably not be viewed positively from the clinic's budget perspective. More broadly, what is viewed as saving money for society may be viewed differently by private third-party payers, administrators, health providers, governmental agencies, or even the individual patient. It is generally agreed among health economists that the societal perspective should always be discussed in an evaluative report, even though the focus of the report might deal with other segments such as hospitals or insurance agencies. In the United States, with many different health care delivery and payer approaches, this can be complicated, and analyses are often done from multiple perspectives to assist adjudication by multiple stakeholders.

1.3 CODE OF ETHICS

The International Society for Pharmacoeconomics and Outcomes Research (ISPOR) has published a code of ethics that is vital to the honesty and transparency of the discipline.[12] The code encourages pharmacoeconomists to maintain the highest ethical standards because the academy recognizes that activities of its members affect a number of constituencies. These include but are not limited to: (1) Patients who are ultimately going to experience the greatest impact of the research; (2) practitioners who will be treating or not treating patients with therapies, medications, and procedures made available or not made available because of the research; (3) governments, employers, decision-makers, and payers who must decide what is covered so as to optimize the health of the patient and resource utilization; (4) professional outcomes researchers; (5) colleagues, where relationships in conducting research and related activities are particularly critical; (6) research employees concerned about how they are regarded, compensated, and treated by the researchers for whom they work; (7) students who work for researchers, where respect and lack of exploitation are important because they are the future of the discipline; and (8) clients for whom the research is conducted, and the researchers' relationships with them.

The ISPOR code of ethics lists many standards for researchers, but a sample section of the code related to "design and research practices" is as follows:

1. Maintain a current knowledge of research practices.
2. Adhere to the standards of practice for their respective fields of research and identify any official guidelines/standards used.

3. Research designs should be defined a priori, reported transparently, defended relative to alternatives, and planned to minimize all types of bias.
4. Respect the rights of research subjects in designing and conducting studies.
5. Respect the reputations and rights of colleagues when engaged in collaborative projects.
6. Maintain and protect the integrity of the data used in their studies.
7. Not draw conclusions beyond those which their data would support.

1.4   OVERVIEW OF ECONOMIC EVALUATION METHODS

This section will introduce the reader with a brief overview of the methodologies based on the two core pharmacoeconomic approaches, namely cost-effectiveness analysis (CEA) and cost-utility analysis (CUA). Table 1.1 provides a basic comparison of these methods with cost-of-illness, cost-minimization, and cost-benefit analysis. One can differentiate between the various approaches according to the units used to measure the inputs and outcomes, as shown in the table. In general, the outputs in CEA are related to various natural units of measure, such as lives saved, life-years added, disability-days prevented, blood pressure, lipid level, and so on. Cost-benefit analysis (CBA) uses monetary values (e.g., euros, dollars, pounds, yen) to measure both inputs and outputs of the respective interventions. Further discussion and examples of these techniques have been presented elsewhere.[1–3,13–21] It is hoped that the evaluation mechanisms delineated further in this book will be helpful in managing pharmaceutical interventions toward improving societal value and generate greater acceptance by health authorities, administrators, and the public. Using the human papillomavirus (HPV) vaccine as an example for case studies, other chapters in this book will further illustrate the various analytical methodologies related to CEA, CUA, CBA, etc.

1.5   QUALITY OF LIFE AND PATIENT PREFERENCES

Significant components in pharmacoeconomics are patient outcomes and quality of life (QoL) with an expanding list of related factors to consider (Table 1.2).[14,15] Although it is recognized that there are physical, mental, and social impairments associated with disease, there is not always consensus on how to accurately measure many of these factors. Consequently, the concept of satisfaction with care is often overlooked in cost-effectiveness studies and even during the approval process of the U.S. Food and Drug Administration (FDA). Generally, pharmacoeconomic and outcomes researchers consider QoL a vital factor in creating a full model of survival and service improvement. QoL is related to clinical outcomes as much as drugs, practitioners, settings, and types of disease. The question becomes how to select and utilize the most appropriate instruments for measuring QoL and satisfaction with care in a meaningful way.

The quality-adjusted life year (QALY) has become a major concept in pharmacoeconomics. It is a measure of health improvement used in CUA, which combines mortality and QoL gains and considers the outcome of a treatment measured as the number of years of life saved, adjusted for quality.

TABLE 1.1

Comparison of Pharmacoeconomic Methods and Calculations

Method	Abbr	Basic Formula	Discounting Math	Input	Output	Results Expressed	Goal Determine:	Advantage / Disadvantage	Example
Cost of Illness	COI	$(DC+IC)$	$\sum_{t=1}^{n}[C_t/(1+r)^t]$	$	$	Total cost of illness	Total cost of illness	Does not look at TXs separately	Cost of migraine in U.S.
Cost Minimization Analysis	CMA	C_1-C_2 or [Preferred Formula] $(DC_1+IC_1)-(DC_2+IC_2)$	$\sum_{t=1}^{n}[C_t/(1+r)^t]$	$	Assumed Equal	Net cost savings	Lowest cost TX	Assume both TXs have same effectiveness	Assume two antibiotics have the same effects for killing infection but differ on nursing and intravenous cost
Cost-Effectiveness Analysis	CEA	$(C_1-C_2)/(E_1-E_2)$ or [Preferred Formula] $(DC_1+IC_1)-(DC_2+IC_2)/(E_1-E_2)$	$\sum_{t=1}^{n}[C_t/(1+r)^t]/\sum_{t=1}^{n}[E_t/(1+r)^t]$	$	Health Effect	Incremental cost against change in unit of outcome	TX attaining effect for lower cost	Compare TXs that have same type of effect units	Compare two HTN prescriptions for life years
Cost–Benefit Analysis or Net Benefit	CBA	$(B_1-B_2)/(DC_1+IC_1)-(DC_2-IC_2)$ or [Preferred Formula] Net Benefit $= (B_1-B_2)-(DC_1+IC_1)-(DC_2+IC_2)$	$\sum_{t=1}^{n}[B_t/(1+r)^t]/\sum_{t=1}^{n}[C_t/(1+r)^t]$ or $\sum_{t=1}^{n}[(B_t-C_t)/(1+r)^t]$	$	Dollars	Net benefit or ratio of incremental benefits to incremental costs	TX giving best net benefit or higher B/C ratio (or return on investment)	TXs can have different effects, but must be put into dollars	Compare two cholesterol prescriptions and convert life years to wages
Cost-Utility Analysis	CUA	$(C_1-C_2)/(U_1-U_2)$ or [Preferred Formula] $(DC_1+IC_1)-(DC_2+IC_2)/(U_1-U_2)$	$\sum_{t=1}^{n}[C_t/(1+r)^t]/\sum_{t=1}^{n}[U_t/(1+r)^t]$	$	Patient Preference	Incremental cost against change in unit of outcome adjusted by patient preference	TX attaining effect (adjusted for patient preference) for lower cost	Preferences are difficult to measure	Compare two cancer prescriptions and use QoL adjusted life years gained

Note: DC = direct cost; IC = indirect cost; r = discount rate; t = time; HTN = hpertension; QoL = quality of life; TX = treatment or intervention.

TABLE 1.2

Outcomes and Quality of Life Measurement Approaches

    I. Basic Outcomes List -- Six D's
- A. Death
- B. Disease
- C. Disability
- D. Discomfort
- E. Dissatisfaction
- F. Dollars (Euros, Pounds, Yen)

  II. Major Quality of Life Domains
- A. Physical status and functional abilities
- B. Psychological status and well-being
- C. Social interactions
- D. Economic status and factors

 III. Expanded Outcomes List
- A. Clinical End Points
  1. Symptoms and Signs
  2. Laboratory Values
  3. Death
- B. General Well-being
  1. Pain/Discomfort
  2. Energy/Fatigue
  3. Health Perceptions
  4. Opportunity (future)
  5. Life Satisfaction
- C. Satisfaction with Care/Providers
  1. Access
  2. Convenience
  3. Financial Coverage
  4. Quality
  5. General

One approach to conceptualizing QoL and outcomes data collected in clinical trials is to consider the source of the data. There are several potential sources of data to evaluate the safety and efficacy of a new drug. Potential sources and examples are listed below:

- Patient-reported outcomes (PROs)[16]—e.g., global impression, functional status, health-related QoL (HRQoL), symptoms
- Caregiver-reported outcomes—e.g., dependency, functional status
- Clinician-reported outcomes—e.g., global impressions, observations, tests of function
- Physiological outcomes—e.g., pulmonary function, blood glucose, tumor size

1.6 DECISION ANALYSIS AND MODELING

Decision analysis is defined as "… a systematic approach to decision making under conditions of uncertainty." Decision analysis is an approach that is explicit, quantitative, and prescriptive.[1]

It is explicit in that it forces the decision maker to separate the logical structure into its component parts so that they can be analyzed individually, then recombined systematically to suggest a decision. It is quantitative in that the decision maker is compelled to be precise about values placed on outcomes. Finally, it is prescriptive in that it aids in deciding what a person should do under a given set of circumstances. The basic steps in decision analysis include identifying and bounding the decision problem; structuring the decision problem over time; characterizing the information needed to fill in the structure, and then choosing the preferred course of action.

Pharmacoeconomic models can involve decision trees, spreadsheets, Markov analyses, discrete event simulation, basic forecasting, and many other approaches.[17]

In a simplified form, a decision tree can double as an educational tool for presenting available therapeutic options and probable consequences to patients and decision makers.[18,19] Wennberg and others have explored ways to involve patients in a shared decision-making process.[19] One of his projects involved a computer interactive program on prostate surgery education. The program explains to patients the probability of success, the degree of pain that might be encountered at each step, and what the procedure actually entails. After viewing this program with visual graphic depictions of the surgery, many of the patients changed their decisions about wanting surgery rather than watchful waiting. This reduction in a major procedure resulted from a greater focus on QoL and patient satisfaction. With further evaluation and perhaps modification of the computer program, it should also produce more cost-effective care. Wennberg's work is an application of outcomes research that helped to weigh costs, utilities, and QoL for the patient.

1.7 RANKING PRIORITIES: DEVELOPING A FORMULARY LIST

Table 1.3 illustrates how cost–utility ratios can be used to rank alternative therapies as one might do for a drug formulary. The numbers in the second column of the table list the total QALYs for all of a decision maker's patient population that is expected to benefit from the treatment options in each row. The numbers in the third column detail the total cost of treatment for all of one's targeted patient population for each treatment option in each row. For the next step in the selection process, rank the therapy options by their cost–utility ratios. Options have already been ranked appropriately in this table. For the final selection step, add each therapy option into one's formulary, moving down each row until your allocated budget (using the cost column) is exhausted. In other words, if you have only $420,000, you would be able to fund therapies A, B, and C. These options have the best cost-utility for one's population given one's available budget. Cost-effectiveness and cost–utility ratios are sometimes presented in similar fashion and are called League Tables. Tengs et al.[20] have published an extensive list of interventions and Neumann and colleagues[21] maintain a website with a substantial list of cost–utility ratios based on health economic studies,

TABLE 1.3
Health Economic Selections* with Fixed Budget

Therapy or Program	QALYS [a]	Cost [b] ($thousand)	Cost–Utility Ratio ($thousand)
A	50	100	2
B	50	200	4
C	20	120	6
D	25	200	8
E	10	120	12
F	5	80	16
G	10	180	18
H	10	220	22
I	15	450	30

[a] Total Quality-Adjusted Life Years (QALYs) for all of patient population benefiting.

[b] Total cost of treatment for all of targeted patient population.

[*] Selection procedure: first, rank therapies by cost–utility ratios, then add therapeutic options until budget is exhausted.

with a sample in Table 1.4. These listings must be used with caution because there are a number of criticisms of rankings with league tables, including:

- Different reports use different methods
- What the comparators were (e.g., which drugs, which surgeries)
- Difficult to be flexible about future comparators
- Orphan and rare disease versus more prevalent diseases
- Randomized prospective trials versus retrospective studies
- Regional and international differences in clinical resource use
- Regional and international differences in direct and indirect costs of treatment
- Statistical confidence intervals of cost and outcomes results
- Difficult to test statistical significance between the pharmacoeconomic ratios of treatments listed

1.8   INCREMENTAL ANALYSIS AND QUADRANTS

Whether one is dealing with cost analyses or decision analysis, it is important to properly compare one treatment with another, and one should understand the concepts in incremental analysis. Incremental analysis does not mean that one is adding a second therapy to the patient's regimen, but it is a technique for comparing one therapy with another. The basic incremental formulas are as follows:

$$\text{CEA: } (\text{Cost}_1 - \text{Cost}_2) / (\text{Effectiveness}_1 - \text{Effectiveness}_2)$$

or

$$\text{CUA: } (\text{Cost}_1 - \text{Cost}_2) / (\text{QALYs}_1 - \text{QALYs}_2)$$

TABLE 1.4
Selected Cost–Utility Ratios from the CEA Registry

Intervention vs. Comparator in Target Population	C/U Ratio in 2002 US$
Elective cesarean section vs. vaginal delivery in 25-year-old HIV-infected women with detectable HIV RNA	Cost-saving
Treatment with interferon alpha for 6 months vs. no treatment (conventional management only) in 40-year-old patients with chronic hepatitis C infection	$ 5,000/QALY
Initial screen for presence of protective antibody with vaccination against hepatitis A if susceptible vs. no vaccination in 2-year-old healthy children in developed countries	$ 8,100/QALY
Combined outreach initiative for pneumococcal and influenza vaccination vs. usual vaccine availability in people 65 years and older	$ 13,000/QALY
Statin therapy vs. usual care in patients aged 75–84 with a history of myocardial infarction	$ 21,000/QALY
Intensive school-based tobacco prevention program—over 50-year period, assumes 30% smoking reduction, dissipates in 4 years vs. status quo (current average national tobacco educational practices) in every 7th and 8th grade in the United States	$ 22,000/QALY
Driver side air bag vs. no air bags in driving population and car passengers	$ 30,000/QALY
Systematic screening for diabetes mellitus vs. none (usual practice) for all individuals aged 25 and older	$ 67,000/QALY
Tamoxifen chemoprevention vs. surveillance in women at high risk for breast cancer	$ 84,000 - 160,000/ QALY
Annual screen of primary care patients for depression vs. no screening in 40-year-old primary care patients	$ 210,000/QALY
Bisphosphonates vs. no treatment in women aged 50 with average risk of hip fracture	$ 300,000/QALY
National regulation against using a cellular telephone while driving vs. no regulation in United States population in 1997	$ 350,000/QALY
Varicella vaccination without testing vs. Varicella antibody testing followed by vaccination if negative in 20–29-year-old adults with no history of chickenpox	$ 2,300,000/QALY
Examination and culture for herpes virus vs. examination only in pregnant women with a history of genital herpes, active disease during pregnancy, or sexual partners with a proven history of genital herpes	$57 million/QALY
Thrombolysis vs. surgery in 65-year-old patients presenting with acute lower extremity ischemia	Dominated

Source: Reprinted with permission from Neumann, P and Olchanski, N. A Web-based Registry of Cost-Utility Analyses. *ISPOR Connections* Vol.10 No. 1: February 15, 2004.[22]

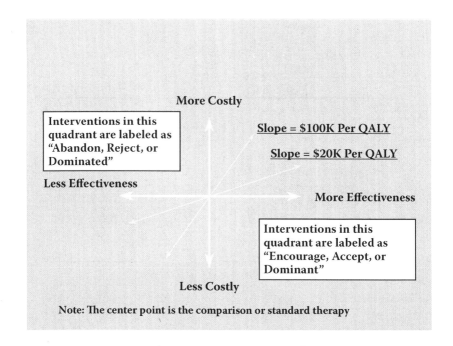

FIGURE 1.2   Incremental ratios and quadrants.

An interesting way of displaying this information is illustrated in Figure 1.2. By displaying this information in quadrants, one can more easily visualize the relationship between therapies. Drugs that are cheaper and more effective would fall in the "accept" or "dominant" sector, while drugs that are more expensive and less effective would be "dominated." The slopes of the lines represent the incremental cost–effectiveness ratios and, in general, therapies between $20,000 to $100,000 per life year saved (or per QALY) are often considered acceptable in public policy reports.

A classic paper involving incremental analysis deals with the comparison of tissue plasminogen activator (TPA) to streptokinase.[23] In this study, the important question did not involve looking at the CEA ratio of each drug individually; instead, it analyzed the incremental differences of the new drug, TPA, over the standard therapy at the time. The analysis demonstrated that TPA, when compared with streptokinase, had an incremental cost per life year saved of about $40,000, which was considered a socially acceptable value.[23]

1.9   FOURTH HURDLE AND DRUG APPROVALS

The classic basic elements required for approval of new drugs are (1) therapeutic efficacy, (2) drug safety, and (3) product quality. But more recently, with the realization of limited national and global financial resources, another drug approval step has been added that considers factors related to pricing and reimbursement. Therefore, in at least two dozen countries, there is an additional jump before the marketing of pharmaceuticals that is often called "the fourth hurdle." This criterion, usually involving cost-effectiveness and pharmacoeconomic analyses, is required even when efficacy, safety, and quality have been demonstrated. Such a fourth hurdle was initially introduced in Austria for the reimbursement of new drugs. Despite the extra development costs to conduct these studies, and concern from the pharmaceutical industry, this fourth step can also be viewed as a positive opportunity to better support more innovative medicines over me-too drugs. Pharmacoeconomic analyses can provide quantitative evidence for more rational new drug approvals. And with post-marketing surveillance and patient registries, pharmacoeconomics should be able to help sustain cost-effective drug utilization throughout the life cycle of the therapy.

1.10   FROM BOARD ROOM TO BEDSIDE

Figure 1.3 provides a basic consult form that suggests a framework for pharmacoeconomic assessments. If a decision between alternative treatments needs to be made, this form could help structure the calculations and considerations related to pharmacoeconomics. With the current technology and resources in most facilities, at an individual patient level, certainly, it would be impossible to have sufficient time with each patient to individually apply detailed calculations. Evolving e-health technologies and the Internet may facilitate patient applications in the future. This consult worksheet is a basic template, then, for evaluating therapeutic options for a drug formulary, framing a formal pharmacoeconomic study. In an ideal pharmacoeconomic world, it could be used for a basic calculation sheet to be discussed with a physician or patient and maintained in a patient's medical record.

Although a pharmacoeconomic analysis of a new treatment may indicate that the intervention is cost-effective versus existing therapy, the continued clinical success of the new treatment is paramount. The least cost-effective drug, from an individual patient perspective, is the drug that does not work. Substantially more research remains to be performed not only on future drugs in the pipeline but also on existing interventions in the marketplace so that we can maximize patient outcomes and enhance cost-effectiveness. Computer technology and the Internet are tremendous resources for disseminating and applying pharmacoeconomic techniques, and then continually documenting outcomes for practitioners and patients.[24] It is expected that reimbursement plans will include more incentives (paying for performance) for improvements in these economic, clinical, and humanistic outcomes.[25] Thus, pharmacoeconomics reaches from the societal (macro) and board room level out to the clinical and patient (micro) level, as envisioned in Figure 1.4.

Even health practitioners will be increasingly expected to allocate scarce resources based on pharmacoeconomic principles. Using pharmacoeconomics and disease management concepts, health providers can produce more cost-effective outcomes in a number of ways.[26] For example:

- Decrease drug–drug and drug–lab interactions.
- Increase the percentage of patients in therapeutic control.

I. ID NUMBER:

II. TREATMENT OBJECTIVES:

III. PERSPECTIVE:

☐ Society ☐ Patient ☐ Payer ☐ Provider ☐ Hospital ☐ Other

IV. TYPE OF ANALYSIS

☐ COI ☐ CMA ☐ CBA ☐ CEA ☐ CUA ☐ Other

V. TREATMENT OPTIONS:

	Treatment A	Treatment B
Names of Treatment:		
Disease/Symptom:		
Major Outcome Measure:		

VI. COST FACTORS

	Treatment A	Treatment B	Incremental
A. DIRECT COSTS: (HEALTH CARE RESOURCES)			
Practitioner			
Clinic/Hospital			
Acquisition			
Administration			
Monitoring			
Managing			
ADRs			
B. DIRECT COSTS: (NON-HEALTH CARE RESOURCES)			
Transport			
Telephone			
C. INDIRECT COSTS			
Morbidity Costs (time lost from work in dollars)			

	Treatment A	Treatment B	Incremental

D. INTANGIBLE COSTS (difficult to put into dollars)

Discomfort/Pain

Emotional

QoL Quality of Life Index (as percentage of full health)

                  TOTAL COST

VII. MEASUREMENT CONSIDERATIONS of effectiveness, benefit, or utility.

Unit of measurement

COI   (direct and indirect costs of illness)

CMA   (input costs only, outcomes assumed equivalent)

CBA & NB (input = $, outcomes all in dollars)

CEA   (input = $, outcomes in natural units, mmHg, etc.)

CUA   (input = $, outcomes in utiles, QALYs)

Other

	Treatment A	Treatment B	Incremental

VIII. CALCULATED RESULTS: (Ratios are results of Inputs divided by Outcomes.)

COI   (direct & indirect costs of illness)

CMA   (total direct & indirect costs)

CBA   (benefit over cost ratio)

NB   [benefit minus cost]

CEA   (cost over effectiveness ratio)

CUA   (cost over utility ratio)

Other

FIGURE 1.3 Pharmacoeconomic consult template. See Table 1.1 for definitions. Developed by McGhan, W.F. and Smith. M.D. Reprinted with permission. Interactive version available through www.healthstrategy.com

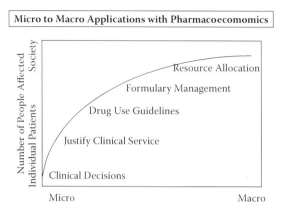

FIGURE 1.4   Micro to macro applications with Pharmacoeconomics.

- Reduce the overall costs of the treatment by utilizing more efficient modes of therapy.
- Reduce the unnecessary use of emergency rooms and medical facilities.
- Reduce the rate of hospitalization attributable to or affected by the improper use of drugs.
- Contribute to better use of health manpower by utilizing automation, telemedicine, and technicians.
- Decrease the incidence and intensity of iatrogenic disease, such as adverse drug reactions.

By improved monitoring and assessment of drug therapy outcomes, practitioners can provide early detection of therapy failure and provide cost-effective prescribing.

1.11   CONCLUSIONS

In this chapter, a general introduction to pharmacoeconomics has been provided. There are many reports in the literature that demonstrate that the benefit of medicines is worth the cost to the payer(s) for numerous disease states. Still, it must be realized that even though most research is positive, there is a need to continue to develop interventions and services that maximize the benefit-to-cost ratio to society. Even though new drugs can demonstrate positive ratios of benefit to cost, society or agencies will ultimately invest their resources in programs that have the higher benefit-to-cost or the best cost–utility ratio. Similarly, the health system must be convinced that any new therapy is worth utilizing, with a resultant modification or even deletion of other, less effective, therapeutic options, if necessary. All sectors of society, and certainly the pharmaceutical arena, must fully understand pharmacoeconomics if everyone around the globe is to have optimal health care and a better future.[27]

REFERENCES

1. Berger, ML et al. *Health Care Cost, Quality, and Outcomes. ISPOR Book of Terms.* International Society for Pharmacoeconomics and Outcomes Research 2003.
2. Kosma, CM et al. Economic, clinical, and humanistic outcomes: A planning model for pharmacoeconomic research. *Clin. Ther.* 1993;15:1121–32.
3. Rascati, K. *Essentials of Pharmacoeconomics.* Philadelphia: Lippincott, Williams & Wilkins. 2008.
4. McGhan, WF. Pharmacoeconomics and the evaluation of drugs and services. *Hosp. Form.* 28(1993):365–378.
5. McGhan, W, Rowland, C, and Bootman, JL. Cost-Benefit and Cost-Effectiveness: Methodology for Evaluating Clinical Pharmacy Service. *Am. J. Hosp. Pharm.* 35 (1978): 133–140.
6. Gold, MR et al. *Cost-Effectiveness in Health and Medicine.* New York: Oxford University Press. 1996.
7. Ray, M. Administration Direction for Clinical Practice. *Am. J. Hosp. Pharm.* 36 (1979): 308.
8. Bootman, JL, McGhan, WF, and Schondelmeyer, SW. Application of cost-benefit and cost-effectiveness analysis to clinical practice. *Drug Intell. Clinical Pharm.* 16 (1982): 235–243.
9. McGhan, WF and Lewis, NJ. Guidelines for pharmacoeconomic studies. *Clinical Therapeut.* 1992;3:486-494.
10. Enright, SM. Changes in health-care financing resulting from the 1984 federal budget. *Am. J. Hosp. Pharm.* 40 (1983): 835–838.
11. Curtiss, FR. Current concepts in hospital reimbursement. *Am. J. Hosp. Pharm.* 40 (1983): 586–591.
12. Palumbo, F, Barnes, R, Deverka, M, McGhan, W, Mullany, L, Wertheimer, A. ISPOR Code of Ethics for Researchers background article—Report of the ISPOR Task Force on Code of Ethics for Researchers. Value Health 2004;7:111–117.
13. Weinstein, MC and Stason, B. Foundations and cost/effectiveness analysis for health and medical practitioners. *NEJM* 296 (1977): 716–721.
14. Ellwood, PM. Outcomes management: A technology of patient experience. *NEJM* 318 (1988): 1549–1556.
15. MacKeigan, LD and Pathak, DS. Overview of health-related quality-of-life measures. *AJHP.* 49 (1992): 2236–2245.
16. Valderas, JM et al. The impact of measuring patient-reported outcomes in clinical practice: A systematic review of the literature. *Qual Life Res.* Mar;17(2) (2008): 179–193. Epub 2008 Jan 4.
17. Briggs, A, Claxton, K, and Sculpher, M. *Decision modeling for health economic evaluation.* New York: Oxford University Press. 2006.
18. Einarson, TR, McGhan, WF, Bootman, JL. Decision analysis applied to pharmacy practice. *AJHP* 42 (1985): 364–371.
19. Wennberg, JE. The paradox of appropriate care. *JAMA* 258 (1987): 2568–2569.
20. Tengs, TO, Adams, ME, Pliskin, JS, Safran, DG, Siegel, JE, Weinstein, MC, and Graham, JD. Five-hundred life-saving interventions and their cost-effectiveness. *Risk Anal.* 15(3) (1995): 369–389.
21. Center for the Evaluation of Value and Risk in Health. The Cost-Effectiveness Analysis Registry [Internet]. (Boston), ICRHPS, Tufts Medical Center. Available from: www.cearegistry.org [accessed on January 5, 2008].
22. Neumann, P and Olchanski, N. A Web-based Registry of Cost-Utility Analyses. *ISPOR Connections* Vol.10 No. 1: February 15, 2004.

23. Mark, DB. et al. Cost effectiveness of thrombolytic therapy with tissue plasminogen activator as compared with streptokinase for acute myocardial infarction. *NEJM* 332 (1995): 1418–24.

24. McGhan, W. Evaluation criteria for pharmacoeconomic and health economic internet resources. *Expert Rev. Pharmacoecon. Outcomes Res.* 2(4) (2002):89–96.

25. Anon. AHRQ Resources on Pay for Performance (P4P) http://www.ahrq.gov/qual/pay-4per.htm (accessed October 6, 2008).

26. Nierenberg, D. et al. Contemporary issues in medicine: Education in safe and effective prescribing practices. *AAMC.* July 2008.

27. McGhan WF, Smith MD. Improving the cost-benefits of pharmaceutical services: Pharmacoeconomics 101. *Pharm. Bus.* (Spring) (1993): 6–10.

2 Decision Modeling Techniques

Mark S. Roberts and Kenneth J. Smith

CONTENTS

2.1 INTRODUCTION

The fundamental purpose of a pharmacoeconomic model is to evaluate the expected costs and outcomes of a decision (or series of decisions) about the use of a pharmacotherapy compared with one or many alternatives. Decision modeling provides an excellent framework for developing estimates of these outcomes in a flexible analytic framework that allows the investigator to test many alternative assumptions and scenarios. In addition to providing an "answer" to a specific pharmacoeconomic decision, one of the major advantages of having a model of a particular decision is that the model can provide significant information regarding how the answer changes with different basic assumptions, or under different conditions. It is this ability to evaluate multiple "what if" scenarios that provides a substantial amount of the power of pharmacoeconomic modeling.

This chapter provides a brief introduction to the many methods of constructing decision models for the purpose of pharmacoeconomic analyses. After describing the basic methods of decision analysis, basic branch and node decision trees are described in the context of an actual pharmacoeconomic problem. Many of the techniques used to make these models more clinically detailed and realistic are detailed in other chapters in this book, and these chapters are referenced where appropriate.

2.2   DECISION MODELING PARADIGM

The most important aspect of the decision modeling process is that it must represent the choice that is being made. When constructing a model of a clinical or pharmacological decision, a series of characteristics of the actual problem must be represented in the model structure and method. First, the model should represent the set of reasonable choices between which the decision maker must choose. Leaving out reasonable potential or common strategies subjects the model to criticisms of bias and selecting comparators that make the superiority of a particular strategy more likely. Even if "doing nothing" is not a viable clinical alternative, it is often useful to include such a strategy as a baseline check of the model's ability to predict the outcomes of the natural history of untreated disease.

Once the strategies are outlined, the modeler must enumerate the possible outcomes implied by each strategy. These outcomes are not always symmetric; a surgical therapy may have an operative mortality whereas a medical therapy may not. However, all potential outcomes that can occur and are considered relevant to clinicians taking care of the problem should be included. Pharmacoeconomic models are characterized by their simultaneous assessment of the clinical and cost consequences of various strategies, so even clinically insignificant outcomes that incur significant costs may need to be modeled. To make an appropriate decision regarding what consequences and outcomes to include, the modeler must make decisions regarding four characteristics: the perspective of the analysis, the setting or context of the analysis, the appropriate level of detail or granularity, and the appropriate time horizon.[1]

Perspective: The perspective of the analysis determines from whose point of view the decision is being made. Defining the perspective of the analysis is especially important in pharmacoeconomic analyses because the costs that are incurred depend heavily on the perspective. The most typical perspectives used in pharmacoeconomic analyses are that of the payer (insurance companies, HMOs, Medicare), in which only those costs incurred by the payer are included, a provider (hospital, health system, provider group) in which the costs and reimbursements for providing a particular service are included, and society, in which all costs and effects are included,

TABLE 2.1
Characteristics of Potential Perspectives

Perspective	Characteristics
Societal	Broadest perspective includes all costs and benefits, regardless of who bears them. Considered the appropriate perspective for a reference case from the U.S. Panel on Cost Effectiveness in Health Care
Payer	Typical perspective for payment/coverage decisions
Health Plan/HMO	
Individual	Appropriate perspective for understanding optimal decisions or strategies for individual patients or groups of patients

irrespective of who has borne them (see Table 2.1). A more detailed description of perspective is provided in standard texts.[2] For example, an analysis conducted from the payer perspective on a particular treatment for a neurological condition might not take into account the differential effects of the various therapies being studied on the patients' ability to return to work, as these are not costs or benefits that are borne by the payer. However, these costs and benefits should be included if the analysis is being conducted from the perspective of society.

Setting: The setting defines the characteristics for which a particular decision is being made. Just as any study design needs to define the population, the study will evaluate (by inclusion and exclusion criteria in randomized controlled trials or by case and control definition in many observational designs), a decision model must explicitly state the type of patient(s) to which the decision will be applied. For example, in developing a pharmacoeconomic model of the use of statins in hypercholesterolemia, the modeler must decide the distribution of age, gender, lipid levels, comorbid disease, and other variables that are important and need to be represented in the model. A model that demonstrated a particular result in one group of patients is not likely to have the same result in populations with different characteristics.

Granularity: The correct amount of detail to include in a model of a given clinical situation is one of the most difficult decisions a modeler must make in the development of a representation of a particular decision and its consequences. Albert Einstein once said: "Things should be made as simple as possible ... but not simpler." Although this concept is directly translatable to building decision models, it provides little actual guidance; the clinical and pharmacoeconomic characteristics of the problem dictate the level of detail required to represent the problem. For example, in many analyses of medications, the modeler must represent side effects of the medication. Should a model contain all of the individual potential side effects and their likelihoods of occurring, or can they be grouped into side effects of various severities such as mild (which might only be assumed to change the quality of life of the patient and perhaps decrease medication adherence) and major (which might be assumed to require some form of medical intervention)? One of the best methods to decide the appropriate level of detail is to engage in discussions and collaborations with clinicians who treat the particular condition in question such that the areas of importance to them can be sufficiently detailed. The model itself can sometimes be used to test whether more detail is necessary. Conducting sensitivity analysis (see Chapter 12) on a particular aspect of the model can indicate whether more detail is required. If multiple sensitivity analyses on the parameters of a more aggregated or simplistic section of a model do not have a significant impact on the results, it is not likely that expanding the detail of that section of the model will provide new or important insights.

Time horizon: The time horizon indicates the period of time over which the specific strategies are chosen and the relevant outcomes occur. This time frame is generally determined by the biology of the particular problem. If an analysis is being done comparing different treatments for acute dysuria in young women, the time frame of the analysis may be as short as a week, as long-term sequelae are extremely uncommon in this condition. In contrast, in an analysis of the effects of various interventions to alter cardiovascular risk, the time frame might very likely be the entire lifetime of the patient. It is important to remember that the time frame does not include only those events directly related to the various strategies, but all of the future events implied by choosing each strategy. If a particular intervention increases the risk of a life-changing complication (stroke, heart attack, pulmonary embolism), the long-term effects of the complications need to be taken into account as well.

2.2.1 Types of Decision Modeling Techniques

Many methodologies and modeling types can be used to create and evaluate decision models, and the modeler should use the method most appropriate to the particular problem being addressed. The choice is dependent upon the complexity of the problem, the need to model outcomes over extended periods of time, and whether resource constraints and interactions of various elements in the model are required. We will describe in detail the development of simple branch and node decision trees, which set the context for many of the other techniques. A brief review of several methodologies is then provided; more detailed descriptions of many of these techniques can be found in other chapters in this book.

2.2.2 Decision Trees

The classic decision analysis structure is the branch and node decision tree, which is illustrated in Figure 2.1. The decision tree has several components that are always present and need to be carefully developed. A decision model comprises the modeling structure itself (the decision tree), which represents the decision that is being made and the outcomes that can occur as the result of each decision, the probabilities that the various outcomes will occur, and the values of the outcomes if they do occur. Similar to any other research problem, the decision tree should start with a specific problem formulation, which in the figure is a choice between therapy A and therapy B in a particular condition. In pharmacoeconomic models, these should represent the actual choice being made, and should include the necessary descriptors of the population in which the decision is being made to allow the reader to understand the context of the choice. The context is followed by a decision node (represented in the

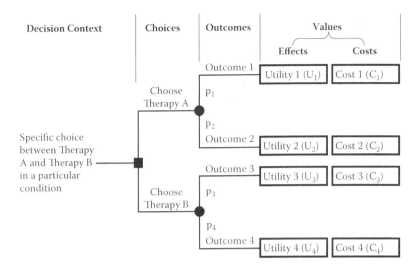

FIGURE 2.1 Basic structure of a branch and node decision tree, illustrating two choices in a particular clinical situation. After each choice is made, outcomes occur with specific probabilities, these outcomes are associated with values, which may be measured in clinical or cost metrics.

figure as a square), and should include as comparators the relevant, real choices the decision maker has at his or her disposal. In the figure, this particular decision has only two choices represented by the branches off the decision node labeled Choose Therapy A and Choose Therapy B. Each choice is followed by a series of chance nodes (represented in the figure by circles), which describe the possible outcomes that are implied by making each of the respective choices. Each outcome occurs with a specific probability (p_1 through p_4 in the figure). Each outcome is also associated with one or more values (represented in the figure by the rectangles), which describe the clinical effects and costs of arriving at that particular outcome. We will use this figure in the following description of the basic steps that should be conducted each time a decision analysis or pharmacoeconomic model is developed.

2.2.2.1 Steps in Conducting a Decision Analysis

In the following sections, we describe the basic steps through which the modeler should proceed in the construction of a model of a pharmacoeconomic decision. The basic question should be framed and the perspective chosen, the structure of the problem should be developed, the probabilities and values for the outcomes should be estimated, the tree should be analyzed to obtain the expected value of the outcomes, and sensitivity analysis should be conducted to evaluate the effect of assumptions on the results. These are not necessarily linear; often evaluation of the tree or sensitivity analysis will indicate that a particular part of the structure of the model needs either more or less detail. Often, several of these steps are cycled through many times during the development of a model. We illustrate a specific example of these steps for the development of a published pharmacoeconomic model of the use of low molecular weight heparin as prophylaxis for thromboembolism in patients with cancer in Section 2.4.

2.2.2.2   Step 1: FRAME the Question

As in any study design, the modeler must decide several basic details regarding for whom and from whose perspective the decision is being made. Deciding for whom the decision is being made is similar to the development of inclusion and exclusion criteria for a typical randomized controlled trial; the decision problem must specify exactly who would be affected by the decision. The description should be as detailed as necessary to describe the problem at hand, and should specify, if important, the age and gender of the population being studied, the specific disease and comorbid conditions that the patients may have, and the specific treatments or strategies that are being evaluated.

Choosing the perspective of the decision maker is also very important, as it determines the appropriate metric in which to measure the outcomes and costs of the analysis. As described in Section 2.2, typical perspectives from which to conduct analysis are society, the payer, or the patient.

2.2.2.3   Step 2: STRUCTURE the Clinical Problem

The structuring of the problem entails diagramming the branches and nodes that represent the particular problem being modeled. Several aspects of the process are important to remember. The first is that the choices one makes from the decision node must be mutually exclusive; one and only one of the choices (branches of the decision node) can be made. If there are several aspects to the choice, then these aspects should be described as a series of mutually exclusive options, rather than described as sequential or embedded decisions. This is illustrated in Figure 2.2, which describes a decision to treat a particular cancer with surgery, medical therapy, or both, and also investigates the order in which the two therapies are applied. The structure on the top of the panel describes all of the possibilities, but at a decision node, all of the decisions should be listed as branches of the initial decision node itself, as in the bottom panel of the figure. This allows for a comparison between all of the specific choices individually, and allows for direct comparisons across each of the choices. However, the appropriate construction for chance nodes is different. For example, Figure 2.3 describes a portion of a model of a surgical therapy that has several possible outcomes; for example, the patient may die or have a major surgical complication, a minor surgical complication, or no surgical complication. In the top panel of Figure 2.3 all possible outcomes are drawn as branches of the root node. As shown, the probabilities of each complication are indicated separately and the probabilities of all four branches must sum to one. If this structure is used it becomes somewhat complicated to conduct sensitivity analysis on the probability of surgical death or major or minor surgical complications. However, if this same tree is drawn as a series of binary chance nodes, as shown in the lower panel of Figure 2.3, sensitivity analysis and the ability to vary prospective probabilities becomes easier. The first chance node indicates whether the patient dies or survives. If the patient survives, whether he or she has a complication or not. If the patient has a complication, it is either a major or minor complication. In this setting, it is much

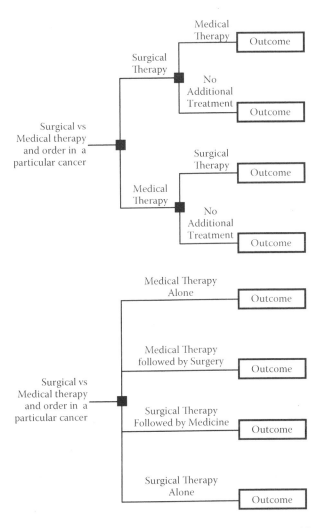

FIGURE 2.2 Embedded decisions. It is very difficult to analyze trees with embedded or sequential decisions, as drawn in the top panel. Each strategy should be its own choice, as shown in the lower panel.

easier to directly model the relationships between complication rates, survival rates, and normal outcomes.

It is important to remember that the structure drawn into a decision tree represents the disease process, treatments, and outcomes that the modeler has decided are important in this particular representation of the disease. Any particular model represents a specific version of the reality that the modeler is trying to represent. The art of modeling is the ability to have the model, as created in software, depict the version of reality that the modeler is hoping to represent.

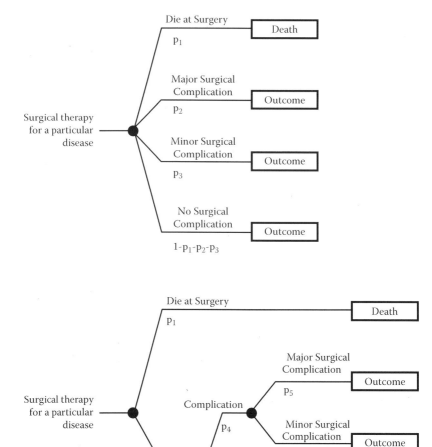

FIGURE 2.3 Superiority of binary chance nodes. It is generally preferable to make complex chance nodes a sequence of individual binary nodes (bottom panel) rather than a complex multi-branch node (top panel).

2.2.2.4   Step 3: Estimate the PROBABILITIES

Once the structure of the decision tree has been developed, the probabilities must be estimated for the various chance nodes in the tree. Modelers can use several sources to find and estimate probabilities for various parameters in a decision model. It is important to understand that the typical hierarchy of evidence-based grading does not necessarily apply to all of the various parameters that are necessary to calibrate a decision analysis or a pharmacoeconomic model. For example, the typical hierarchy for evidence-based medicine ranks randomized controlled trials as the best type of evidence for efficacy. However, as mentioned in Chapter 5, Retrospective Database Analysis, randomized controlled trials are very poor at estimating many other types of the parameters that are important in a decision model. For example, the incidence of a particular disease cannot be estimated by a randomized controlled trial, nor can the complication rate of a particular therapy when it is applied in general practice. Therefore, the quality of the evidence that a modeler uses to calibrate a decision model is entirely dependent upon the type of data necessary for a particular parameter in the model. Indeed, parameters on effectiveness of therapy may well be best derived from the reports of randomized controlled trials or meta-analyses of randomized controlled trials, whereas incidence and prevalence data may best come from observational studies and large cohort or administrative database analyses, and medication use data may best come from claims databases maintained by large health insurance plans. The important concept is that a model requires the best unbiased estimates of the specific parameters in the model; these parameters do not need to come from the same source nor do they all need to be of the same type of study or accuracy of data. These sorts of differences can be investigated in sensitivity analysis.

2.2.2.5   Step 4: Estimate the VALUES of the Outcomes

Similar to estimating the probabilities of various events, the modeler needs to assess the values for the outcomes that occur as a consequence of each one of the choices. The appropriate outcome measure will have previously been determined in the framing of the question when the perspective of the analysis is decided. This will direct the modeler to choose the appropriate outcome measure for the analysis. For example, in an analysis conducted from a societal point of view, the appropriate outcome measure is usually QALYs (see Introduction, Chapter 1). The choice of outcome is also determined by the particular disease the treatment is designed to ameliorate. For example, in a pharmacoeconomic model of a treatment for depression, it may be that the appropriate outcome measure is depression-free days or a similar disease-related outcome metric. In a model of a particular intervention for oral hygiene, the appropriate outcome might simply be the number of cavities avoided. The outcomes used must be those that are clinically relevant to the particular decision makers involved in the decision. One of the advantages of developing a model of a pharmacoeconomic problem is that clinical and cost outcomes may be evaluated and modeled simultaneously. Therefore, in most economic models, the model will simultaneously account for the clinical and cost consequences of each potential decision.

2.2.2.6   Step 5: ANALYZE the Tree (Average Out/Fold Back)

The evaluation of the decision tree is conceptually quite simple. The overall goal is to calculate the expected value of the outcomes implied by choosing each branch of the root decision node. For example, in Figure 2.1 there are two choices: Therapy A and Therapy B. If therapy A is chosen a portion of the population (indicated by p_1) will experience Outcome 1, which has a utility U_1 and another portion of the population (indicated by p_2) will experience Outcome 2, which has a utility U_2. Assume the utilities represent life expectancies, then the expected value of choosing Therapy A represents the life expectancy of a cohort of people who would be given that therapy, p_1 of them living U_1 years, p_2 of them living U_2 years. Mathematically, the expected value of choosing Therapy A is:

$$E(\text{Therapy A}) = (p_1 * U_1) + (p_2 * U_2)$$

Similarly, the expected value of choosing Therapy B is:

$$E(\text{Therapy B}) = (p_3 * U_3) + (p_4 * U_4)$$

The choice that has the highest expected value is then chosen as superior.

Essentially, no matter how complicated the tree becomes, the process of finding the expected value is the same. Starting with the terminal nodes, each chance node is replaced by the expectation of that chance node (the expected value of the outcome at that chance node), and that process is continued until one is left with the expected value of each branch of the initial decision node. Pragmatically, a modeler is never required to do this calculation by hand; there are several decision analysis software packages that do the analysis and calculations automatically.

2.2.2.7   Step 6: TEST ASSUMPTIONS (Sensitivity Analysis)

After the model has been developed, calibrated, and the initial analyses completed, one of the most useful steps in modeling is conducting sensitivity analyses. In its simplest form, the definition of sensitivity analysis is the evaluation of the outcomes of the model for various different levels of one or more input variables. Sensitivity analyses have several purposes. They can be used to "debug" a model to make sure that the model behaves as it is designed to behave. It is often the case that the modeler and the content experts with whom the modeler has developed a model will be able to predict the optimal choice under certain specified conditions. By using basic theoretical principles or knowledge of the given disease process the modeler may be able to make predictions about the direction the value of a particular strategy should move under different assumptions. For example, in a decision between surgical and medical therapy, it seems obvious that the relative value of the medical therapy choice should increase compared with the surgical therapy choice as the mortality from surgery increases. If a sensitivity analysis on surgical mortality is conducted and the expected finding does not occur, this may indicate programming or structural errors in the development of the model.

Another important use of sensitivity analysis is in the determination of which variables in the model have the most impact on the outcomes. This is the traditional use of sensitivity analysis and is the basis for many initial valuations of the stability of a particular decision modeling result over a wider range of underlying assumptions and probabilities. There are many types of sensitivity analyses, the simplest of which is a one-way sensitivity analysis in which the changes in the outcomes are evaluated as the value of a single variable is changed. Slightly more complicated is a two-way sensitivity analysis, which plots the optimal choice implied with various combinations of two different input variables, and a multiway sensitivity analysis is conducted by changing and evaluating the results across many input variables simultaneously. Finally, probabilistic sensitivity analyses are used to test the stability of the results over ranges of variability in the input parameters. We describe a simple sensitivity analysis from published work in Section 2.3.6. A more complete description of sensitivity analysis in pharmacoeconomic analyses is provided in Chapter 12.

2.2.2.8 Step 7: INTERPRET the Results

Once the analysis has been completed, the stability of the model has been tested with sensitivity analysis, and a modeler is convinced that the model represents the clinical and pharmacoeconomic characteristics of the problem adequately, the results must be interpreted and summarized. It is often the case that a specific answer that the model gives under one particular set of conditions is not the most important attribute of the model itself. Oftentimes, it is the manner in which the answer varies with changes in underlying parameter estimates and underlying probabilities and values for outcomes that are the most interesting aspect of the interpretation of an analysis.

However, most pharmacoeconomic analyses will result in an estimate of a cost-effectiveness ratio or similar metric of each choice as its major finding.

2.2.3 Markov Models

In a traditional branch and node decision tree, as illustrated in Figure 2.1, the terminal nodes are all single outcomes. For example, the value of the outcome might be measured as a life expectancy and quality-adjusted life expectancy or a cost. However, for any model, the outcomes that are expected to occur after each choice are actually quite complex combinations of events that happen in the lives of the people proceeding down that path. Many times, the intervention being modeled at a decision node affects the risks of future events, such as heart attacks and strokes in the case of cholesterol-modifying therapy, or might affect the rate of recurrence of a particular event, such as asthma episodes in an analysis of the use of corticosteroids in patients with reactive airway disease. When a model must consider events that occur over time or events that may recur in time, the traditional branch and node structure is an inefficient method for representing these events. Standard decision analytic methods typically use a Markov process to represent events that occur over time. As illustrated in Figure 2.4, a simple decision tree would terminate in single values such as a life expectancy shown in the upper panel of Figure 2.4. However, that life expectancy is actually determined by the average life histories of many people who would proceed down that choice. This can be represented as seen in the lower half of Figure 2.4 by replacing the single life expectancy value with a Markov process that represents the events the modeler wants to detect that occur after the decision is made and certain outcomes occur. A Markov process is simply a mathematical representation of the health states in which a patient might find him- or herself and the likelihood of transitioning between those states. The Markov process itself, when it is evaluated, calculates the average life expectancy of a cohort proceeding through the Markov process. Markov processes are described in much more detail in Chapter 4.

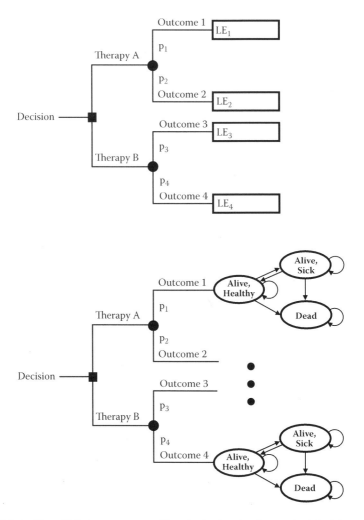

FIGURE 2.4 Use of Markov processes. The terminal node of a standard decision tree typically represents life expectancy, which is a complex summary of many possible paths and
events. These can often be represented by a Markov process, in which the actual events that
occur over time are specifically modeled. The dots in the lower model represent the same
health states and transitions as outcome 1 for outcomes 2 and 3. See Text and Chapter 4 for
details.

2.2.4 SIMULATION MODELS

Over the past 10 to 15 years, the decision analytic and pharmacoeconomic investigators have started to rely more on simulation methodologies to create progressively
more complicated and clinically realistic models of disease processes and treatments. Although a detailed exposition of these methods is beyond the scope of this
chapter, we will briefly describe the three most common simulation methodologies
used in current pharmacoeconomic analysis. They differ by their ability to model

progressively more complicated clinical situations as well as interactions between individual patients in the model.

2.2.4.1 Microsimulation

The term microsimulation has come to represent those models in which individual patients are modeled, one at a time, as they proceed through the model. The advantage of microsimulation is that it eliminates a problem with standard Markov process models in that it releases the assumption of path-independent transition probabilities. Although this is discussed in more detail in Chapter 4, the basic problem is that in standard Markov decision models, transition probabilities are dependent only upon the state the patient is in; information regarding where the patient was in the prior time period is lost. Because only one patient is in the model at any given time in a microsimulation, the patient's specific history can be recorded and transition probabilities can be made to depend on those variables, allowing for remarkable clinical complexity in the development of a model. There are several examples of the use of microsimulation in the current literature: Freedberg has used microsimulation to evaluate the cost-effectiveness of various treatment and prevention strategies in HIV disease.[3] Details of simulation methodology can be found in several texts.[4,5]

2.2.4.2 Discrete Event Simulation

One of the problems with many of the modeling systems previously discussed is that they cannot easily model the competition for resources. Therefore, although a decision analysis or a cost-effectiveness analysis might be able to determine that a particular diagnostic or therapeutic strategy should be adopted, these analyses cannot tell whether the resources, delivery systems, geographic constraints, or other problems allow for the optimal strategy to actually be implemented. Discrete event simulation, which was originally developed over 50 years ago by industrial engineering to model production processes in factories, provides the modeler with a set of tools that can represent queues, resource limitations, geographic distribution, and many other physical structures or limitations that constrain the implementation of a particular strategy or therapy.

In health care, discrete event simulation has been used for many years to allow for understanding flows and bottlenecks in operating room scheduling, emergency vehicle distribution and response time, throughput in emergency rooms, and many other resource constraint problems. More recently, as the ability to blend highly detailed clinical data with discrete event simulation models has improved, discrete event simulation has been used to address and evaluate more clinically interesting problems. For example, we have used discrete event simulation to model the U.S. organ allocation process and evaluate the effects of various organ allocation policy changes prior to their implementation.[1,6] The advantage of discrete event simulation, in this case, is that it has specific structures to allow for the formation of queues, waiting lists, and arrival of both patients and donated organs.

2.2.4.3 Agent-Based Simulation

One of the purposes of making models more complex is to represent more realistic physiological or biological systems. Many components of biological systems act entirely independently and simply respond to their environments based on internal sets of processes that govern their behavior. Cells respond to cytokines, hormones, and other biological signals; organs (the pancreas) respond to levels of hormones (insulin) and a myriad of other factors and signals. Agent-based models, in which each "agent" or component of the model independently contains all of the information it needs to interact with and respond to the actions of the other agents in the model, have been increasingly used to understand and model complex biological systems, from individual cells and organs to populations. One fundamental concept of agent-based models is that the aggregated behavior of multiple individual autonomous agents can replicate and predict very complex social and group behaviors. In the realm of medicine and public health, agent-based models have been used recently in the modeling of epidemics and population reactions to epidemics.[7–9]

2.2.5 DETERMINISTIC (MECHANISTIC) MODELS

Deterministic models seek to capture and characterize specific biological relationships and causes and effects directly through a series of equations. Some of the first medical problems to be evaluated using deterministic models were what are termed "compartment models" that represented the spread of infectious diseases in a community. Also called "susceptible, infected, recovered" (SIR) models, they have been widely used over the past 50 years to model the effects of interventions, such as quarantines and vaccines, on epidemic and pandemic infections. Basically, the relevant population is divided into compartments, and the flows among those compartments are represented as series of differential equations that are related to both the level and rates of flow of each of the compartments.

More recently, these sorts of models have been used to model physiological processes. At their highest level of abstraction, these models represent physiology and disease as one might see in a physiology textbook, with diagrams that indicate how one hormone or cytokine, or level of some electrolyte or other substance, affects the production and level of another. These typically form feedback loops; examples might be that thyroid stimulating hormone (TSH) is produced in response to low thyroid hormone levels and TSH acts on the thyroid to produce more thyroid hormone. Recent examples of the application of deterministic modeling to health care have been the development of complex systems models of sepsis and injury.[10–13] More physiologically complex, and more directly applicable to problems in pharmacoeconomics, the Archimedes model of disease uses a very complex system of mathematical and differential equations in the concept of an agent-based model to represent multiple metabolic processes and diseases that include diabetes, heart disease, and some cancers.[14,15] It has been recently used to compare and evaluate the cost-effectiveness of different strategies for the prevention of diabetes.[16]

2.2.6 SUMMARY OF MODELING TYPES

A wide variety of mathematical modeling types are available to the modeler to represent disease, treatments, and costs. There is a tradeoff between complexity of the process being modeled and the type of model that should be used to represent the problem. In general, the simplest modeling technique that accurately represents the components of the problem according to a clinical expert is sufficient. It is our experience that most problems can be addressed with either simple branch or node decision trees or standard Markov process-based state transition models. In the next section, we will illustrate the development and analysis of a simple branch and node decision tree model to evaluate a clinical treatment problem.

2.3   EXAMPLE

To illustrate the seven steps used to conduct a decision analysis, we will use an analysis performed by Aujesky et al.[17] examining the use of low molecular weight heparin as secondary prophylaxis for venous thromboembolism in patients with cancer.

2.3.1   STEP 1: FRAMING THE QUESTION

Venous thromboembolism frequently occurs in patients with cancer and carries a poor prognosis. In addition, cancer patients who have had an episode of venous thromboembolism are prone to recurrent episodes. Because of this recurrence risk, prolonged use of anticoagulants as secondary prophylaxis has been advocated, typically for 6 months or longer. Recent data suggest that low molecular weight heparin (LMWH) is more effective than warfarin for this patient group, leading to recommendations for LMWH as first line therapy in this clinical scenario. However, the costs of LMWH and the potential need for home nursing to administer daily subcutaneous injections raises questions about whether effectiveness gained through LMWH use is worth its significantly increased cost.

Thus, the question this analysis seeks to answer is: what are the costs and benefits of using LMWH compared with warfarin for secondary prophylaxis of venous thromboembolic disease in cancer patients. In the base case analysis, patient cohorts were 65 years old, based on the mean patient age in studies of cancer-related venous thromboembolism. Because venous thromboembolism can recur throughout the remaining life span of cancer patients, a lifetime time horizon was chosen for the analysis. However, the life expectancy of cancer patients with venous thromboembolism averages only 1–2 years, due to venous thromboembolism itself, the high prevalence of advanced cancer in patients with thromboembolism, and the age of the patient group.

This analysis sought to inform physicians and policy makers about the incremental value, defined broadly, of LMWH use compared with warfarin use. For decisions framed in this fashion, cost and effectiveness metrics should be as comprehensive and generalizable as possible. With this in mind, the analysis took the societal perspective, where costs include both direct medical costs and the costs of seeking and receiving care, and used life expectancy and quality-adjusted life expectancy for the effectiveness measures.

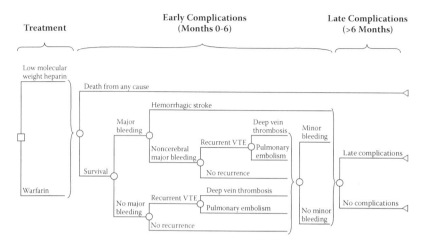

FIGURE 2.5 Basic decision tree for low molecular weight heparin as secondary prevention for cancer-induced thromboembolism. Reproduced with permission.

2.3.2 Step 2: Structuring the Clinical Problem

A decision tree model was chosen to depict this problem, based on the relatively short time horizon of the model and the concentration on outcomes related to venous thromboembolism and its treatment. If a longer time horizon or more outcomes had been required to adequately model the problem, another model structure, such as a Markov process, could have been used. The decision tree model is shown in Figure 2.5. This model assumes that all events that are not related to venous thromboembolism or its treatment are unaffected by the choice between LMWH and warfarin.

In the decision tree, the square node on the left depicts the decision to use either LMWH or warfarin. Circular nodes depict chance nodes, where events occur based on their probabilities. All patients are at risk for early complications, whose probabilities differ based on treatment choice. Patients who survive the first 6 months after a venous thromboembolism episode are at risk for later complications. The triangular nodes on the right represent the cost and effectiveness values associated with that particular path through the model. In addition, the model assumes that patients suffering a hemorrhagic stroke had anticoagulation permanently discontinued, with only transient interruption of anticoagulation with noncerebral bleeding, and that a second venous thromboembolic episode resulted in permanent inferior vena cava filter placement.

2.3.3 Step 3: Estimate the Probabilities

Probabilities for the model were obtained from a variety of sources. A large clinical trial of cancer patients with venous thromboembolism provided data on mortality, recurrent thromboembolism, and major bleeding associated with LMWH or warfarin use.[18] Anticoagulation-related intracranial bleeding rates, which could not be reliably estimated from single trials, were obtained from a meta-analysis of venous thromboembolism therapy in a wide variety of patient groups;[19] its base case value (9%) was varied over a broad range (5–30%) in sensitivity analyses to account for the possibility of greater risk in cancer patients. Intracranial bleeding risk was assumed to be the same with either anticoagulation regimen. In the model, an estimated 20% of patients receiving LMWH required daily home nursing, and 50% of patients with deep venous thrombosis received outpatient treatment.

2.3.4 STEP 4: ESTIMATE THE VALUES OF THE OUTCOMES

Model outcomes were cost and effectiveness. U.S. Medicare reimbursement data were used to estimate costs for hospitalization, emergency department, physician and home nursing visits, laboratory tests, and medical procedures. Anticoagulant drug costs were 2002 average wholesale prices; base case daily pharmacy costs for LMWH and warfarin averaged $48 and $1, respectively. Costs related to intracranial bleeding and late complications were obtained from medical literature sources. Because the analysis took the societal perspective, patient costs for seeking and receiving care were incorporated into the analysis, including patient transportation expenses for care visits and anticoagulation monitoring and patient time costs related to continuing care needs.

Effectiveness was measured as life expectancy and quality-adjusted life expectancy. Life expectancy was estimated using 6- and 12-month mortality data from randomized trials of secondary venous thromboembolism prophylaxis in cancer patients[18–20] and longer-term survival data from a cohort study of cancer patients with venous thromboembolism.[21] Quality-adjusted life expectancy was calculated by multiplying quality of life utility values (see Chapter 11, Patient-Reported Outcomes) for chronic health states by the length of time spent in those states. These utilities were obtained from the medical literature. In addition, decreases in utility from acute complications were accounted for by subtracting days of illness, based on U.S. average hospital length of stay data, from quality-adjusted life expectancy totals.

TABLE 2.2
Example Analysis Results

	Low Molecular Weight Heparin	Warfarin	Difference
Life expectancy, years	1.442	1.377	0.066
Quality-adjusted life expectancy, years	1.097	1.046	0.051
Total costs	$15,239	$7720	$7609
Incremental cost-effectiveness ratio, $/life-year	—	—	$115,847
Incremental cost-effectiveness ratio, $/QALY	—	—	$149,865

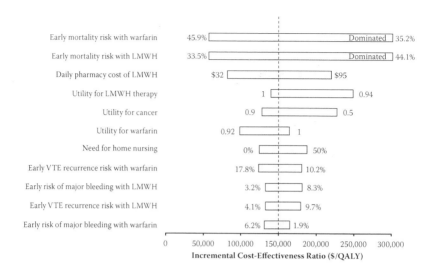

FIGURE 2.6 Tornado diagram of multiple one-way sensitivity analyses of the important variables in the low molecular weight heparin example. Reproduced with permission.

2.3.5 STEP 5: ANALYZE THE TREE

Averaging out and folding back the tree results in Table 2.2, the LMWH strategy was more effective than warfarin, whether in terms of life expectancy or quality adjusted life expectancy, while also being nearly twice the cost of the warfarin strategy. Effectiveness differences between strategies translated to about 24 days in the unadjusted life expectancy analysis or about 19 quality-adjusted days in quality-adjusted life expectancy. Two incremental cost-effectiveness ratios resulted, because two effectiveness metrics were used, both of which were more than $100,000 per effectiveness unit gained.

2.3.6 STEP 6: TEST ASSUMPTIONS (SENSITIVITY ANALYSIS)

In a series of one-way sensitivity analyses, varying parameter values over clinically plausible ranges, individual variation of 11 parameters was found to change base case results by 10% or more. These parameters and the incremental cost-effectiveness ratios resulting from their variation are shown in Figure 2.6 as a tornado diagram, where the range of incremental cost-effectiveness results that occur with variation of that parameter are shown as horizontal bars arranged from the greatest range to the least. Results were most sensitive to variation of parameters at the top of the figure; low values for early mortality with warfarin or high values for early mortality with LMWH caused the LMWH strategy to be dominated, i.e., to cost more and be less effective than the warfarin strategy. Variation of an individual parameter did not cause cost per QALY gained for the LMWH strategy to fall below $50,000. However, when simultaneously varying both early mortality due to LMWH and to warfarin in a two-way sensitivity analysis, cost per QALY gained was < $50,000 if mortality differences between the two agents were > 8%. The LMWH strategy cost <

$100,000/QALY gained if the utility for warfarin was <0.93, daily pharmacy cost for LMWH was < $41, or if the early mortality difference between agents was > 3%.

A probabilistic sensitivity analysis was also performed, where all sensitive parameters were varied simultaneously over distributions 1000 times. In this analysis, warfarin was favored in 97% of model iterations if the societal willingness-to-pay threshold was $50,000/QALY, or in 72% when the threshold was $100,000/QALY gained.

2.3.7 STEP 7: INTERPRET THE RESULTS

The results of this analysis suggest that treatment with LMWH in cancer patients with a history of venous thromboembolism is relatively expensive when compared with warfarin therapy, with gains in effectiveness and decreased costs resulting from fewer early complications with LMWH offset by its much higher pharmacy costs. These results were relatively robust in sensitivity analyses when parameters were varied individually and collectively over clinically reasonable ranges. A key exception was when the cost of LMWH was varied; this agent became more economically reasonable when its daily cost was in the range of $40 or less. Interestingly, in many countries other than the United States, LMWH costs are well below this range ($10–13 per day in Europe and Canada).

Thus, we can conclude that LMWH for secondary prophylaxis of venous thromboembolism in U.S. cancer patients is expensive, calling into question whether the documented improvement in outcomes is worth the added cost. However, the added expense of the newer intervention is largely driven by the cost of the agent itself, making LMWH a much more economically reasonable strategy when (and where) it costs less.

REFERENCES

1. Roberts MS, Sonnenberg FA. Decision modeling techniques. In: Chapman GB, Sonnenberg FA, Eds. *Decision making in health care. Theory, psychology, and applications*. Cambridge, UK: Cambridge University Press. 2000. 20–64.
2. Drummond MF, Sculpher MJ, Torrance GW, O'Brien BJ, Stoddart GL. *Methods for the economic evaluation of health care programmes*. Oxford, UK.: Oxford Medical Publications, Oxford University Press. 2005.
3. Freedberg KA, Losina E, Weinstein MC, et al. 2001. The cost effectiveness of combination antiretroviral therapy for HIV disease. *N Engl J Med.* 344(11):824–31.
4. Bratley P, Fox BL, Schrange LE. 1987. *A guide to simulation*, 2nd ed. New York: Springer.
5. Law AM. *Simulation modeling and analysis*, 4th ed. 2007. Columbus, OH: McGraw-Hill.
6. Shechter SM, Bryce CL, Alagoz O, et al. 2005. A clinically based discrete-event simulation of end-stage liver disease and the organ allocation process. *Med Decis Making* 25(2):199–209.
7. Burke DS, Epstein JM, Cummings DA, et al. 2006. Individual-based computational modeling of smallpox epidemic control strategies. *Acad Emerg Med* 13(11):1142–9.

8. Halloran ME, Ferguson NM, Eubank S, et al. Modeling targeted layered containment of an influenza pandemic in the United States. *Proc Natl Acad Sci USA.* 2008;105(12):4639–44.

9. Longini IM, Jr., Halloran ME, Nizam A, et al. Containing a large bioterrorist smallpox attack: A computer simulation approach. 2007. *Int J Infect Dis* 11(2):98–108.

10. Clermont G, Neugebauer EA. 2005. Systems biology and translational research. *J Crit Care* 20(4):381–2.

11. Vodovotz Y, Chow CC, Bartels J, et al. 2006. In silico models of acute inflammation in animals. *Shock* 26(3):235–44.

12. Vodovotz Y, Clermont G, Hunt CA, et al. 2007. Evidence-based modeling of critical illness: An initial consensus from the Society for Complexity in Acute Illness. *J Crit Care* 22(1):77–84.

13. Kumar R, Chow CC, Bartels JD, Clermont G, Vodovotz Y. 2008. A mathematical simulation of the inflammatory response to anthrax infection. *Shock* 29(1):104–11.

14. Eddy DM, Schlessinger L. 2003. Validation of the Archimedes diabetes model. *Diabetes Care* 26(11):3102–10.

15. Eddy DM, Schlessinger L. Archimedes: A trial-validated model of diabetes. 2003. *Diabetes Care* 26(11):3093–101.

16. Eddy DM, Schlessinger L, Kahn R. 2005. Clinical outcomes and cost-effectiveness of strategies for managing people at high risk for diabetes. *Ann Intern Med* 143(4):251–64.

17. Aujesky D, Smith KJ, Cornuz J, Roberts MS. 2005. Cost-effectiveness of low-molecular-weight heparin for secondary prophylaxis of cancer-related venous thromboembolism. *Thromb Haemost* 93(3):592–9.

18. Lee AY, Levine MN, Baker RI, et al. 2003. Low-molecular-weight heparin versus a coumarin for the prevention of recurrent venous thromboembolism in patients with cancer. *N Engl J Med* 349(2):146–53.

19. Linkins LA, Choi PT, Douketis JD. 2003. Clinical impact of bleeding in patients taking oral anticoagulant therapy for venous thromboembolism: A meta-analysis. *Ann Intern Med* 139(11):893–900.

20. Lee AY, Rickles FR, Julian JA, et al. 2005. Randomized comparison of low molecular weight heparin and coumarin derivatives on the survival of patients with cancer and venous thromboembolism. *J Clin Oncol* 23(10):2123–9.

21. Cook N, Thomas DM. 2002. Retrospective survey of unselected hospital patients with and without cancer comparing outcomes following venous thromboembolism. *Intern Med J*;32(9-10):437–44.

3 Cost of Illness

Renée J.G. Arnold

CONTENTS

3.1 INTRODUCTION

Cost-of-illness (COI) analysis measures the economic burden of disease and illness on society. It is often called burden-of-illness (BOI). The components of a pharmacoeconomic or cost-effectiveness analysis include costs and consequences. Costs can be divided into direct and indirect costs. Direct medical costs are those related to providing medical services, such as a hospital stay, physician fees for outpatient visits, and drug costs (including the cost of the medication itself and any downstream adverse events that may arise as a result of drug administration). Direct nonmedical costs are those related to expenses, such as transportation costs, that are a direct result of the illness. Direct costs are most frequently included in a COI study, whereas indirect costs, those associated with changes of individual productivity, are often not included in a COI study, because they are difficult to obtain. Examples of indirect costs are lost time from work (absenteeism) and unpaid assistance from a family member. In addition, intangible costs, such as pain and suffering, may be included in the analysis. Analyses can be done from one or several perspectives, which will help in determining the distribution of disease costs across multiple stakeholders.[1] The societal perspective typically includes indirect, as well as direct, medical costs because these are costs to society, that is, as previously mentioned, lost time from work. The payer perspective typically includes only direct costs (see Chapters 1 and 2 for more on perspective).

COI analyses are used to aid in policy making; resource allocation—that is, prioritizing resource use for disease treatment and prevention—and as baseline research from which to determine the potential benefit of new therapies.

3.1.1 APPROACHES

There are two approaches to conducting COI analyses, the prevalence-based approach and the incidence-based approach. The prevalence-based approach considers the cost of disease within a specified time period. The prevalence-based approach is most appropriate for diseases or illnesses that are measured within the time period of analysis and that do not change much over time (e.g., migraine) or acute diseases (e.g., asthma, eczema).

This is in contrast to the incidence-based approach, which calculates the life-time costs of disease. This approach is most appropriate for chronic diseases, such as hypertension, or diseases that take a long time to progress, such as diabetes. This approach considers disease progression and survival probability. The disease is first defined using existing disease definitions or classification systems, such as International Classification of Diseases--Ninth Revision (ICD-9-CM) codes. To accurately capture the disease COI over the appropriate timeframe, depending on the aforementioned approaches, one must take into consideration the epidemiology of the disease under study and the demographic profiles of the typical patient population.

3.1.2 METHODS

A micro-costing method has been used in many studies to examine COI. The direct costs included in this method typically comprise out-of-pocket expenses for non-insured items (over-the-counter medications, visits to out-of-plan health practitioners, laundry/clothing, and specialty items) and co-payments for prescription medications and clinic visits determined from insurance claims databases as well as the usual direct cost items previously outlined.

Two examples of COI studies, atopic dermatitis (AD) and human papillomavirus (HPV), will now be examined.

3.2 ATOPIC DERMATITIS

AD is a chronic disease that affects the skin of children and adults. It results in itchy, flaky skin and demonstrates a considerable impact on patient QoL, as well as a sub-stantial monetary burden.[2–13] Direct and indirect costs for AD have been measured in various countries and are substantial from both a patient and a societal perspec-tive. The direct costs have been reported to range from $71 to $2,559 per patient per year.[14] This variation in cost is due to differences in study methodology as well as differences in health care systems of the various countries. Most of the costs of AD consist of indirect costs associated with time lost from work, lifestyle changes, and non-traditional or over-the-counter treatments for AD.[14] The financial burden on the health care system and on society is expected to grow because the prevalence of the disease is increasing.

Indeed, studies in the past 7 years, using a prevalence-based approach to calculate COI, have demonstrated direct costs ranging from US$150[5] (using the approximate US$ equivalent in 2005) to US$580[6] per patient per year, with differences vary-

TABLE 3.1
Selected References of Cost of Illness of Atopic Dermatitis

Reference	Year	Direct	Indirect	Perspective (Payer)	Total[1]
Ehlken (5)	2005	$150[1]	$1589	Societal	$1739
Ellis (6)	2002	$580	Not measured	Private insurer	
Ellis (6)	2002	$1250	Not measured	Medicaid	
Fivenson (8)	2002	$167	$147	Health plan	$609
Emerson (7)	2001	$73[2]	$42	Societal	$115
Jenner (11)	2004		$281[2]	Patient	
Ricci (31)	2006		$1540	Patient	
Verboom (13)	2002	$71		Country	

[1] If both direct and indirect available.
[2] US$ equivalent for 2005 calculated using www.gocurrency.com historic EU to US$ converter.

ing due to different cost-accounting methods. Table 3.1 lists numerous references in which US$ (or equivalent) per patient COI were calculated.

Typically, outpatient visits and medications composed the majority of direct costs,[8,13] ranging from approximately 62% to >90%.[8] The distribution of AD-associated direct costs from Fivenson and colleagues is shown in Figure 3.1.[8] In those studies that examined indirect costs (e.g., the patient out-of-pocket costs for co-pays, medications, household items, loss of productivity) they made up substantial percentages of the total, e.g., 36%[7] or 73%.[8] Several studies showed increasing costs with worsening disease severity in adults. Using a micro cost-accounting approach, whereby costs of hospitalizations, consults, drug therapy, treatment procedures, diagnostic tests, laboratory tests, clinic visits, and urgent care visits were summed, Fivenson, Arnold, and colleagues (Table 3.2) reported an average annual per patient direct cost ranging from $435 in mild patients to $3229 in severe patients.

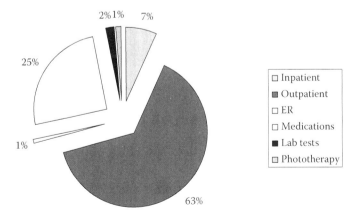

FIGURE 3.1 Distribution of atopic dermatitis-associated direct costs in a U.S. health plan.

TABLE 3.2
Total Annual Costs for Adults by Provider-Assessed Severity

	Mild (N=55)		Moderate (N=31)		Severe (N=3)		Unknown (N=18)	
	Total $	Mean per patient $ ± SE	Total $	Mean per patient $ ± SE	Total $	Mean per patient $ ± SE	Total $	Mean per patient $ ± SE
Direct Costs								
Inpatient	1,082	19.68 ± 19.68	0	0	0	0	0	0
Outpatient	4,947	89.95 ± 7.54	3,605	116.29 ± 15.7	884	294.67 ± 49.67	1,406	78.11 ± 11.56
Emergency room	0	0	0	0	0	0	0	0
Medications	1,873	.06 ± 9.86	1,765	56.95 ± 14.14	1,189	396.40 ± 349.59	764	42.44 ± 11.57
Labs	24	0.44 ± 0.44	0	0	0	0	0	0
Phototherapy	0	0	63	2.03 ± 1.44	0	0	0	0
Subtotal	**7,926**	**144.13 ± 23.97**	**5,433**	**175.27 ± 25.84**	**2,073**	**691.07 ± 389.36**	**2,170**	**120.55 ± 17.08**
Indirect Costs								
Practitioner visits	575	10.45 ± 6.75	100	3.23 ± 2.29	0	0	1,510	83.89 ± 58.39
Visit copays	380	6.91 ± 0.59	280	9.03 ± 1.28	70	23.33 ± 4.41	110	6.11 ± 0.86
Medications	3,740	68.00 ± 25.83	1,306	42.13 ± 13.52	357	119.00 ± 55.32	1,808	100.44 ± 48.73
Medication copays	316	5.74 ± 0.99	254	8.21 ± 1.73	88	29.33 ± 19.06	83	4.61 ± 1.25
Household items	1,024	18.62 ± 10.37	1,863	60.10 ± 29.52	620	206.67 ± 206.67	1,000	55.56 ± 25.66
Child care	0	0	0	0	0	0	0	0
Subtotal	**6,035**	**109.72 ± 35.34**	**3,803**	**122.70 ± 34.49**	**1,135**	**378.33 ± 244.31**	**4,511**	**250.61 ± 84.65**
Productivity								
Days lost from work	9,983	181.51 ± 120.62	8,705	280.82 ± 113.89	6,476	2,159.65 ± 1,033.12	4,138	229.90 ± 93.63
Subtotal	9,983	181.51 ± 120.62	8,705	280.82 ± 113.89	6,476	2,159.65 ± 1,033.12	4,138	229.90 ± 93.63
TOTAL	**23,944**	**435.35 ± 156.40**	**17,941**	**578.79 ± 131.27**	**9,684**	**3,229.05 ± 1,306.96**	**10,819**	**601.06 ± 137.26**

Indirect costs also increased by worsening disease severity—by more than two-fold[3,12] to threefold[11] to as much as almost tenfold.[8] Similarly, Ehlken and co-authors showed a greater than twofold increase in total (both direct and indirect) costs for patients with mild vs. severe disease.[5]

3.2.1 THERAPY-SPECIFIC COST

Several studies have compared the cost of different uses of topical corticosteroids (TCS) vs. topical immunomodulators (i.e., pimecrolimus and tacrolimus) and of the topical immunomodulators against each other. Some of these are detailed below.

3.2.1.1 Topical Corticosteroids

Green and colleagues undertook a systematic review of 10 randomized controlled trials (RCTs) in patients with AD.[9,10] Their literature search at the time revealed no published studies of this nature. The authors noted a wide variation in price and product availability, with the lowest price being generic hydrocortisone (£0.60 [approximately US$1.09]) to the highest at that time being mometasone furoate (Elocon) of £4.88 (approximate US$8.80 equivalent).

Six of the RTC studies favored the once-daily option as the lowest-cost treatment and four favored a twice-daily option, with successful outcome being defined by overall response to treatment, relapse or flareup rate, adverse effects, compliance, tolerability, patient preference measures, and impact on quality of life. One of the twice-daily-favored studies achieved a greater benefit (number of successful treatment responders) at a greater cost. However, it was felt that this greater cost would still likely be very cost-effective, given the relatively low prices of TCS. The limitations noted in the review were that of potentially low generalizability due to 80% of the RCTs' referring to potent TCS in patients with moderate-to-severe disease, whereas the majority of patients with AD have mild disease and lack of information on quantity of product usage.

3.3.2.2 Topical Immunomodulators

Clinical data show that topical immunomodulators are effective in AD, yet do not cause the significant adverse effects associated with TCS.[3] Delea and colleagues[4] retrospectively compared 157 pimecrolimus patients with 157 tacrolimus patients previously receiving TCS in a large claims database of managed care patients in terms of resource utilization (concomitant medications) and AD-related follow-up costs. They used propensity matching to control for differences between the groups in baseline demographic and clinical characteristics and utilization of AD-related services prior to assessment of disease severity. Patients in the pimecrolimus group had fewer pharmacy claims for TCS (mean 1.37 vs. 2.04, $P = 0.021$); this occurred primarily in the high-potency topical corticosteroid category. Fewer patients in the pimecrolimus group also received antistaphylococcal antibiotics during the follow-up period (16% vs. 27%, $P = 0.014$) and total AD-related costs during this time were lower in this group than in the tacrolimus group (mean $263 vs. $361, $P = 0.012$).

3.4   HPV

Persistent infection with cancer-associated HPV (termed oncogenic or high-risk HPV) causes the majority of squamous cell cervical cancer, the most common type of cervical cancer, and its histologic precursor lesions, the low-grade cervical dysplasia Cervical Intraepithelial Neoplasia-1 (CIN1) and the moderate-to-high-grade dysplasia CIN 2/3. Multiple HPV strains cause varying degrees of invasive cervical cancer (ICC) and its CIN precursors. HPV strains 16 and 18 cause approximately 70% of all cervical cancers[15,16] and CIN3, specifically, and 50% of CIN2 cases. In addition, HPV 16 and 18 cause approximately 35 to 50% of all CIN1. Low-oncogenic HPV risk types 6 and 11 account for 90% of genital wart cases.[17] Unfortunately, cytological and histological examinations cannot reliably distinguish between those patients who will progress from cervical dysplasia to ICC from those whose dysplasias will regress spontaneously, the latter being the vast majority of cases.[18] This inability to definitely ascertain the natural history of HPV infection is one of the primary reasons for the dilemma with HPV vaccination.

Although cervical cancer screening programs, such as the use of routine screening via the Papanicolaou (Pap) cervical smear, have substantially reduced the incidence and mortality of ICC in developed countries over the past 50 years,[17,19] there has been a slowing of these declines in recent years due to poor sensitivity of cervical cytology, anxiety and morbidity of screening investigations, poor access to and attendance of screening programs, falling screening coverage, and poor predictive value for adenocarcinoma, an increasingly common cause of ICC.[19] HPV is the most common sexually transmitted disease in the United States and virtually 100% of cervical cancer is due to HPV. HPV is also linked to head and neck cancer in men. There are more than 100 HPV strains (thereby potentially reducing vaccine efficacy for oncogenic strains not covered by the vaccine); HPV infection is often self-limited. A mitigating factor for the argument against using the vaccine is the fact that the cost-effectiveness of screening with Pap smears is reduced (improves) from USD1 million/QALY if patients continue to be screened annually, as is the common current recommendation, to USD150,000/QALY if patients are screened every 3 years, the latter a likely scenario if the vaccine is used.[15,20–22]

Worldwide, the incidence of cervical cancer is 470,000 new cases and 233,000 deaths per year; it is the second-leading cause of cancer deaths,[23] with 80% of these cases observed in developing countries.[24] Women in developing countries are especially vulnerable as they lack access to both cervical cancer screening and treatment. The demographics of cervical cancer in the United States show that 9710 new cases of ICC were expected to be diagnosed in 2006 and about 3700 deaths in women were expected from ICC.[25] The National Cancer Institute estimates an annual incidence of new genital HPV infections of 6 million.[26] Quadrivalent Human Papillomavirus (HPV) Vaccine recombinant (Gardasil®), the vaccine recently approved for use in the United States and Europe, covers the two major oncogenic HPV strains (16 and 18) for cervical cancer. In addition, it covers HPV strains 6 and 11, the primary causes of genital warts. Therefore, the vaccine does not offer full protection against cervical cancer, because it does not protect against HPV strains 31 and 45, which are also implicated in ICC and cervical dysplasia. To significantly reduce the rate of cervical cancer in the population as a whole, 70% of girls need to be vaccinated to achieve what is called "herd immunity"—when the vaccine's impact goes beyond just people who are inoculated. So far, it is unknown if HPV strains will mutate as the vaccine is introduced, although this is not very likely, seeing that HPV is a DNA-based virus.[18]

Insinga and colleagues used administrative and laboratory data from a large U.S. health plan to examine costs, resource utilization, and annual health plan expenditures for cervical HPV-related disease.[27] An episode of care was defined as beginning with a routine cervical smear, that is, one that required no evidence of follow-up for a previous Pap smear abnormality or ICD-9 diagnosis of a cervical abnormality during the previous 9 months. If CIN or cancer was not detected during an episode of care, biopsy results were termed false-positive. Because the data source was a prepaid health plan without direct billing for procedures or services, service-specific costs were assigned from the Medstat Marketscan database as a proxy for the health plan costs. Because of the small number of cervical cancer cases in the data set, costs were assigned on an age- and stage-specific basis using the Surveillance Epidemiology and End Results Program (SEER; National Cancer Institute; U.S. Department of Health and Human Services, Bethesda, MD) and an Agency for Healthcare Research and Quality evidence report. All cost estimates were converted to 2002 dollars using the Medical Care component of the Consumer Price Index.

The authors found that episodes of care after an abnormal routine cervical smear were $732 on average, compared with $57 for visits with negative results, with a statistically significant trend toward higher costs with increasing grade of initial cytologic abnormality. False-positive cervical smears cost $376 annually, while incomplete follow-up was $79. Regardless of age group, cervical HPV-related disease annual health care costs were $26,415 per 1000 enrollees, with the greatest costs of $51,863 being observed in the 20- to 29-year-old age group. The largest cost contribution was that of routine screening at 63.4% of total costs (range by age group of 54.1% to 70.8%), followed by cost of CIN 2/3, then cancer, false-positive smear, CIN 1 and incomplete follow-up (see Figure 3.2). [27,28]

Insinga and co-authors extrapolated their results to the general U.S. population to derive a total health care cost for HPV-related disease in 1998 of $3.4 billion, with

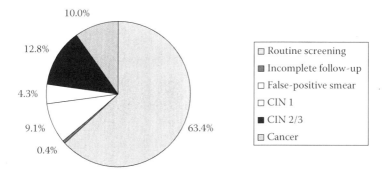

FIGURE 3.2   Distribution of cervical HPV-related disease direct costs in a commercial U.S. health plan.

expenditures for routine screening accounting for $2.1 billion, false-positive Pap test $300 million, CIN 1 $150 million, CIN 2/3 $450 million, and IC $350 million in 2002 dollars. A follow-up study by the same authors estimated the annual direct costs of abnormal cervical findings and treating cancer at $3.5 billion in 2005 US$.[29] Annual direct cost estimates in 2005 US dollars have been as high as $4.6 billion[29] and adding in costs of anogenital warts and other cancers associated with oncogenic HPV strains raises the total estimated economic burden to as high as US$5 billion in 2006 US$.[27,28]

Insinga and colleagues also estimated indirect costs, assuming that there were 130,377 women who would have been alive during 2000 had they not died from cervical cancer during that or a previous year, >75% of these women died before age 60, with >25% dying prior to age 40, and that 37,594 (29%) of these women would have had labor force earnings during 2000. Using these data, the total productivity loss in 2000 owing to cervical cancer mortality was estimated at $1.3 billion, several times higher than recent estimates of the annual U.S. direct medical costs of US$300 to $400 million associated with cervical cancer.[30] As in the AD studies, therefore, indirect costs are thought to account for a much greater burden than direct costs of HPV.

3.5 SUMMARY

In summary, COI or BOI lays the foundation on which to frame the different types of analyses (see Chapters 4 through 9) that are used to make decisions in allocation of healthcare resources. As indirect costs, that is, productivity, often account for a substantial portion of the burden, these should be assessed as part of the COI computation whenever possible.

REFERENCES

1. Honeycutt AA, Segel JE, Hoerger TJ, Finkelstein EA. Comparing cost-of-illness estimates from alternative approaches: An application to diabetes. 2009. *Health Serv Res.* 44(1):303–20.
2. Arnold R, Kuan R. Quality-of-life and costs in atopic dermatitis. *Handbook of Disease Burdens and Quality of Life Measures.* Heidelberg: Springer; 2008.
3. Abramovits W, Boguniewicz M, Paller AS, et al. 2005. The economics of topical immunomodulators for the treatment of atopic dermatitis. *Pharmacoeconomics.* 23(6):543–66.
4. Delea TE, Gokhale M, Makin C, et al. 2007. Administrative claims analysis of utilization and costs of care in health plan members with atopic dermatitis who had prior use of a topical corticosteroid and who initiate therapy with pimecrolimus or tacrolimus. *J Manag Care Pharm.* 13(4):349–59.
5. Ehlken B, Mohrenschlager M, Kugland B, Berger K, Quednau K, Ring J. 2005. Cost-of-illness study in patients suffering from atopic eczema in Germany. *Hautarzt.* 56(12):1144–51.
6. Ellis CN, Drake LA, Prendergast MM, et al. 2002. Cost of atopic dermatitis and eczema in the United States. *J Am Acad Dermatol.* 46(3):361–70.
7. Emerson RM, Williams HC, Allen BR. 2001. What is the cost of atopic dermatitis in preschool children? *Br J Dermatol.* 144(3):514–22.

8. Fivenson D, Arnold RJ, Kaniecki DJ, Cohen JL, Frech F, Finlay AY. 2002. The effect of atopic dermatitis on total burden of illness and quality of life on adults and children in a large managed care organization. *J Manag Care Pharm.* 8(5):333-42.

9. Green C, Colquitt JL, Kirby J, Davidson P. 2005. Topical corticosteroids for atopic eczema: Clinical and cost effectiveness of once-daily vs. more frequent use. *Br J Dermatol.* 152(1):130–41.

10. Green C, Colquitt JL, Kirby J, Davidson P, Payne E. 2004. Clinical and cost-effectiveness of once-daily versus more frequent use of same potency topical corticosteroids for atopic eczema: A systematic review and economic evaluation. *Health Technol Assess.* 8(47):iii,iv, 1–120.

11. Jenner N, Campbell J, Marks R. 2004. Morbidity and cost of atopic eczema in Australia. *Australas J Dermatol.* 45(1):16–22.

12. Kemp AS. 2003. Cost of illness of atopic dermatitis in children: A societal perspective. *Pharmacoeconomics.* 21(2):105–13.

13. Verboom P, Hakkaart-Van L, Sturkenboom M, De Zeeuw R, Menke H, Rutten F. 2002. The cost of atopic dermatitis in the Netherlands: An international comparison. *Br J Dermatol.* 147(4):716–24.

14. Carroll CL, Balkrishnan R, Feldman SR, Fleischer AB, Jr., Manuel JC. 2005. The burden of atopic dermatitis: Impact on the patient, family, and society. *Pediatr Dermatol.* 22(3):192–9.

15. Kulasingam SL, Myers ER. 2003. Potential health and economic impact of adding a human papillomavirus vaccine to screening programs. *JAMA.* 290(6):781–9.

16. Van de Velde N, Brisson M, Boily MC. 2007. Modeling human papillomavirus vaccine effectiveness: quantifying the impact of parameter uncertainty. *Am J Epidemiol.* 165(7):762–75.

17. Brisson M, Van de Velde N, De Wals P, Boily MC. 2007. The potential cost-effectiveness of prophylactic human papillomavirus vaccines in Canada. *Vaccine.* 25(29):5399–408.

18. Woodman CB, Collins SI, Young LS. 2007. The natural history of cervical HPV infection: Unresolved issues. *Nat Rev Cancer.* 7(1):11–22.

19. Adams M, Jasani B, Fiander A. 2007. Human papilloma virus (HPV) prophylactic vaccination: Challenges for public health and implications for screening. *Vaccine.* 25(16):3007–13.

20. Goldie SJ, Kohli M, Grima D, et al. 2004. Projected clinical benefits and cost-effectiveness of a human papillomavirus 16/18 vaccine. *J Natl Cancer Inst.* 96(8):604–15.

21. Sanders GD, Taira AV. 2003. Cost-effectiveness of a potential vaccine for human papillomavirus. *Emerg Infect Dis.* 9(1):37–48.

22. Taira AV, Neukermans CP, Sanders GD. 2004. Evaluating human papillomavirus vaccination programs. *Emerg Infect Dis.* 10(11):1915–23.

23. Food and Drug Administration. GARDASIL® Questions and Answers. http://www.fda.gov/cber/products/hpvmer060806qa.htm. Accessed 5/15/09.

24. Cox T, Cuzick J. 2006. HPV DNA testing in cervical cancer screening: from evidence to policies. *Gynecol Oncol.* 103(1):8–11.

25. Arnold RJ. 2007. Cost-effectiveness analysis: Should it be required for drug registration and beyond? *Drug Discov Today.* 12(21–22):960–5.

26. US National Institutes of Health/National Cancer Institute. National Cancer Institute FactSheet: Human Papillomavirus (HPV) Vaccines: Questions and Answers. http://www.nci.nih.gov/cancertopics/factsheet/prevention/HPV-vaccine. Accessed 2/10/09.

27. Insinga RP, Glass AG, Rush BB. 2004. The health care costs of cervical human papillomavirus-related disease. *Am J Obstet Gynecol.* 191(1):114–20.

28. Lipsy RJ. 2008. Assessing the short-term and long-term burden of illness in cervical cancer. *Am J Manag Care.* 14(6 Suppl 1):S177–84.

29. Insinga RP, Dasbach EJ, Elbasha EH. 2005. Assessing the annual economic burden of pre-venting and treating anogenital human papillomavirus-related disease in the US: Analytic framework and review of the literature. *Pharmacoeconomics.* 23(11):1107–22.
30. Insinga RP. 2006. Annual productivity costs due to cervical cancer mortality in the United States. *Women's Health Issues.* 16(5):236–42.
31. Ricci G, Bendandi B, Pagliara L, Patrizi A, Masi M. 2006. Atopic dermatitis in Italian children: evaluation of its economic impact. *J Pediatr Health Care.* 20(5):311–5.

4 Markov Modeling in Decision Analysis

J. Robert Beck

CONTENTS

4.1 INTRODUCTION

A pharmacoeconomic problem is attacked using a formal process that begins with constructing a mathematical model. In this book a number of pharmacoeconomic constructs are presented, ranging from spreadsheets to sophisticated numerical approximations to continuous compartment models. For more than 40 years the decision tree has been the most common and simplest formalism, comprising choices, chances, and outcomes. As discussed in Chapter 2, the modeler crafts a tree that represents near-term events within a population or cohort as structure, and attempts to balance realism and attendant complexity with simplicity. In problems that lead to long-term differences in outcome, the decision model must have a definite time horizon, up to which the events are characterized explicitly. At the horizon, the future health of a cohort must be summed and averaged into "subsequent prognosis." For problems involving quantity and quality of life, where the future natural history is well characterized, techniques such as the Declining Exponential Approximation of Life Expectancy[1,2] or differential equations may be used to generate outcome measures. Life tables may be used directly, or the results from clinical trials may be adopted to generate relevant values. Costs in decision trees are generally aggregated, collapsing substantial intrinsic variation into single monetary estimates.

Most pharmacoeconomic problems are less amenable to these summarizing techniques. In particular, clinical scenarios that involve a risk that is ongoing over time, competing risks that occur at different rates, or costs that need to be assessed incrementally lead to either rapidly branching decision trees or unrealistic pruning of possible outcomes for the sake of simplicity. In these cases a more sophisticated mathematical model is employed to characterize the natural history of the problem and its treatment. Dasbach, Elbasha, and Insinga reviewed the types of models used in the human papillomavirus (HPV) vaccination problem, and identified cohort, population dynamic, and hybrid approaches.[3] This chapter explores the pharmaco-economic modeling of cohorts using a relatively simple probabilistic characterization of natural history that can substitute for the outcome node of a decision tree. Beck and Pauker introduced the Markov process as a solution for the natural history modeling problem in 1983, building on their and others' work with stochastic models over the previous 6 years.[4] During the ensuing 25 years, more than 1,000 articles have directly cited either this paper or a tutorial published a decade later,[5] and more than 1,700 records in PubMed can be retrieved using (Markov decision model) OR (Markov cost-effectiveness) as a search criterion. This chapter will define the Markov process model by its properties and illustrate its use in pharmacoeconomics by exploring a simplified HPV vaccination example.

4.2   THE MARKOV PROCESS AND TRANSITION PROBABILITIES

4.2.1   STOCHASTIC PROCESSES

A Markov process is a special type of stochastic model. A stochastic process is a mathematical system that evolves over time with some element of uncertainty. This contrasts with a deterministic system, in which the model and its parameters specify the outcomes completely. The simplest example of a stochastic process is coin flipping. If a fair coin is flipped a number of times and a record of the result kept (H = "heads"; T = "tails"), a sequence such as HTHHTTTHTHHTHTHTHHTHTHTTTT might arise. At each flip (or trial), either T or H would result with equal probability of one half. Dice rolling is another example of this type of stochastic system, known as an independent trial experiment. Each flip or roll is independent of all that have come before, because dice and coins have no memory of prior results. Independent trials have been studied and described for nearly 3 centuries.[6]

4.2.2   MARKOV PROCESSES

The Markov process relaxes this assumption a bit. In a Markov model the probability of a trial outcome varies depending on the current result (generally known as a "state"). Andrei Andreevich Markov, a Russian mathematician, originally characterized such processes in the first decade of the 20th century.[7] It is easy to see how this model works via a simple example. Consider a clerk who assigns case report forms to three reviewers: Larry, Maureen, and Nell. The clerk assigns charts to these readers using a peculiar method. If the last chart was given to Larry, the clerk assigns the current one to Larry, Maureen, or Nell with equal probability. Maureen never gets two charts in a row; after Maureen, the clerk assigns the next chart to Larry with probability one quarter and Nell three quarters. After Nell gets a chart, the next chart goes to Larry with probability one half, and Nell and Maureen one quarter. Thus, the last assignment (Larry, Maureen, or Nell) must be known to determine the probability of the current assignment.

4.2.2.1 Transition Probabilities
Table 4.1 shows this behavior as a matrix of *transition probabilities*. Each cell of Table 4.1 shows the probability of a chart's being assigned to the reviewer named at the head of the column, if the last chart was assigned to the reviewer named at the head of the row. An nXn matrix is a *probability matrix* if each row element is non-negative, and each row sums to 1. Because the row headings and column headings refer to states of the process, Table 4.1 is a special form of probability matrix—a transition probability matrix.

This stochastic model differs from independent trials because of the *Markov Property*: the distribution of the probability of future states of a stochastic process depends on the current state (and only on the current state, not the prior natural history). That is, one does not need to know what has happened with scheduling in the past, only who was most recently assigned a chart. For example, if Larry got the last review, the next one will be assigned to any of the three readers with equal probability.

4.2.2.2 Working with a Transition Probability Matrix
The Markov property leads to some interesting results. What is the likelihood that, if Maureen is assigned a patient, that Maureen will get the patient after next? This can be calculated as follows:

After Maureen, the probability of Larry is one quarter and Nell three quarters. After Larry the probability of Maureen is one third, and after Nell it is one quarter. So, the probability of Maureen–(anyone)–Maureen is one quarter × one third + three quarters × one quarter, or 0.271. A complete table of probabilities at two assignments after a known one is shown in Table 4.2. This table is obtained using matrix multiplication, treating Table 4.1 as a 3 × 3 matrix and multiplying it by itself.* Note

TABLE 4.1
Chart Assignment Probability Table

Current	Next		
	Larry	Maureen	Nell
Larry	0.333	0.333	0.333
Maureen	0.250	0.000	0.750
Nell	0.500	0.250	0.250

---
* Matrix multiplication can be reviewed in any elementary textbook of probability or finite mathematics, or at http://en.wikipedia.org/wiki/Matrix_multiplication.

that the probability of Maureen's going to Maureen in two steps is found in the corresponding cell of Table 4.2.

This process can be continued, because Table 4.2 is also a probability matrix, in that the rows all sum to 1. In fact, after two more multiplications by Table 4.1, the matrix is represented by Table 4.3.

The probabilities in each row are converging, and by the seventh cycle, after a known assignment the probability matrix is shown in Table 4.4. This is also a probability matrix, with all of the rows identical, and it has a straightforward interpretation. Seven or more charts after a known assignment, the probability that the next chart review would go to Larry is 0.380, to Maureen 0.225 and to Nell 0.394. Or, if someone observes the clerk at any random time, the likelihood of the next chart's going to Larry is 0.380, etc. This is the limiting Markov matrix, or the steady state of the process. This particular scheduler, despite the idiosyncratic behavior, gives a little less than 40% of the charts each to Larry and Nell over time, and assigns Maureen only 22.5%.

TABLE 4.2
Two-Step Markov Probabilities

Current	Chart After Next		
	Larry	Maureen	Nell
Larry	0.361	0.194	0.444
Maureen	0.458	0.271	0.271
Nell	0.354	0.229	0.417

TABLE 4.3
Assignment Model after Four Cycles

Current	After Four Cycles		
	Larry	Maureen	Nell
Larry	0.377	0.225	0.398
Maureen	0.386	0.225	0.390
Nell	0.380	0.226	0.393

TABLE 4.4
Steady-State or Limiting Markov Matrix

	Larry	Maureen	Nell
Larry	0.380	0.225	0.394
Maureen	0.380	0.225	0.394
Nell	0.380	0.225	0.394

4.2.3   ABSORBING MARKOV MODELS

The chart review example is known as a *regular* Markov chain. The transition probabilities are constant, and depend only on the state of the process. Any state can be
reached from any other state, although not necessarily in one step (e.g., Maureen
cannot be followed immediately by Maureen, but can in two or more cycles). Regular
chains converge to a limiting set of probabilities. The other principal category of
Markov models is *absorbing*. In these systems the process has a state that it is possible to enter, in a finite set of moves, from any other state, but from which no movement is possible. Once the process enters the absorbing state, it terminates (i.e.,
stays in that state forever). The analogy with clinical decision models is obvious; an
absorbing Markov model has a state equivalent to death in the clinical problem.

4.2.3.1   Behavior of the Absorbing Model

This is shown in Figure 4.1, a simplified three-state absorbing clinical Markov model.
In a clinical model the notion of time appears naturally. Assume that a clinical process is modeled where definitive disease progression is possible, and that death often
ensues from progressive disease. At any given month the patient may be in a Well
state, shown in the upper left of Figure 4.1, the Progressive state in the upper right,
or Dead in the lower center. If in the Well state, the most likely result for the patient
is that he or she would remain well for the ensuing month, and next be found still in
the Well state. Alternatively, the patient could become sick and enter the Progressive
state, or die and move to the Dead state. If in Progressive, the patient would most
likely stay in that state, but could also die from the Progressive state, presumably at
a higher probability than from the Well state. There is also a very small probability
of returning to the Well state.

A possible transition probability matrix for this model is shown in Table 4.5. In
the upper row a Well patient remains so with probability 80%, has a 15% chance of
having progressive disease over one cycle, and a 5% chance of dying in the cycle.
A sick patient with progressive disease is shown with a 2% chance of returning to
the Well state, a 28% chance of dying in 1 month, and the remainder (70%) staying

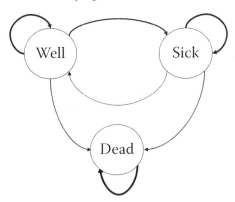

FIGURE 4.1   Simple three-state absorbing Markov model.

TABLE 4.5
Transition Probability Matrix for Clinical Example

Current	Next		
	Well	Progressive	Dead
Well	0.80	0.15	0.05
Progressive	0.02	0.70	0.28
Dead	0.00	0.00	1.00

in the Progressive state. Of course, the Dead state is *absorbing*, reflected by a 100% chance of staying Dead.

Table 4.5 is a probability matrix, so it can be multiplied as in the prior example. After two cycles the matrix is shown in Table 4.6. Thus, after two cycles of the Markov process, someone who started in the Well state has slightly less than a two-thirds chance of staying well, and a 22.5% chance of having Progressive disease. By the 10th cycle, the top row of the transition matrix is:

Well	Progressive	Dead
0.124	0.126	0.750

So, someone starting well has a 75% chance of being dead within 10 cycles, and of the remaining 25%, roughly an even chance of being well or having Progressive disease. This matrix converges slowly because of the moderate probability of death in any one cycle, but eventually this matrix would end up as a set of rows:

0	0	1

Everyone in this process eventually dies.

Clinical Markov models offer interesting insights into the natural history of a process. If the top row of the transition matrix is taken at each cycle and graphed, Figure 4.2 results. This graph can be interpreted as the fate of a cohort of patients beginning together at Well. The membership of the Well state decreases rapidly, as the forward transitions to Progressive and Dead overwhelm the back transition from Progressive to Well. The Progressive state grows at first, as it collects patients

TABLE 4.6
Two Cycle State Matrix for Clinical Example

	Well	Progressive	Dead
Well	0.643	0.225	0.132
Progressive	0.030	0.493	0.477
Dead	0.000	0.000	1.000

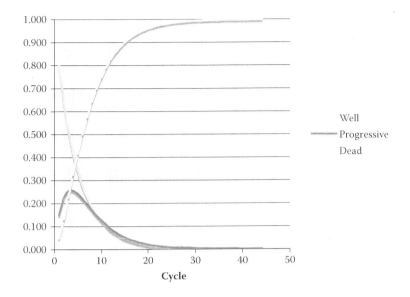

FIGURE 4.2   Absorbing Markov chain natural history.

transitioning from Well, but soon the transitions to Dead, which, of course, are permanent, cause the state to lose members. The Progressive state peaks at Cycle 4, with 25.6% of the cohort. The Dead state actually is a sigmoid (S-shaped) curve, rising moderately for a few cycles because most people are Well, but as soon as the 28% mortality from the Progressive state takes effect, the curve gets steeper. Finally it flattens, as few people remain alive. This graph is typical of absorbing Markov process models.

4.2.3.2   Use of Absorbing Markov Models in Clinical Decision Analysis

The Markov formalism can substitute for an outcome in a typical decision tree. The simplest outcome structure is life expectancy. This has a natural expression in a Markov cohort model: Life expectancy is the summed experience of the cohort over time. If we assign credit for being in a state at the end of a cycle, the value of each state function in Figure 4.2 represents the probability of being alive in that state in that cycle. At the start of the process, all members of the cohort are in the Well state. At Cycle One (Table 4.5), 80% are still Well and 15% have progressive disease, so the cohort would have experienced 0.8 average cycles Well, and 0.15 cycles in Progressive disease. At Cycle Two (Table 4.6), 64.3% are Well and 22.5% have Progressive disease. So, after two cycles, the cohort experience is 0.8+0.643, or 1.443 cycles Well and 0.15+0.225, or 0.375 cycles in Progressive disease. Summing the process over 45 cycles, until all are in the Dead state, the results are 4.262 cycles Well and 2.630 cycles in Progressive. So the life expectancy of this cohort, transitioning according to the probability matrix in Table 4.5, is 6.892 cycles, roughly 2:1 in Well versus Progressive disease. Refinements to this approach, involving correction for initial state membership, can be found in Sonnenberg and Beck.[5]

Whereas a traditional outcome node is assigned a value, or in Chapters 9 or 11 a *utility*, the Markov model is used to calculate the value by summing adjusted cohort membership. For this to work, each Markov state is assigned an incremental utility for being in that state for one model cycle. In the example above, the Well state might be given a value of 1, the Progressive state a value of 0.8. That is, the utility for being in the Progressive state is 80% of the value of the Well state for each cycle in it. In most models Dead is worth 0. Incremental costs can also be applied for Markov cost-effectiveness or cost-utility analysis. For this tutorial example, assume the costs of being in the Well state are $5000 per cycle, and in the Progressive state $8000 per cycle. Summing the cohort over 45 cycles leads to the results in Table 4.7. Thus, in this tutorial example, the cohort can expect to survive 6.892 cycles, or 6.366 quality-adjusted cycles, for a total cost of more than $42,000. These values would substitute for the outcomes at the terminal node of a decision tree model, and could be used for decision or cost-utility analysis.

An alternative way to use a Markov model is to simulate the behavior of a cohort of patients, one at a time. This approach is known as a Monte Carlo analysis. Each patient begins in the starting state (Well, in this example), and at the end of each cycle the patient is randomly allocated to a new state based on the transition probability matrix. Life expectancy and quality adjustments are handled as in the cohort solution. When the patient enters the Dead state, the simulation terminates and a new patient is queued. This process is repeated many times, and a distribution of survival, quality-adjusted survival, and costs results. Modern approaches to Monte Carlo analysis incorporate probability distributions on the transition probabilities, to enable statistical measures such as mean and variance to be determined.[8]

Two enhancements to the Markov model render the formalism more realistic for clinical studies; both involve adding a time element. First, although the Markov property requires no memory of prior states, it is possible to superimpose a time function on a transition probability. The most obvious example of this is the risk of death, which rises over time regardless of other clinical conditions. This can be handled in a Markov model by modifying the transition probability to death using a function: in the tutorial example time could be incorporated as p (Well->Dead) = 0.05 + G(age), where G represents the Gompertz mortality function[9] or another well-characterized actuarial model.

Second, standard practice in decision modeling discounts future costs and benefits to incorporate risk aversion and the decreasing value of assets and events in the future. Discounting (see Chapter 10) may be incorporated in Markov models as simply another function that can modify (i.e., reduce) the state-dependent incremental utilities.

TABLE 4.7
Markov Cohort Costs and Expected Utilities

	Well (Q = 1.0)	Progressive (Q = 0.8)	Total
Expected Cycles	4.262	2.630	6.892
Quality-Adjusted	4.262	2.104	6.366
Cost/Cycle	$5,000	$8,000	
Total Costs	$21,311	$21,043	$42,354

Note: Q = utility

4.3 MARKOV MODEL EXAMPLE: CERVICAL CANCER

Figure 4.3 depicts a simplified model of the progression from mild CIN 1 to invasive cervical cancer or recovery to normal. This model and its attendant data are drawn from the Goldie et al. study of the costs and projected benefits of an HPV vaccine (2004), to which the reader is referred for the complete model and cost-effectiveness analysis.[10] For this chapter the model and data are simplified in favor of didactic value.

In Figure 4.3 states are represented for Well, persistent HPV infection, CIN 1, CIN 2,3, invasive cervical CA, and death. For clarity, arrows from states to themselves have not been drawn, and a few rare transitions and non-cancer deaths are also omitted. The figure thus depicts the principal transitions in the model. The largest state-to-state transition is from CIN 1 to HPV. The basic 1-year cycle transition probability matrix for a 35-year-old woman is presented in Table 4.8. In this table the baseline or favorable range estimates from Goldie et al. are used.

Note that from CIN 1, the most likely transition is to HPV, although remaining in CIN 1 is also frequent. Cervical Cancer (CVX CA) is reached only from CIN 2,3

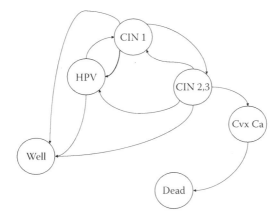

FIGURE 4.3 Principal transitions in Cervical Cancer Model. Transitions to same state (e.g., Well–Well) not shown.

TABLE 4.8
Transition Probability Matrix for the CIN Model

	Well	HPV	CIN 1	CIN 2,3	CVX CA	Dead
Well	0.9960	0.0040	0.0000	0.0000	0.0000	0.0000
HPV	0.1900	0.7881	0.0140	0.0080	0.0000	0.0000
CIN 1	0.2079	0.4400	0.2795	0.0726	0.0000	0.0000
CIN 2,3	0.0020	0.0199	0.0000	0.9661	0.0120	0.0000
CVX CA	0.0000	0.0000	0.0000	0.0000	0.9651	0.0349
DEAD	0.0000	0.0000	0.0000	0.0000	0.0000	1.0000

TABLE 4.9
Expected State Membership of Markov Cohort over 10 Years

	CIN 1	Well	HPV	CIN 2,3	CVX CA	Dead
35	10000					
36	2778	2079	4400	726	0	17
37	845	3479	4696	937	9	34
38	315	4527	4083	1002	20	54
39	163	5341	3369	1022	31	75
40	114	5982	2741	1023	42	98
41	94	6489	2225	1016	52	124
42	83	6889	1810	1004	63	152
43	76	7204	1479	988	72	182
44	70	7450	1214	968	81	215

and has an annual risk of death of 3.5%. If this table were used as depicted, both Well and Dead would be absorbing Markov states. Therefore, a time-dependent general population risk of death must be added. At 35, the annual risk of death is 0.17%, rising annually according to the Gompertz exponential function. At 84, the risk of death is 10%. Table 4.9 shows the experience over 10 years of 10,000 women aged 35 with CIN 1, according to the Markov model with the rising general death rate. In 1 year many women are well or have persistent HPV; none has cervical cancer because the model forces a transition to CIN 2,3 beforehand. CVX CA begins to appear at 37 and rises slowly.

Over an expected lifetime, the Markov model yields a probability of being in each state as shown in Figure 4.4. The Well cohort rises rapidly, and falls slowly as the natural death rate rises over time. The Well and Dead cohorts show the typical sigmoid functions. CIN 2,3 peaks at age 40, whereas CVX CA peaks at age 60 (149 prevalent cases). This is due to the relatively small excess mortality of CVX

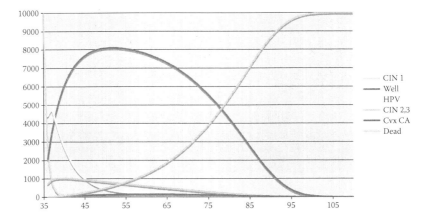

FIGURE 4.4   Natural history of CIN 1 example.

CA, and the structural assumptions in the Markov model in Figure 4.3 that has a patient remain in the CVX CA state until death. New cases of cervical cancer peak at age 41. One could extend the model by incorporating a state reflecting long-term survival from cervical cancer, but this would necessitate keeping track of how long each cohort member had had the cancer diagnosis. Modeling software can handle such issues, but the stochastic process becomes a semi-Markov model with attendant complexity.

Baseline results from this model are presented in Table 4.10. Averaged over a cohort, the patient with CIN 1 in this model can expect to live 1.63 years in that state, 33 years well, 3.56 years with persistent HPV, 3 years with CIN 2,3, and 0.55 years with CVX CA. Of course, no single patient has precisely this experience. A Monte Carlo simulation of 10,000 patients shows that the average number of cancer cases in this cohort is 356, with 95% of the simulations ranging between 335 and 378.

Sensitivity analysis (see Chapter 12) can be conducted on Markov transition probabilities, and modern software easily supports this. A linked sensitivity analysis, moving probability estimates to the upper end (worst case) of their ranges, generates the results found in Table 4.11. In this formulation the transition from CIN 1 to CIN 2,3 is much higher, the 5-year survival from CVX CA is 63% vs. a baseline of 84%, and the transition from CIN to cancer is doubled. Monte Carlo analysis shows a mean 1147 invasive cancers (95% range 1126 to 1161).

Goldie et al.'s more complete Markov formulation incorporates quality adjustments, effects of screening, and a primary focus on the role of vaccination to prevent persistent HPV and resulting CIN and downstream sequelae. It also has an extensive cost model. Later chapters in this text will illustrate how costs and structural interventions can modify Markov and other stochastic models to generate sophisticated analyses of pharmacoeconomic problems.

TABLE 4.10
Expected Results of CIN 1 Model

CIN 1	Well	HPV	CIN 2,3	CVX CA	Total
1.63	33.33	3.56	2.97	0.55	42.04

TABLE 4.11
Worst Case Results from CIN 1 Model

CIN 1	Well	HPV	CIN 2,3	CVX CA	Total
1.73	17.85	2.59	9.56	3.43	35.15

ENDNOTE

Some of the didactic material concerning regular and absorbing Markov chains has been adapted from "Markov Models (Introduction, Markov Property, Absorbing States)," an entry in *Encyclopedia of Medical Decision Making*, Sage Publications, 2009, in press.

REFERENCES

1. Beck JR, Kassirer JP, Pauker SG. 1982. A convenient approximation of life expectancy (the "DEALE"). I. Evaluation of the Method. *Am J Med* 73:883–888.
2. Beck JR, Pauker SG, Gottlieb JE, Klein K, Kassirer JP. 1982. A convenient approximation of life expectancy (the "DEALE"). II. Use in medical decision making. *Am J Med* 73:889–897.
3. Dasbach EJ, Elbasha EH, Insinga RP. 2006. Mathematical models for predicting the epidemiologic and economic impact of vaccination against human papillomavirus infection and disease. *Epidemiol Rev* 28:88–100.
4. Beck JR, Pauker SG. 1983. The Markov process in medical prognosis. *Med Decis Making* 3:419–458.
5. Sonnenberg FA, Beck JR. 1993. Markov models in medical decision making: A practical guide. *Med Decis Making* 13:322-338.
6. Bernoulli J. *Ars Conjectandi*, Op. Posthum. Accedit Tractatujs de Seriebus infinitis, et Epistola Gallice scripta de ludo Pilae recticularis, Basileae, 1713. (Ch. 1–4 trans. Bu Sung B. Technical Report No. 2, Dept. of Statistics, Harvard University, 1966).
7. Basharin GP, Langville AN, Naumov VA. The life and work of A. A. Markov. In, Grassman W, Meyer C, Stewart B, Szyld D. *Special Issue on the Numerical Solution of Markov Chains 2003, Linear Algebra and Its Applications* 2004; 386:3–26.
8. Briggs A, Sculpher M. 1998. An introduction to Markov modeling for economic evaluation. *Pharmacoeconomics* 13:397-409.
9. Gompertz B.1825. On the nature of the function expressive of the law of human mortality, and on a new mode of determining the value of life contingencies. *Philos Tran R Soc* 115:513–585.
10. Goldie SJ, Kohli M, Grima D, Weinstein MC, Wright TC, Bosch FX, Franco E. 2004. Projected clinical benefits and cost-effectiveness of a human papillomavirus 16/18 vaccine. *JNCI* 96:604–615.

5 Retrospective Database Analysis

Renée J.G. Arnold and Sanjeev Balu

CONTENTS

5.1 INTRODUCTION

Retrospective databases, whether created de novo from pre-existing sources, such as patients' written charts, or from preexisting electronic datasets, such as medical and pharmacy claims databases, electronic medical records, national insurance administrative data, hospital medical records, disease-specific patient registries, and patients and provider survey data, are a rich source of data for pharmacoeconomic analyses.[1–5] A listing of some population-based data sources (Table 5.1) and data sources available commercially or from the U.S. government (Table 5.2) is provided. In addition to health economic analyses, the data collected from these datasets can be used for outcomes research (such as analysis of healthcare practice patterns, epidemiologic analysis of disease progression, prevalence and characteristics of patient populations), evaluation of populations for prediction of future events, for formulary evaluation and to supplement prospective datasets, among other uses. When evidence

TABLE 5.1
Databases Available for Retrospective Analyses

Database Name	Inpatient Data	Outpatient Data	Major Advantage(s)	Major Limitation(s)	Cost
Claims					
PharMetrics	√ (limited)	√	Large database. Potentially more generalizable. Single–record layout (rather than multiple databases)	Limited hospital drug data	$75,000
General Practice Research Database (GPRD)*	√ (very limited)	√ (in U.K.)	Comprehensive outpatient data	U.K. only. Limited inpatient	$60,000–$100,000
THIN	√ (very limited)	√ (in U.K.)	Extension of GPRD	Extension of GPRD	$60,000–$100,000
Claims + Hospital					
Geisinger	√	√	Comprehensive inpatient and outpatient/lab data. Information on all payer types	Regional (rural Pennsylvania). takes approximately 16–20 weeks to obtain data	Approximately $100,000
Medicare 5% Datasets	√	√	Inpatient and outpatient data	Patients>65 years old	MEDPAR $3655/year of data. HOPPS $3000. Denominator file $250/year. SAF $3100
Thomson/Medstat MarketScan Hospital/Drug	√	√	Hospital drug information	Unsure about viability of linking inpatient and outpatient data. They will not license data to independent third party	Approximately $75,000
Premier/i3 Innovus	√	√	Comprehensive	Cost/exclusivity	Unattainable?

Hospital only

Cerner	√	√ (limited)	Comprehensive inpatient/ICU LOS/labs	Limited outpatient	Approximately $100,000–$125,000
Premier	√	√ (very limited)	Comprehensive inpatient/ICU LOS	Very limited outpatient	Very expensive
Ingenix/IHCIS	√	√ (limited)	Large cohort of Medicare beneficiaries	Standardized financials	?

* not really claims, since payer is NHS, but outpatient data

TABLE 5.2
U.S. Survey Databases

Dataset	Description	Comment	Patient–Level Data	Cost Data	Source	Media	Current Year	Basis for Release of Data
National Center for Health Statistics								
National Health Care Survey (NHCS)	National Ambulatory Medical Care Survey (NAMCS) National Hospital Ambulatory Medical Care Survey (NHAMCS) National Hospital Discharge Survey (NHDS[1]) National Nursing Home Survey (NNHS) National Health Provider Inventory[2] National Home and Hospice Care Survey	Statistical support re: adequate sample size. Extrapolation to U.S. Listing of nursing homes, residential care facilities, hospices, and home health agencies	No – encounter data	No	Providers	Internet for NAMCS, NHAMCS CD and download–able (FTP) for NHDS	2006	Annual
National Health Interview Survey (NHIS)	Nationwide survey by U.S. Bureau of Census	Productivity data Modified ICD–9	Yes	No	Patients	CD	2006	Annual

Agency for Healthcare Research and Quality (AHRQ)[3]

Medical Expenditure Panel Survey[4] (MEPS)	Series of surveys of healthcare utilization and costs last conducted in 2002 Projected 2008	Modified ICD-9 codes (CCS[5])	Yes	Yes	Patients	CD, diskette, Internet for projected 1998	2006	Longitudinal, roughly every 2 yrs
Healthcare Cost & Utilization Project (HCUP)	20% sample of U.S. community hospitals 1988–97	Inpatient data only Uses nonspecific CCS codes	Yes	Yes	Hospitals	CD	1998–97	Periodically

[1] Now also includes National Survey of Ambulatory Surgery (NSAS)
[2] Also includes National Employer Health Insurance Survey (NEHIS)
[3] Formerly Agency for Health Care Policy and Research (AHCPR)
[4] Formerly National Medical Expenditure Survey (NMES)
[5] Clinical Classification Software; condenses >12,000 ICD-9-CM codes into 260 categories

is not available for a decision that is imminent, analyses utilizing retrospective data-bases can provide decision support that is real-time, relevant, and comprehensive, providing that precautions are taken to address statistical considerations that may be inherent in these data sources. Indeed, several studies have found that treatment effects in observational studies were neither quantitatively nor qualitatively differ-ent from those obtained in "well-designed" randomized, controlled trials (RCTs).[6,7] Advantages of retrospective analyses in comparison to, for example, RCTs, include the fact that they are relatively inexpensive, quickly done, reflective of different pop-ulations, encompass a realistic time frame, organizationally specific, can be used for benchmarking purposes, include large sample sizes, and can capture real-world prescribing patterns.[1–4,8]

5.2   CLAIMS AND MEDICATION DATABASES

Health care administrative claims data, generally developed and maintained by third-party payers, offer a convenient and unique approach to studying health care resource utilization and associated cost. These databases represent a convenient alternative because data already are collected and stored electronically by health insurance companies. Claims data include outpatient, inpatient, and emergency room services, along with cost of outpatient prescription drugs. Computerized health insurance claims databases are maintained largely for billing and administrative purposes. Unlike studies with primary data collection, claims data are not collected to meet specific research objectives. Nevertheless, these databases are useful for describing health care utilization, patterns of care, disease prevalence, drug and dis-ease outcomes, medication adherence, and cost of care. Administrative claims data are thus an important source of information about major processes of care.

Administrative claims databases tend to be highly representative of a large, defined population. Large sample sizes permit enhanced precision and are particu-larly useful for studying rare events. As the data already are collected and comput-erized, data analysis is inexpensive, particularly in relation to prospective studies. Claims data also include outpatient drug information for patients younger than 65 years and, in some instances, for patients aged 65 years or older. This is very useful for studying drug outcomes and drug safety. An added benefit of using claims data is that it precludes any imposition on the patient, physician, or other provider.

However, claims data are affected by certain biases that may compromise the internal validity and, thereby, the robustness of the data (see Section 5.7).

The most important benefit of using claims databases to analyze clinical and eco-nomic outcomes is ease and convenience. The need to examine clinical, economic, and humanistic outcomes usually is limited by practical considerations, such as financial and time constraints, as well as concerns about patient privacy. Given these practical realities, the use of a claims database for some or all data collection offers an attractive alternative. Claims databases offer a number of important advantages for conducting health outcomes research. As mentioned, unlike RCTs, they reflect routine clinical "real world" practice. RCTs include carefully selected populations of particular ages and disease severity with few or no comorbidities. In addition, the procedures and protocols are not often representative of routine clinical care. Patient compliance typically is greater in RCTs than in the "real world" because of the support services available to treat adverse effects and the tendency of RCT participants to be more compliant than the population at large. In addition, they are unobtrusive and relatively inexpensive to use once the information system is in place. Further, databases provide a timely means of analyzing a problem. Answers can be found in days or weeks, rather than months or years. Finally, databases offer a great deal of flexibility. Rare diseases or specific subpopulations can be researched, or a problem can be approached in a number of different ways.

Claims databases allow for the measurement of clinical and economic outcomes (e.g., hospital and emergency room visits). Beyond such high-level outcome measures, the availability of the diagnosis, procedure, and revenue codes allow for further specification of a patient's outcome. ICD-9-CM (*International Classification of Diseases*, 9th Revision) codes provide diagnostic information allowing for identification of patients with a particular diagnosis or combination of diagnoses. *Physicians' Current Procedural Terminology*, 4th Edition (CPT-4 codes) identifies procedures that are used to bill physician and other professional services. For example, CPT-4 codes could be used to determine whether a depressed patient received hypnotherapy. The Healthcare Common Procedure Coding System (HCPCS) can be used to provide further information on physician and non-physician services that are not included in the CPT-4, such as whether a patient obtaining care in a physician's office for asthma received an injection of epinephrine.[9]

The processes of care also can be assessed from a claims database. For example, the number of outpatient physician visits might be considered a good measure of the quality of care received by hypertension patients. Procedure codes allow for the measurement of additional processes of care such as whether or not atrial fibrillation patients are receiving annual electrocardiograms or electrical cardioversion. A typical example of using medical databases for human papillomavirus (HPV) vaccine-associated studies would be to get a preliminary estimate of the burden of cervical cancer within a particular region. One such study by Watson M et al used multiple databases to estimate the burden of cervical cancer in the United States.[10] This study used data from two federal cancer surveillance programs, the Centers for Disease Control and Prevention (CDC)'s National Program of Cancer Registries, and the National Cancer Institute's Surveillance, Epidemiology, and End Results (SEER) Program to estimate cervical cancer incidence among different sub-populations. Identification of the study patients through diagnosis codes obtained in medical databases, incidence and prevalence rates among different age populations, race and gender mix, and across various geographical regions[11] can be easily accomplished through such databases. Another example would be a study examining the cervical cancer incidence before the HPV vaccine was introduced in the United States market.[12] Patients who are provided HPV vaccines for prevention of certain cancers and those who are not could also be studied to evaluate the incidence of future complications and associated total health care costs through most medical databases that provide clinical and economic data. However, most measures of the structure of care are not found in the database itself but within the patient benefit manual or other records held by the managed care organization (MCO). Important examples include copayment amount, formulary coverage of specific drugs, prescription quantity limits, and limits on mental health benefits.

Although databases offer a number of advantages for conducting outcomes management, they are not without their limitations. It is widely recognized that the diagnosis found in databases is not always valid or reliable. While some overcoding does occur, in most cases undercoding of actual diagnoses is more common. Undercoding is an even bigger problem with chronic diseases, which are notoriously underreported.[13,14] The principal finding in the Kern study was that identification of veteran diabetes patients with comorbid chronic kidney disease with a low glomerular filtration rate was severely underreported in Medicare administrative records.[13] Similarly, the Icen study found misclassification of patients diagnosed with psoriasis.[14] Several potential reasons for this misclassification would include the psoriasis diagnosis being differential in initial and follow-up physician visits, wrong initial diagnosis followed by actual psoriasis treatment, and the use of a nonspecific psoriasis code that does not specify the type of psoriasis.[14] Given these limitations, it is helpful to know for which disease states the coding is insufficient, calling for a review of the medical record. Unfortunately, there is no published research to provide guidance on this issue.

Another important consideration is patients' severity of illness. The goal often is to compare the outcomes of care for persons receiving different treatments or receiving care from different types of providers. Zhao et al.[15] used a claims database to analyze the prevalence of diabetes-associated complications and comorbidities and its impact on health care costs among patients with diabetic neuropathy. This study identified the various complications and comorbidities through diagnosis codes and health care costs in the claims data. However, there may be important differences in the patients being compared that cannot be measured or controlled when using the information in the database. Other significant indicators of a patient's disease severity, including smoking status, alcohol consumption status, laboratory values, and results of other diagnostic tests, are sometimes not available for analysis in the database. Pharmacy use described in the claims databases usually provides information about prescription medications. However, over-the-counter medications that are being used are generally not captured in such databases.

5.2.1 Description of Claims Database Files

Medication or claims databases usually have several files that characterize different patient settings where care is provided. These include, among others, inpatient, outpatient, emergency room, and pharmacy (medication) files. The outpatient file, for example, contains final action claims data submitted by institutional outpatient providers. Outpatient claims provide detailed information on the date of service, site of service (e.g., home care), provider specialty, type of service, and reimbursed charges. These variables allow us to calculate the frequency of health care utilization and its respective cost. Among several variables listed in outpatient files, the variables that are discussed in this data file are date of service, amount billed and amount paid, and provider information. Each outpatient visit record in the outpatient file usually includes the following information: date of visit, whether the respondent/patient saw a physician, type of care received, type of services received, medicines prescribed, flat-fee information, imputed sources of payment, total payment, and total charge, among others.

Similarly, claims data for hospitalizations can be an extremely valuable source for evaluating health outcomes in terms of incidence and frequency of hospitalization episodes, severity of the hospitalization episode in terms of length of stay and hospitalization costs. Inpatient claims data are also useful to assess the hospitalization costs associated with a condition or disease in a population. For each claim during a hospitalization episode, the file contains fields such as patient identification number, provider number, ICD-9 code of diagnosis for which the service was provided, CPT code for procedures and services provided, Diagnosis-Related Group (DRG) codes, date of hospital admission, date of discharge, location of service (outpatient, emergency room, or inpatient), total amount billed, and total amount paid.

The prescription drug file in a claims dataset contains useful information on medications prescribed and taken by patients. Information is captured when the patient fills the prescription and a claim is then filed by the pharmacy. Importantly, the primary focus of the claim is the fill transaction; claims will show the activity of when the fills occur, but they will not show whether the patient actually took the medications. Thus, while claims serve as a proxy for compliance and adherence due to their ability to show fills, primary research may be used as an adjunct to determine if the patient actually used the medications when at home. Each record in the prescription drug file represents one reported prescribed medicine that was purchased for a particular episode. Only prescribed medicines that were purchased for a particular episode are usually represented in this file. Medication refills are also usually captured in this file, which allows for tracking medication usage by the patient longitudinally. The typical descriptors for medications on record include an identifier for each unique prescribed medicine; detailed characteristics associated with the event (e.g., national drug code (NDC), medicine name, etc.); conditions, if any, associated with the medicine; the date on which the person first used the medicine; total expenditure and sources of payments; and the types of pharmacies that filled the household's prescriptions.

Similarly, information provided by the emergency room visits file includes date of the visit, whether the patient saw the doctor, type of care received, type of services (i.e., lab test, sonogram or ultrasound, x-rays, etc.) received, medicines prescribed during the visit, cost information, imputed sources of payment, total payment, and total charge.

5.3 ELECTRONIC MEDICAL RECORDS AND MEDICAL CHARTS

5.3.1 MEDICAL CHART/MEDICAL RECORD IN GENERAL

A medical chart or a record is a confidential document that contains detailed, comprehensive, and current information about a patient's health care experience, including diagnoses, treatment, tests, and treatment responses, in addition to other factors that might play a significant role in his or her health condition. This document summarizes the overall collected information of an individual related to health status. Once a patient enters a health care setting, be it a hospital or a clinic, documentation in a medical chart or record begins. Different medical settings follow different types of such documentation practices; however, there are certain aspects of such a document that remain universal.

Some of the most common entries in a medical chart or record include the following: admission information, medical history and physical information, medication and treatment orders, medications and other treatments received, procedures, diagnostic and other tests, insurance, consultations, patient consents, and discharge information.[16] Documentation in the chart or record is usually done by the physician or the nurse.

5.3.2 Electronic Medical Records (EMRs) or Charts

With recent advances in technology, written medical charts or records are gradually being converted to computerized or electronic versions. The electronic version, similar to the paper version of the medical record or chart, serves the same purpose of communication and documentation of an individual's contact with a health care provider and the decisions made by the provider regarding the patient, including diagnoses and treatments provided.

5.3.2.1 Advantages/Disadvantages

Several advantages of EMRs over print medical records or charts could recommend their use by a medical institution. These include ease of chart or record accessibility, reduction of medical errors and task automation, legible medical notes, continuity of care and accountability, availability of an organized chart, and increased security.[17] Other advantages include patient report generation for certain screening methods, including mammography and cholesterol screening, patients taking medications that have been recalled, computerized practice or treatment guidelines that can be easily accessible, adequate alert systems that would notify the health care provider about certain adverse results that require prompt action, improved documentation and care management, and potential cost savings.[18–21] However, certain disadvantages of EMRs also should be noted. There have been instances where a patient's laboratory and other clinical data have not been integrated with the computerized system. This affects the comprehensiveness of the medical record, as key elements pertaining to the patient's health are missing. Efforts must be made to integrate all detailed and pertinent patient information. Another significant disadvantage would be system crashes during a patient visit that render unavailability of patient information during that period. Appropriate measures should ensure adequate back-up measures in the event of such crashes or system malfunction.[17]

5.3.2.2 Current Use of EMRs

Though EMRs show potential benefits for healthcare organizations to adopt them into their systems, according to a recent study, only 4% of U.S. physicians have had access to an EMR system.[22] Moreover, primary care physicians and those working in large groups are more likely than physicians in other medical specialties and smaller size practices, respectively, to use EMRs.[22] In another study that researched the use of EMRs in ambulatory care practices in the state of Massachusetts, only 18% of the surveyed office practices reported using one.[23] Some prominent reasons for this low uptake of technology include, among others, the significant direct and indirect cost for licensing the EMR software. Indirect costs include staff training to use the software and system maintenance. Cost is also a factor points to the fact that large physician practices have greater financial and technological resources than smaller practices and solo physician practice and, thus, the higher adoption rate of technological advances, including EMRs in large practices. Other factors include data entry obstacles, lack of trained staff, lack of uniformity, legal issues, and patient confidentiality and security concerns.[24] Similarly, another study found a higher adoption of EMRs among physicians owned by health maintenance organizations (HMOs).[25]

Some specific examples of how EMRs have been used as databases to provide insights into various therapeutic areas are provided below. The main advantages of using EMRs as databases to conduct pharmacoeconomic analyses include the richness and comprehensiveness of the data to estimate prevalence, incidence, physician treatment patterns, and cost of various prevention and treatment strategies available to medical practitioners. One example would be a study that estimated the tobacco-use prevalence using EMRs.[26] The availability of data needed to analyze the study objective eliminates the need to do expensive multiple surveys of different sub-populations to get the needed answer. This particular study used the EMR database of a large medical group in Minnesota. The study showed that out of the overall included population, 19.7% were tobacco users during the year March 2006 to February 2007, of which 24.2% were aged 18–24 years, 16% were pregnant women, 34.3% were Medicaid enrollees, 40% were American Indians, and 9.5% were Asians.

Another study used an EMR to analyze associations between cardiometabolic risk factors and body mass index based on diagnosis and treatment codes.[27] This particular study used the General Electric (GE) Centricity research database, which is a rich source of data used by more than 20,000 physicians to manage about 30 million patient records in 49 states. The availability of data, including clinical data captured in the practice setting, such as diagnoses, patient complaints, medication orders, medication lists, laboratory orders and results, and biometric readings, was a significant factor in the appropriateness of this dataset for the particular study. The Kaiser Permanente EMR was used to evaluate the complications associated with dysglycemia and medical costs associated with non-diabetic hyperglycemia.[28] The EMR database used for this study provided information on all inpatient admissions, outpatient visits, pharmacy medication dispenses, and results of laboratory tests. As the study was based on diabetes patients, clinical information on isolated impaired fasting glucose (available in the database) was the primary factor used in classifying the study diabetes patients. The study found that more than half of the studied dysglycemia patients had at least one associated complication as compared with only 34% of normoglycemic patients (p<0.001). The study also found that macrovascular and microvascular complications had an incremental annual cost of $3,863 (p<0.0001) and $1,874 (p<0.0001) for dysglycemic patients versus normoglycemic patients. A final example would be a study evaluating the acceptance of HPV vaccine by gynecologists in an urban setting.[29] This study found that the overall vaccination rate was 28% (6%–55.8%) for the initial 3-month period when the vaccine became available to the health plan.

5.4   PATIENT REPORTED OUTCOMES

A patient-reported outcome (PRO) is a measurement and assessment of a patient's health status coming directly from the patient rather than from a physician or any other health care provider.[30] The Food and Drug Administration refers to a PRO as any report coming from patients about a health condition and its treatment.[30] An important feature that differentiates a PRO from any other measurement is that the measurement is done directly from the patient. A PRO thus provides a patient's perspective on treatment effectiveness,[31,32] adverse events, etc. Health-related quality of life (HRQoL), a term closely related to PRO, specifically refers to measures that are not only patient reported, but also include the impact of the disease and its treatment on the patient's well-being and functioning (see Chapter 11 on PROs).[31] A PRO measure includes various facets of disease treatment and its effectiveness as reported directly by the patient. These include, among others, reports of symptoms such as pain, fatigue, physical functioning, and well-being in the physical, mental, and social domains of life.[33] Many health behaviors, including use of tobacco and alcohol, participation in exercise programs, etc., are also included in a typical PRO. Other end points captured in a PRO include patient preferences for a particular treatment and treatment satisfaction.[33] A PRO measure can include patient satisfaction with treatment, medication adherence, and other aspects of disease treatment, functional status, psychological well-being, and health status in addition to HRQoL.[34,35]

5.4.1   USE OF PRO INSTRUMENTS IN PHARMACOECONOMIC STUDIES: FOCUS ON HPV VACCINE STUDIES

Although PROs usually consist of specific health-related questionnaires or instruments, providing a simple survey questionnaire for patient response also makes up a simpler form of PRO. This section provides examples of how such PRO questionnaires have been used in HPV vaccine-related issues and studies. Gerend and Magloire assessed the awareness, knowledge, and beliefs about HPV in a racially diverse sample of young adults.[36] The authors used a survey to get respondent-reported responses among 124 students aged 18–26 years from two southeastern universities. The survey assesses demographics, sexual history, awareness and knowledge of HPV, HPV-related beliefs, and interest in the HPV vaccine (women only). This study reported some interesting findings that could be used for further economic studies on HPV vaccine, including great knowledge of HPV, greater awareness among women of HPV as compared with men, and a greater interest in HPV education among blacks and sexually active respondents.[36] Another study examined the stage of adoption of the HPV vaccine among college women aged 18–22 years at a New England University.[37] This study used an online survey as a means to complete the PRO instrument. The survey examined knowledge of HPV, perceived susceptibility, severity, vaccine benefits or barriers, and stage of vaccine adoption. The use of such PRO measures provides a useful means to get responses directly from patients (in this case, women) who have used HPV vaccine or have potential to use one in the future. The analyzed results indicated that the acceptance of the vaccine was high among the study respondents and that the importance of Pap smears was also high.[37] Yet another study analyzed the acceptance of HPV vaccine among mid-adult women.[38] This particular study used a convenience sample of 472 mid-adult women who completed a survey that examined the demographic, knowledge, and behavioral variables associated with HPV vaccine acceptance. This study assumes clinical significance, as some of the variables that were found to be associated with vaccination among the study respondents could be useful to clinicians to identify potential female patients who might be more receptive to the vaccine.[38] These variables included women who were younger than 55 years, had had an abnormal Papanicolaou test, understood the association of HPV and cervical cancer, and those who felt at risk for HPV infection.

Though HPV-related diseases are more common among women, men are also exposed to the virus in varying forms and severity. A study similar to the Ferris study based on women examined the variables associated with HPV vaccine acceptance among men.[39] Similar results were obtained from this study in that the (male) respondents with a higher education and knowledge about HPV were more likely to accept HPV vaccination than others.[39]

5.5   ALTERNATIVE POPULATION-BASED DATA SOURCES

As mentioned in Table 5.1, numerous datasets are available either commercially or from the U.S. government. These include:

1. Thomson/Medstat

- MarketScan claims database
- Hospital/drug database (formerly Solucient)

MarketScan contains claims and encounters data representing commercially insured, Medicare supplemental (Medigap), and Medicaid patients. It covers approximately 17 million lives in any given year. Longitudinal tracking, across health plans and across payers, is possible. Subsets of patients may be linked to laboratory test results. Approximately 350,000 discharges have been linked between the Hospital/drug (inpatient) and MarketScan (outpatient) databases. Intensive care unit (ICU) length of stay (LOS) is also available.

2. IMS/PharMetrics

The PharMetrics Patient-Centric Database comprises medical and pharmaceutical claims for a very large number of patients from more than 90 health plans across the United States. The database includes both inpatient and outpatient diagnoses (in ICD-9-CM format) and procedures (in CPT-4 and HCPCS formats), as well as both retail and mail order prescription records. Available data on prescription records include the NDC code, as well as quantity dispensed. Charges, allowed and paid amounts are available for all services rendered, as well as dates of service for all claims. The inpatient data are less comprehensive than the Thomson Hospital/drug database, as drug-specific data and ICU LOS are not available. However, full Medicare data are available.

3. Medicare Datasets

Available from the Centers for Medicare and Medicaid Services (CMS), a benefit of using the Medicare databases is that they include inpatient and outpatient data for most U.S. hospitals, with the exception of VA (Veterans Affairs) and military hospitals. These data are readily available for transformation to a usable form for comparative purposes. A limitation is that they are primarily constituted by an elderly sector of the population (approximately 40 million patients), so are not generalizable to younger populations.

There are several types of encrypted general-use Medicare datasets, available in 5% or 100% segments, which are described below:

- LDS (Limited Dataset) Standard Analytical Files (SAFs): contain payment information for each institutional (inpatient, outpatient, skilled nursing facility, hospice, or home health agency) and non-institutional (physician and durable medical equipment providers) claim type
- LDS MEDPAR (Medicare Provider Analysis and Review) Files: contain inpatient hospital "final action stay" records, summarizing all services received by a patient from admission through discharge
- LDS Denominator File: contains demographic and enrollment data about each beneficiary in the Medicare and Medicare Managed Care Organizations
- LDS Outpatient Hospital Prospective Payment System (PPS): contains select claim level data from the Hospital Outpatient PPS claims

4. Geisinger

Data from Geisinger hospitals and physicians, both general practice and specialists, comprise data available from MedMining, a Geisinger Health System business. It has 7-plus years of longitudinal, full clinical data on over 3 million patients and 10-plus years of lab results that are captured electronically in an electronic health record, as well as other clinical, financial, and administrative systems. The data include an associated reason code for every prescription. Dispensing information and drug cost are not available. Being from hospitals and community-based physicians throughout rural Pennsylvania, the data may not be generalizable to all U.S. patients. In addition, patient co-payment information is not available.

5. Cerner

Cerner Health Facts™ contains inpatient and hospital outpatient data on over 12 million patients; the Cerner dataset also contains lab results data. However, no longitudinal (claims) data are available from community-based outpatient settings.

6. Premier

Premier's Perspective Hospital Database is a comprehensive hospital utilization database that includes patient-level clinical and financial data reflecting an accurate national representation of the U.S. hospital market in over 6 million patients. It contains hospital drug data and some patient subsets have inpatient and outpatient hospital data; laboratory test results are currently not available. Premier also can combine its inpatient records with i3 Innovus, which provides an integrated database of enrollment, inpatient and outpatient medical claims, pharmaceutical claims, and laboratory results. However, this database combination appears to be proprietary.

7. Ingenix/IHCIS

The former IHCIS business, now part of Ingenix, constructs a database comprising commercial plan payers and contains a large number of Managed Medicare beneficiaries. Although it has data for approximately 3 million lives from community-based labs, there are no patient co-pay data or original paid amounts, as they have standardized, rather than actual, financials.

8. General Practice Research Database

The General Practice Research Database, or GPRD, dataset is a near-complete electronic record of all care for 5.5% of the United Kingdom, containing more than 3 million active patients. The most current format of GPRD is termed FF-GPRD. Because these are data collected by general practitioners (GPs), while the community data are very detailed (labs, medications), the hospital data are not very comprehensive.

9. THIN (The Health Improvement Network)

For The Health Improvement Network, or THIN, data collection commenced in January 2003, using information extracted from Vision, a widely used general practice management software package developed by In Practice Systems. The database is regularly updated and currently contains data on over 5 million individuals living in the U.K. THIN was developed as a replacement for the GPRD, because the EPIC version of the GPRD was discontinued from April 2002. Meanwhile, the GPRD is maintained by the U.K. Medicines and Healthcare Products Regulatory Agency (MHRA) in London. THIN's pluses and minuses are the same as GPRD.

10. General Electric Centricity Research Database

GE Centricity is an EMR. The database comprises de-identified electronic patient records from users of the EMR software and currently consists of data from over 8 million unique patients. A potential positive to this database is the availability of patient-reported over-the-counter medication use, while a potential negative to this database is its lack of inpatient data.

11. Framingham Offspring Study (FOS) Database

The Framingham Study is a longitudinal population-based observational study that began in 1948 in Framingham, MA. In 1971, a second-generation cohort was recruited into the Framingham Offspring/Spouse (FOS) study.[40] Cohort members are examined in the clinic every 4 years, on average, where they undergo a standardized protocol for data collection approved by the Boston University Institutional Review Board. This database provides a rich source of information related to cardiovascular disease, including coronary heart disease, stroke, hypertension, peripheral arterial disease, and congestive heart failure.

12. Atherosclerosis Risk in Communities (ARIC) Database

Atherosclerosis Risk in Communities (ARIC) Study, sponsored by the U.S. National Heart, Lung, and Blood Institute (NHLBI) National Institute of Health, is a prospective observational biracial follow-up of 15,792 men and women between the ages of 45 and 64, recruited from Forsyth County, North Carolina; Jackson, Mississippi; suburbs of Minneapolis, Minnesota; and Washington County, Maryland. This database provides key clinical information on the etiology and risk factors associated with atherosclerosis, along with differences in medical care obtained by patients of different race and gender as well as those residing in different locations.

5.6   ISSUES AND CHALLENGES

Although numerous advantages exist with use of retrospective databases over RCTs, considerations of internal validity (reproducibility of results) and external validity (generalizability of results) must be addressed. For example, with RCTs, because they are protocol-based, it is relatively easy to reproduce the results of a trial of a hypertension drug using an identical protocol in a patient population following the same inclusion and exclusion criteria. With retrospective databases, however, confounding factors (see Section 5.7), such as a center effect or regional variation in the prevalence of hypertension, may limit the ability to duplicate these results between different populations, such as between two MCOs or even between two locations of the same MCO. However, the very measure that helps to ensure reproducibility, namely, the protocol, may reduce the study's use in the real world, as any analysis would have to consider protocol-induced (artificial) resource use and costs. Generalizability refers to the ability to extrapolate results across health care settings or even countries. A pharmacoeconomic analysis must provide segregated healthcare resource units (e.g., numbers of MRIs) and costs per unit (e.g., cost of an individual MRI), so that if a resource is not used the same way in the United States and Canada or the costs are very dissimilar, each country can use the resource data, but customize it to its own cost structure. The caveat here, of course, is to determine whether the resource utilization itself is similar across the two countries.

To determine if a dataset is appropriate to answer a pharmacoeconomic question, key attributes of the population (such as demographics), covered services, benefit design (e.g., nationalized or private insurance, deductibles, patient co-payments), formulary design (e.g., open [allowing any drug], closed [allowing only specific drugs]) and any special programs (e.g., physician detailing, disease management initiatives) that might affect its generalizability should be enumerated. Johnson outlines a six-step process for conducting outcomes analyses using administrative databases, as seen in Table 5.3.[41] Since practice, including available treatments and procedures, changes over time, it is essential to use retrospective data to continuously inform health policy decisions.[42] An example of use of data from a pharmacy benefits

---

TABLE 5.3
Steps to Designing a Database Study

- Define the study objective
- Extract key data elements
- Apply inclusion, exclusion criteria
- Perform initial data analyses
- Create "calculated" analysis variables
- Compare groups

---

management claims database to evaluate two decision-analytic models regarding the cost-effectiveness of therapeutic regimens to eradicate *Helicobacter pylori* in ulcer patients is a case in point.[43] The authors found that model results overstated the cost-effectiveness of the previously more cost-effective regimen and underestimated the cost-effectiveness of the other regimen such that the model assumptions and, ultimately, the outcomes, were not supported by the data.

Regardless of how the data are used, issues of data quality must be addressed. A checklist detailing many of these issues was published as a result of an International Society for Pharmacoeconomics and Outcomes Research (ISPOR) Task Force's being convened to examine the quality of published studies using retrospective databases.[4] It is important to have plans to examine a representative number or percentage of source documents (e.g., patient charts) to determine that diagnosis and procedure codes are reasonably accurate. For example, Fivenson, Arnold, and colleagues determined that approximately 10% of diagnosis codes in an atopic dermatitis study utilizing a claims dataset were inaccurate.[3] Moreover, coding may change over time, such as use of different versions of the ICD-9-CM coding set, differing frequencies of use of codes according to reimbursement policies or varying regional codes (e.g., HCPCS codes).[44] In a study to evaluate the coding data quality of the Healthcare Cost & Utilization Project (HCUP) National Inpatient Sample, claims data failed to identify more than 50% of patients with prognostically important conditions, and miscoding of diagnoses resulted in nonspecific disease identification or coexisting conditions.[45] Coding error rates were found to vary widely among states, hospitals within states, geographic location, and hospital characteristics. Coding errors were significantly different among patient demographic groups and whether the state used billing versus abstract data.

In addition, services may not be captured in the database because they are administered elsewhere (e.g., carved out, such as mental health services).[4] It is important to minimize missing and out-of-range values, ensure consistency of data (e.g., no menopausal men), control duplication of records, assure continuous enrollment, ascertain the availability of the continuum of care, and make certain that data have been recorded uniformly because if there is inconsistency in coding, there is inconsistency in the resulting judgments derived from that data.[46] Sax[47] mentions the pharmacy field "days supply" as potentially problematic as an indicator of patient adherence to a medication regimen due to dose titrations (e.g., gradual reductions in prednisone "burst" during asthma exacerbation,[48–50] unknown actual use, as-needed medications, and possible unknown sources of additional medication, such as from an unrelated pharmacy. As with prospective data collection, benchmarking values against established norms, such as the SF-36 for quality of life, will assure researchers that the data are representative of the population at large.[51]

It is also important that data links across relational databases be consistent. For example, there should be unique identifiers for each family member. Many times, data must be concatenated (or joined) from several fields in a database to make sure that this is the case.[21] Moreover, events may not be recorded at the same time that they actually occurred for the patient, as with provider charges occurring perhaps 6 months to a year after a procedure for a Medicare patient, so it is essential that this lag time is considered when evaluating an episode of care.[47–52]

In addition, temporal factors may play a role in analyses using preexisting data, either in terms of hypothesis testing or as a confounder. For example, Arnold and colleagues used clinical trials, published literature, and a modified Delphi panel to establish the effect of timing of administration of a thrombin inhibitor, argatroban, on its cost-effectiveness in patients with heparin-induced thrombocytopenia (that is, heparin hypersensitivity).[53] It is also necessary to define and identify disease-related costs. For example, in patients with asthma, should claims be related only to the various ICD-9 diagnosis codes for the various types of asthma[54] or should there be the added requirement of an asthma medication or diagnostic testing sometime during the index or eligibility period? It is useful to be able to "tease out" costs during a hospitalization related specifically to the diagnosis of interest; however, this is often not possible because of potential overlap between the diagnosis of interest and concomitant illness, e.g., pneumonia in the case of asthma. It is also important to account for natural history of disease progression and medical and technological advances that may have impacted on the course of the disease in terms of the index date (beginning of data collection) and duration of data inclusion. Indeed, Motheral and colleagues discuss the idea of censoring or the time limits placed at the beginning (left censoring, period prior to initiation of therapy of interest) or end (right censoring, follow-up time) of the study period.[4]

5.7   STATISTICAL ISSUES

Bias is a significant problem that must be addressed. The types of biases include selection bias, measurement bias, length of measurement bias, misspecification bias, interdependence of observations, diagnostic ascertainment bias, autocorrelation, omitted variables, quasi-omitted variables, investigator bias, obsolescence bias, vintage bias (human and physical capital), claims vs. encounter bias and recall bias. The reader is referred to a lengthy review of these types of bias by Sackett and colleagues.[55]

The previously discussed ISPOR checklist has categorized many of the statistical issues facing users of retrospective databases in general.[4] These are reviewed below. The first is control variables. It is important to account for the effects of all variables so that biased estimates of treatment effects, or confounding bias, do not occur. For example, it is important to control for the likelihood of prescribing certain compounds given a patient's history of comorbid conditions. Common approaches to adjust for confounding bias include stratification of the cohort by different levels of the confounding variables with comparison of the treatments within potential confounders, such as demographic variables; the use of multivariate statistical techniques; cohort matching and propensity adjustment.[4,56] Multivariate regression can be used to estimate the association among the intervention, confounders, and the outcome of interest.[56,57] Stratification divides the study population into subgroups on the basis of confounding characteristics to reduce confounding. With cohort matching, a comparator cohort is generated based on characteristics associated with confounding bias.[58] A Chronic Disease Score or the Charlson Index can be used to control for comorbidities[59] or disease severity,[60] respectively. Moreover, instrumental variable techniques can be used to group patients by choice of treatment, but without unmeasured confounders.

Selection bias may be introduced by the inclusion and exclusion criteria used in the study design, especially considering that missing data, such as a diagnosis code, may cause records not to be chosen for analysis. Thus, the population selected may not be representative of all patients that should be included.[46] A method that is frequently used to account for potential inherent differences in treatment assignment due to selection bias in retrospective databases is propensity scoring.[61] The propensity score, defined as the conditional probability of being treated given the covariates, or the probability that a patient would have been treated, can be used to balance the covariates in the groups, thereby adjusting the estimate of the treatment effect. To estimate the propensity score, one models the distribution of the treatment indicator variables, considering the observed covariates. The propensity score is then estimated using logistic regression or discriminant analysis. Once estimated, the propensity score can be used to reduce bias through matching, stratification (subclassification), regression adjustment, or some combination of all three. All of these methods are an attempt to effect a "quasi-randomized" treatment allocation.

Since much data in retrospective databases is expected to be skewed in its distribution, techniques such as log-transformation and two-part models should be considered. Methods such as hierarchical linear modeling may be appropriate when using pooled data from several different health plans or multiple sites from a single health plan to account for center (that is, facility) effects.[4]

Outliers are another issue that must be addressed in economic analyses using retrospective databases. As mentioned above and particularly true when using costs rather than the quantity of units, such as hospital days or physician office visits, to measure resource use, just a small number of outliers can greatly skew the analysis. Logarithmic transformations that have been used previously to reduce skewness can create difficulties with non-log-transformed costs. For this reason, it is often prudent to record unit costs and quantities separately and, if a high degree of skewness is present, use the quantities for the statistical calculation, then multiplying by a set dollar amount from a fee schedule.

5.8 NON-U.S. COUNTRIES

As with U.S. data sources, international retrospective databases encompass such sources as national insurance administrative data, hospital medical records, disease-specific patient registries, and provider survey data.[5] Table 5.1 contains two (U.K.) sources of such data from a study[5] that qualitatively reviewed the methodological challenges of using non-U.S. databases to conduct retrospective economic and outcomes research studies. The researchers conducted a MEDLINE search to obtain a sample of literature published after the year 2000 on retrospective analyses incorporating non-U.S. databases using the ISPOR checklist and found that few economic studies included information on indirect cost components because of a lack of relevant data. Moreover, they found that the quality of non-U.S. retrospective database analyses varied, leading to problems of internal validity, that is, study design errors that could compromise conclusions. The economic datasets were from Italy, Australia, United Kingdom, Switzerland, Singapore, seven other European countries, Canada, Japan, and France. Only two of the 12 studies reviewed included indirect costs. Ten of the 12 economic studies reviewed made adjustments for confounders or sampling schemes (i.e., to reduce selection bias), typically with some form of regression model. The authors thought that five studies did not sufficiently address external validity. Sensitivity analysis was the most common approach to dealing with uncertainty in the studies. Five studies extensively discussed study limitations; however, all of the study authors, as well as the review author, advised caution regarding the external validity of the studies.

5.9 THE FUTURE IN USE OF RETROSPECTIVE DATABASES

What is the future for use of retrospective databases to inform pharmacoeconomic analyses? Stallings and colleagues[62] developed a decision-analytic model to test the likely cost impact of a hypothetical pharmacogenomic test to determine a preferred initial therapy in patients with asthma. They compared annualized per patient cost distributions using a "test all" strategy for a nonresponse genotype prior to treating versus "test none." They found that the cost savings per patient of the testing strategy simulation ranged from US$200 to US$767 (95% confidence interval) and concluded that upfront testing costs were likely to be offset by avoided nonresponse costs. This shows the potential use of retrospective database studies in analytic data mining and improved hypothesis testing.

Indeed, there is an increasing likelihood that genomics will play a role in decisions about drug use. For example, a recent theoretical Markov model showed pharmacogenomic-guided dosing for anticoagulation with warfarin not to be cost-effective in patients with nonvalvular atrial fibrillation.[63] Interestingly, another recently published algorithm using logistic regression from international retrospective databases showed that incorporating pharmacogenetic information was more likely to result in a therapeutic international normalized ratio (INR), the major method of determining anticoagulation, than use of clinical data alone.[64] However, the data used to inform the Markov model were published studies that did not include the latter study and the algorithm did not indicate the clinical diagnoses, nor the clinical outcomes, of the patients who were more or less likely to be within a therapeutic INR. Therefore, more research is needed to coordinate these two somewhat conflicting results. Indeed, another potential for the use of such easily available databases is to increase their use in validation studies. Testing the same hypothesis in several databases increases the validity of the study results, thereby increasing the credibility of the findings. However, in the near future, retrospective databases are more likely to continue being used for quick identification of treatment patterns, prevalence, and incidence of a medical condition, medication adherence, and persistence, and health care resource utilization and associated costs related to a particular medical condition. With clinical trials getting more and more time consuming and expensive, retrospective databases offer an attractive alternative to provide this "real-life" medical information.

REFERENCES

1. Arnold R. Use of interactive software in medical decision making. In: Ekins S, Ed. *Computer Applications in Pharmaceutical Research and Development*. Hoboken: John Wiley & Sons, Inc. 2006.
2. Arnold RG, Kotsanos JG. 1999. Panel 3: Methodological issues in conducting pharmacoeconomic evaluations—retrospective and claims database studies. *Value Health* 2(2):82–7.
3. Fivenson D, Arnold RJ, Kaniecki DJ, Cohen JL, Frech F, Finlay AY. 2002. The effect of atopic dermatitis on total burden of illness and quality of life on adults and children in a large managed care organization. *J Manag Care Pharm* 8(5):333–42.
4. Motheral B, Brooks J, Clark MA, et al. 2003. A checklist for retrospective database studies—report of the ISPOR Task Force on Retrospective Databases. *Value Health* 6(2):90–7.
5. Shi L, Wu EQ, Hodges M, Yu A, Birnbaum H. 2007. Retrospective economic and outcomes analyses using non-US databases: A review. *Pharmacoeconomics* 25(7):563–76.
6. Benson K, Hartz AJ. 2000. A comparison of observational studies and randomized, controlled trials. *N Engl J Med* 342(25):1878–86.
7. Concato J, Shah N, Horwitz RI. 2000. Randomized, controlled trials, observational studies, and the hierarchy of research designs. *N Engl J Med* 342(25):1887–92.
8. Arnold R. 1996. Applications of large databases to evaluate cost-effective therapy. *Clinical Ther* 18(suppl A):15.
9. HCPS general information available on: http://www.cms.hhs.gov/MedHCPCSGenInfo/01_ Overview.asp#TopOfPage. Last accessed on January 5, 2009.
10. Watson M, Saraiya M, Benard V, Coughlin SS, Flowers L, Cokkinides V, Schwenn M, Huang Y, Giuliano A. 2008. Burden of cervical cancer in the United States, 1998–2003. *Cancer* 113(10Suppl): 2855–2864.
11. Becker TM, Espey DK, Lawson HW, Saraiya M, Jim MA, Waxman AG. 2008. Regional differences in cervical cancer, incidence among American Indians and Alaska Natives, 1999–2004. *Cancer* 113(5 Suppl): 1234–1243.
12. Saraiya M, Ahmed F, Krishnan S, Richards TB, Unger ER, Lawson HW. 2007. Cervical cancer incidence in a prevaccine era in the United States, 1998–2002. *Obstet Gynecol* 109(2 Pt 1): 360–370.
13. Kern EFO, Maney M, Miller DR, Tseng C-L, Tiwari A, Rajan M, Aron D, Pogach L. 2006. Failure of ICD-9-CM codes to identify patients with comorbid chronic kidney disease in diabetes. *Health Serv Res* 41(2): 564–580.

14. Icen M, Crowson CS, McEvoy MT, Gabriel SE, Kremers HM. 2008. Potential misclassification of patients with psoriasis in electronic databases. *J Am Acad Dermatol* 59(6): 981–985.

15. Zhao Y, Ye W, Boye KS, Holcombe JH, Hall JA, Swindle R. 2008. Prevalence of other diabetes-associated complications and comorbidities and its impact on health care charges among patients with diabetic neuropathy. *J Diabetes Comp* October 17 (Ahead of print).

16. Encyclopedia of Surgery. Medical charts. At http://www.surgeryencyclopedia.com/La-Pa/Medical-Charts.html. Accessed November 25, 2008.

17. Tahil FA. 2003. Hello electronic medical records, farewell paper charts. *Psych News* 38(9): 34.

18. Sujansky WV. 1998. The benefits and challenges of an electronic medical record: Much more than a "word-processed" patient chart. *West J Med* 169: 176–183.

19. Miller H, Sim I. 2004. Physicians' use of electronic medical records: Barriers and solutions. *Health Affairs* 23(2): 116–126.

20. Hillestad R, Bigelow J, Bower A, Girosi F, Meili R, Scoville R, Taylor R. 2005. Can electronic medical record systems transform health care? Potential benefits, savings, and costs. *Health Affairs* 24(5): 1103–1117.

21. Zaid RR. 2008. Electronic medical records: What are you waiting for? *J Am Osteo Assoc* 108(2): 81–82.

22. DesRoches CM, Campbell EG, Rao SR, Donelan K, Ferris TG, Jha A, Kaushal R, Levy DE, Rosenbaum S, Shields AE, Blumenthal D. 2008. Electronic health records in ambulatory care: A national survey of physicians. *NEJM* 359(1): 5060.

23. Simon SR, McCarthy ML, Kaushal R, Jenter CA, Volk LA, Poon EG, Yee KC, Orav EJ, Williamns DH, Bates DW. 2008. Electronic health records: Which practices have them, and how are clinicians using them? *J Eval Clin Pract* 14: 43–47.

24. Wager KA, Lee FW, White AW, Ward DM, Ornstein SM. 2000. Impact of an electronic medical record system on community-based primary care practices. *J Am Board Fam Pract* 13(5): 333–348.

25. Burt CW, Sisk JE. 2005. Which physicians and practices are using electronic medical records? *Health Affairs* 24(5): 1334–1343.

26. Solberg LI, Flottemesch TJ, Foldes SS, Molitor BA, Walker PF, Crain AL. 2008. Tobacco-use prevalence in special populations taking advantage of electronic medical records. *Am J Prev Med* 35(6 Suppl): S501–7.

27. Brixner D, Ghate SR, McAdam-Marx C, Ben-Joseph R, Said Q. 2008. Association between cardiometabolic risk factors and body mass index based on diagnosis and treatment codes in an electronic medical record database. *JMCP* 14(8): 756–767.

28. Nichols GA, Arondekar B, Herman WH. 2008. Complications of dysglycemia and medical costs associated with nondiabetic hyperglycemia. *AJMC* 14(12): 791–798.

29. Jaspan DM, Dunton CJ, Cook TL. 2008. Acceptance of human papillomavirus vaccine by gynecologists in an urban setting. *J Low Genit Tract Dis* 12(2): 118–21.

30. Available at: http://www.fda.gov/downloads/aboutFDA/centersoffices/CDER/UCM1187. Last Accessed December 29, 2008.

31. Revicki DA, Osoba D, Fairclough D, Barofsky I, Berzon R, Leidy NK, Rothman M. 2000. Recommendations on health-related quality of life research to support labeling and promotional claims in the United States. *Qual Lif Res* 9(8): 887–900.

32. Willke RJ, Burke LB, Erickson P. 2004. Measuring treatment impact: A review of patient-reported outcomes and other efficacy endpoints in approved product labels. *Controlled Clinical Trials* 25: 535–552.

33. Fung CH, Hays RD. 2008. Prospects and challenges in using patient–reported outcomes in clinical practice. *Qual Life Res* 17(10): 1297–1302.

34. Lohr KN, Zebrack BJ. Using patient-reported outcomes in clinical practice: challenges and opportunities. *Qual Life Res* November 2008: Ahead of print.

35. Acquadro C, Berzon R, Dubois D, Leidy NK, Marquis P, Revicki D, Rothman M. 2003. For the PRO Harmonization Group. Incorporating the patient's perspective into drug development and communication: An ad hoc task force report of the patient–reported outcomes (PRO) harmonization group meeting at the Food and Drug Administration, February 16, 2001. *Value in Health* 6(5): 522–531.

36. Gerend MA, Magloire ZF. 2008. Awareness, knowledge, and beliefs about human papillomavirus in a racially diverse sample of young adults. *J Adolesc Health* 42(3): 237–242.

37. Allen JD, Mohllajee AP, Shelton RC, Othus MK, Fontenot H, Hanna R. 2008. Stage of adoption of the human papillomavirus vaccine among college women. *Prev Med* December 24 (Ahead of print).

38. Ferris DG, Waller JL, Owen A, Smith J. 2008. HPV vaccine acceptance among mid-adult women. *JABFM* 21(1): 31–37.

39. Ferris DG, Waller JL, Miller J, Patel P, Price GA, Jackson L, Wilson C. 2009. Variables associated with human papillomavirus (HPV) vaccine acceptance by men. *JABFM* 22(1): 34–42.

40. Kannel WB, Feinleib M, McNamara PM, Garrison RJ, Costal W. 1979. An investigation of coronary heart disease in families: The Framingham Offspring Study. *Am J Epidemiol.* 110: 281–290.

41. Johnson N. 2002. The six-step process for conducting outcomes analyses using administrative databases. *Formulary* 37:362–364.

42. Arnold RJ. 2007. Cost-effectiveness analysis: Should it be required for drug registration and beyond? *Drug Discov Today* 12(21–22):960–5.

43. Fairman KA, Motheral BR. 2003. Do decision-analytic models identify cost-effective treatments? A retrospective look at helicobacter pylori eradication. *J Manag Care Pharm* 9(5):430–40.

44. Centers for Medicare and Medicaid Services. Healthcare Common Procedure Coding System (HCPCS) code set. http://www.cms.hhs.gov/MedHCPCSGenInfo/ (accessed 14 November 2008).

45. Berthelsen CL. 2000. Evaluation of coding data quality of the HCUP National Inpatient Sample. *Top Health Inf Manage* 21(2):10–23.

46. Sax MJ. 2005. Benchmarking as a management tool in decision making. *J Manag Care Pharm* 11(1 Suppl A):S3–4.

47. Sax MJ. 2005. Essential steps and practical applications for database studies. *J Manag Care Pharm* 11(1 Suppl A):S5–8.

48. (National Institutes of Heath, National Heart, Lung, Blood Institute). National Asthma Education and Prevention Program Expert panel report 3: Guidelines for the diagnosis and management of asthma. 2007.

49. Bateman ED, Boushey HA, Bousquet J, et al. 2004. Can guideline-defined asthma control be achieved? The Gaining Optimal Asthma Control study. *Am J Respir Crit Care Med* 170(8):836–44.

50. Dolan CM, Fraher KE, Bleecker ER, et al. 2004. Design and baseline characteristics of the epidemiology and natural history of asthma: Outcomes and Treatment Regimens (TENOR) study: a large cohort of patients with severe or difficult-to-treat asthma. *Ann Allergy Asthma Immunol* 92(1):32–9.

51. Arnold RJ, Donnelly A, Altieri L, Wong KW, Sung JC. 2007. Assessment of outcomes and parental effect on quality-of-life endpoints in the management of atopic dermatitis. *Manag Care Interface* 20(2):18–23.

52. Lewis RL, Canafax DM, Pettit KG, et al. 1996. Use of Markov modeling for evaluating the cost-effectiveness of immunosuppressive therapies in renal transplant recipients. *Transplant Proc* 28(4):2214–7.

53. Arnold RJ, Kim R, Tang B. 2006. The cost-effectiveness of argatroban treatment in heparin-induced thrombocytopenia: The effect of early versus delayed treatment. *Cardiol Rev* 14(1):7–13.

54. Marcus P, Arnold R, Ekins S, et al. 2008. A retrospective randomized study of asthma control in the US: results of the CHARIOT study. *Curr Med Res Opin* 24:3443–3452.

55. Sackett DL. 1979. Bias in analytic research. *J Chronic Dis* 32(1–2):51–63.

56. Takemoto S, Arns W, Bunnapradist S, et al. 2008. Expanding the evidence base in transplantation: The complementary roles of randomized controlled trials and outcomes research. *Transplantation* 86(1):1–8.

57. Normand S, Sykora K, Li P, et al. 2005. Readers guide to critical appraisal of cohort studies: 3. Analytical strategies to reduce confounding. *BMJ* 330.

58. Kurth T, Walker A, Glynn R, et al. 2006. Results of multivariable logistic regression, propensity matching, propensity adjustment, and propensity–based weighting under conditions of nonuniform effect. *Am J Epidemiol* 163.

59. Clark D, Von Korff M, Saunders K, et al. 1995. A chronic disease score with empirically derived weights. *Med Care* 33:783–795.

60. Deyo A, Cherkin D, MA C. 1992. Adapting a clinical comorbidity index for use with ICD-9-CM administrative databases. *J Clin Epidemiol* 45:613–619.

61. D'Agostino RB, Jr. 1998. Propensity score methods for bias reduction in the comparison of a treatment to a non–randomized control group. *Stat Med* 17(19):2265–81.

62. Stallings SC, Huse D, Finkelstein SN, et al. 2006. A framework to evaluate the economic impact of pharmacogenomics. *Pharmacogenomics* 7(6):853–62.

63. Eckman MH, Rosand J, Greenberg SM, Gage BF. 2009. Cost-effectiveness of using pharmacogenetic information in warfarin dosing for patients with nonvalvular atrial fibrillation. *Ann Intern Med* 150(2):73–83.

64. The International Warfarin Pharmacogenetics Consortium. 2009. Estimation of the Warfarin Dose with Clinical and Pharmacogenetic Data. *N Engl J Med* 360(8):753–764.

6 What Is Cost-Minimization Analysis?

Alan Haycox

CONTENTS

6.1   INTRODUCTION

The principal issues that are addressed in this chapter are:

1. The circumstances in which cost-minimization analysis (CMA) is an appropriate methodology to undertake health economic evaluations.
2. Steps that can be taken to improve the quality of CMAs and, hence, their reliability as a basis for healthcare decision making.

The appropriateness of any economic methodology depends on the nature and quality of the underlying clinical evidence, with evaluations based on inappropriate or poor quality clinical data's failing to provide a reliable basis for health care decision-making. The primacy of clinical data is particularly evident in the case of CMA in which, conditional on health benefits between two equivalent competing options, the least expensive option is preferred. Perhaps as a consequence of this apparent simplicity, scant attention has been previously paid to the theoretical and practical methods used to inform the analysis or to establish the appropriateness of this choice of methodology.

Many sources of clinical evidence can be used to support economic analyses; however, the "gold standard" is normally considered to be the randomized controlled trial (RCT), which holds everything constant with the exception of the drug being evaluated. Given that, by definition, the results of clinical trials cannot be known in advance, it is impossible to plan to undertake a CMA alongside an RCT because it is not certain that the health outcomes being compared will be equivalent (Donaldson, Hundley et al. 1996). Therefore, no prospective economic evaluation starts out as a CMA; only when the health outcomes generated are empirically demonstrated to be "identical or similar" will the CMA be adopted as an appropriate methodology by the health economist.

CMA is frequently portrayed as being the "poor relation" among health economic methodologies, with its apparent simplicity making it unworthy of being considered alongside more theoretically rigorous health economic methodologies. However, it is important that health economists recognize and acknowledge that the theoretical underpinnings of CMA are just as rigorous as those underpinning other methods of economic evaluation. Perhaps as a consequence of the comparative disdain in which CMA has been held, its use to date appears to have been poorly conceived and frequently inappropriate. In this regard, CMA has been frequently employed as an evaluative tool to support and justify the introduction of cheaper, but potentially less effective, treatments. The usual procedure is for the analyst to simply assume that the benefits of a new health technology are equivalent to the existing "gold standard" therapy without having sufficient evidence to justify such a claim. For example, by assuming a class effect for similar types of drugs (each drug in a class having equivalent outcomes) it then becomes possible to base subsequent analysis solely on a comparison of costs—an attractive strategy if you are introducing a cheaper but less effective drug.

The methods currently used to justify equivalence in outcomes in a CMA therefore appear to be inherently flawed and indicate an urgent need to improve the theoretical rigor underlying this aspect of CMAs if they are to be taken seriously as a method of economic evaluation. The current haphazard approach leads to a situation in which CMA is typically described in health economics textbooks as a form of economic evaluation where "… the decision simply revolves around the costs" (Gold, Siegel et al. 1996 p. 165).

This interpretation ignores the extreme rigor that should be required to ensure equivalence in health benefits prior to deciding on the appropriateness of employing CMA as an economic methodology. The crucial decision relates to the fact that CMA has been defined as being an appropriate methodology. Underpinning this decision is a detailed analysis of clinical data that convinces the analyst that the interventions being compared lead to equivalent health outcomes. Only in these strictly controlled circumstances is it legitimate for CMA to concentrate on costs alone. As such, a crucial and indispensable element underpinning the decision to use CMA as an economic methodology is the need to unambiguously determine the therapeutic equivalence of competing interventions (Newby and Hill 2003). In practice, therefore, the extent to which CMA represents an appropriate methodological structure is entirely determined by the interpretation that can be placed on the available clinical evidence.

6.1.1 WHAT IS MEANT BY THERAPEUTIC EQUIVALENCE?

The extent to which alternative health care technologies are sufficiently similar to justify the use of CMA is an area of theoretical uncertainty and, thus, still open to subjective interpretation, with the majority of published CMAs appearing to be based on assumptions rather than evidence of clinical equivalence. This primacy of hope over experience may cause misleading recommendations to be made for health care resource allocation.

Given this fact, it is perhaps surprising that the exact nature of the evidence base required to support therapeutic equivalence and, hence, the appropriateness of CMA as an economic methodology has not been subject to more intense scrutiny. CMAs are frequently based on the results of clinical trials that have attempted but failed to identify the superiority of a new drug over the existing "gold standard" therapy. This occurs despite the obvious fact that the inability of a health intervention to prove superiority in a superiority trial (ST) in no way indicates that this necessarily implies clinical equivalence. Recent advances in clinical trial design have made it easier to directly compare clinical equivalence in a more meaningful manner with the development of non-inferiority trials (NIs) allowing this issue to be directly addressed. Alternatively, where a trial is initially designed as a ST but such superiority remains unproven, the analysis can be switched from superiority to non-inferiority in appropriate cases. The use of such improvements in trial design should enable CMAs to be more effectively targeted in a manner that ensures that they are undertaken only in appropriate circumstances using rigorous sources of evidence. In this manner, only CMAs that meet minimum standards with regard to clinical equivalence will be accepted; CMAs that fail to meet such criteria will be dismissed. Such an approach would enable health economics to gain enhanced credibility from the use of this potentially valuable economic methodology.

6.1.2 OPTIMIZING EVIDENCE FROM CLINICAL TRIALS

If CMAs are to form a reliable basis for health care decision-making, due consideration must be given to the claims of clinical equivalence that are crucial to the adoption of the CMA methodology. The implications of adopting an inappropriate clinical trial design or misinterpreting the results of a clinical trial are often considerable:

> "… wrongly discounting treatments as ineffective will deprive patients of better care. Wrongly accepting treatments as effective exposes patients to needless risks and wastes." (Tarnow-Mordi and Healy 1999 p. 210).

RCTs typically compare the gold standard existing treatment with a new intervention (Tramer, Reynolds et al. 1998). RCTs can be structured to evaluate ST, therapeutic equivalence (ET) or therapeutic NI. The trial designs differ in terms of their objectives and these differences have significant implications for the use of the CMA methodology. The greatest support for the use of CMA occurs when an ET proves that two health care technologies are clinically equivalent; however, there exists a myriad of "gray" areas that may be indicative of therapeutic equivalence and, hence, require more careful analytical consideration and judgement. Such gray areas are analyzed in detail in the remainder of this chapter.

6.2   SOURCES OF CLINICAL TRIAL EVIDENCE

6.2.1   SUPERIORITY TRIALS

The extent to which clinical evidence can be used to inform CMAs is dependent on the design of the RCT. STs are specifically designed to show a difference in health benefits between two health care technologies. Typically, the primary objective of the research is to determine whether an experimental intervention is more efficacious than the established gold standard treatment. To identify whether there is a difference in health benefits between two health care technologies it is necessary to begin with a null hypothesis that treatment X yields the same health benefits as treatment Y.

The ST estimates the probability that the effect exists when the null hypothesis is true using the test statistic (p-value). The smaller the size of the p-value the more likely it is that the null hypothesis is false and that a difference *does* exist between the health benefits generated by the treatments. P-values, therefore, can identify statistically whether an effect is likely by conveying information about the probability of an incorrect inference given the observed effect but can say nothing about the size of the effect or its clinical relevance.

Newby and Hill (2003) emphasize the inadequacy of using p-values obtained in STs to interpret the results of clinical trials and recommend the use of confidence intervals and personal judgment when determining clinical equivalence before accepting or rejecting an equivalence claim:

> "... leaving it up to the reader to decide whether the confidence interval includes or
> excludes potentially clinically important differences between two treatments. If it does
> not exclude differences ... assume that the two drugs are not the same" (Newby and
> Hill 2003).

When the original objective of an ST is not achieved, there is an obvious incentive to refocus the analysis to support more restricted claims of clinical equivalence. However, STs are specifically designed to demonstrate that there is, indeed, a difference and, thus, to reject the null hypothesis in favor of the alternative hypothesis (i.e., that there is a difference). In STs, it is impossible to prove that the null hypothesis is true, as the aim is to reject it by proving that the observed difference is unlikely to be commensurate with equivalent health outcomes of the competing health care interventions.

In CMAs the clinical evidence from failed STs is often misinterpreted as proving that the health care interventions being compared are clinically equivalent. Such methodological flaws resulting from the misinterpretation of clinical trial results can also "...lead to false claims, inconsistencies and harm to patients" (Greene 2000 p. 715).

However, if appropriately planned for, it is possible to switch the focus of the analysis from superiority to non-inferiority in a single trial. Thus, failed STs that are well designed and have adequate sample size could therefore potentially be used to provide evidence of health equivalence for use in CMAs.

6.2.2 EQUIVALENCE TRIALS

6.2.2.1 Characteristics of Equivalence Trials

ETs are intended to demonstrate that the effect of a new treatment is not worse than the effect of the current treatment by more than a specified equivalence margin. The aim of an ET is, therefore, to specifically rule out significant clinical differences between the treatments by directly evaluating the extent to which two health care interventions have equivalent therapeutic effects. Briggs and O'Brien (2001) argue that CMA should be used only when clinical evidence has been obtained from an ET. They argue that it is inappropriate to use the results of a failed ST to demonstrate clinical equivalence "... unless a study has been specifically designed to show the equivalence of treatments it would be inappropriate to conduct cost-minimization analysis" (Briggs and O'Brien 2001).

However, even where an equivalence trial indicates clinical equivalence in primary outcomes, scrutiny of secondary outcomes may reveal significant differences in safety, cost, or convenience. "... one therapy may offer clinical benefits such as a more convenient administration schedule, less potential for drug interaction or lower cost" (Hatala et al. 1999 p.9).

Reliance on a single clinical measure of effectiveness may potentially be misleading as it may fail to capture an important difference in health outcome between two alternatives. Thus, ideally, clinical equivalence should be established for a range of health outcomes before the use of CMA can be supported. In addition, in evaluating claims of clinical equivalence it is important to acknowledge that:

> "It is never correct to claim that ... there is no difference in effects of treatments....
> There will always be some uncertainty surrounding estimates of treatment effects, and
> a small difference can never be excluded" (Alderson and Chalmers 2003 p.476).

Even if one compared a drug with itself, there would be a difference; therefore, it cannot be unequivocally claimed that two health care technologies are clinically equivalent. Thus, even where the results of ETs indicate no difference, this may simply indicate that the true difference exists outside of the specified probabilities of error.

If clinical equivalence is demonstrated in a good quality ET, there remain two other issues that must be addressed prior to unambiguously supporting the use of the cost-minimization approach. First, the primary health outcome must encompass the main benefit(s) of the treatments being compared. Second, any differences in other health outcomes, e.g., secondary health outcomes, must be sufficiently small so as not to attain clinical significance. If these assumptions cannot be substantiated, then it would not be appropriate to adopt the CMA approach despite the availability of equivalence obtained in an ET.

6.2.2.2   Equivalence Range or Margin

A crucial step in the design of an ET is the definition of clinical equivalence. The equivalence margin attempts to incorporate all values that represent unimportant clinical differences in treatment and must be stipulated in advance of the clinical trial. The equivalence range, therefore, includes the largest difference between treatments that is clinically acceptable before treatments become defined as providing significantly different benefits. The first step in any ET is, therefore, to define the smallest unacceptable degree of inferiority or superiority to ensure that the ET can be appropriately powered. For example:

> "... if the difference between the two groups in respect of change in pulmonary function was within +/– 1.5 units, then the treatments would be considered clinically equivalent" (Huson 2004 p.2).

This means that if treatment A is better or worse than treatment B by more than a 1.5 unit change in pulmonary function, the two treatments cannot be considered to be clinically equivalent. Clinical equivalence can be claimed if the 95% CI around the difference in treatments is found to lie entirely within the predetermined clinical equivalence margin. The setting of the equivalence margin communicates a judgment about what is and what is not clinically and statistically acceptable (Pater 2004).

Clearly, different clinical situations require different equivalence margins and analysts must justify their chosen range with regard to clinician opinion and previous trials comparing active controls with placebo. An equivalence margin that is too wide could mean that significantly different treatments are considered to be clinically equivalent; conversely an equivalence margin that is too narrow could mean that clinically equivalent treatments are mislabeled as being significantly different. It is important that good clinical judgment be combined with sound clinical and statistical reasoning to ensure that the chosen margin is clinically relevant and statistically feasible.

A negative study result from an ET can take two forms. The CI around the treatment difference may lie partially within the equivalence margin or it can lie entirely outside, leading to the conclusion that the probability of a difference between the two treatments has not been rejected (see Figure 6.1).

6.2.3   Non-Inferiority Trials

6.2.3.1   Characteristics of a Non-Inferiority Trial

The rationale behind a NI trial is to demonstrate that the new health care technology is not worse than the current health care technology by a pre-stated clinical margin. This type of trial is useful when the clinical issue relates to the extent to

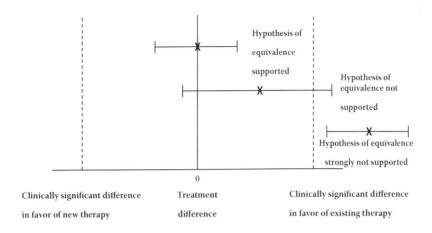

FIGURE 6.1 Interpretation of equivalence trials.

which the new health care technology is as good as current therapy. In NIs, analysis is focused entirely in one direction—typically the new treatment is not worse than the established therapy by more than the non-inferiority margin specified. An improvement of any size fits within the definition of non-inferiority. Span and colleagues published the first paper that acknowledged the link between CMA and NIs:

> "... the most efficient analysis of the clinical effect in a cost minimization study is the non-inferiority analysis" (p.262). They conclude that: "... to obtain valid results from a cost-minimization study, care has to be taken to adapt the correct methodology for non-inferiority testing in clinical outcomes" (Span, TenVergert et al. 2006 p.261).

To ensure a robust interpretation of trial results, some analysts call for both per protocol (PA) and intention to treat (ITT) analyses to be conducted and only if both types of analysis support the hypothesis should non-inferiority be claimed (Snappinn 2000). Therefore, the extent and nature of the evidence of non-inferiority that is required to provide an acceptable platform on which to base a CMA is still open to debate.

6.2.3.2 Non-Inferiority Range or Margin

The non-inferiority range should be set in relation to the clinical notion of a minimally important effect. An acceptable non-inferiority margin depends on defining a difference that has previously been identified as not being clinically significant. To do this, two additional conditions must be met. First, the smallest expected effect of the active control over placebo must exceed this margin to ensure that no positively harmful treatments can be introduced and, second, the margin must be no greater than the difference between active treatments judged clinically important.

In a NI, non-inferiority is demonstrated when the CI around the treatment difference lies entirely to the right of the lower bound of the non-inferiority margin. Non-inferiority is not demonstrated if the lower bound of the CI lies to the left of the non-inferiority margin (see Figure 6.2).

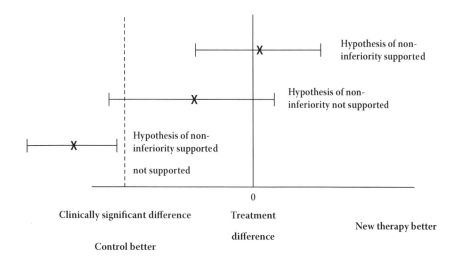

FIGURE 6.2   Interpreting NIs using CIs.

6.3   OTHER ISSUES TO BE ADDRESSED IN EVALUATING EQUIVALENCE

6.3.1   STATISTICAL VERSUS CLINICAL SIGNIFICANCE

One of the failings of statistical analyses undertaken in the context of an ST is that statistical significance may differ from clinical significance. Variables that are identified as exhibiting statistically significant differences may be entirely unimportant from a clinical perspective, whereas clinically crucial differences remain crucial even if they fail to achieve statistical significance. In contrast, in ETs and NIs, statistical and clinical significance are inextricably linked via the setting of equivalence and non-inferiority margins.

6.3.2   EQUIVALENCE IN SINGLE OR MULTIPLE OUTCOMES?

In any clinical trial it is necessary to identify a primary health outcome that is common to the competing alternative interventions. Choice and measurement of such an outcome measure is a crucial step in determining the appropriateness of the trial as an evidence source on which to undertake CMAs. To be of value, the primary health outcomes must be the dominant outcome from the perspective of both patients and clinicians and capture the most clinically relevant benefits of the competing treatments. If not, claims of clinical equivalence, even when based on ETs, are not sufficient to support the use of CMA.

In clinical practice it is highly unlikely that two health care interventions will yield exactly the same health benefits in all dimensions of clinical and patient outcomes. Typically, the design of ETs and NIs identifies a single endpoint for comparison despite the perception that one of the treatments is likely to offer significant advantages in another area. For example, where two treatments have equal efficacy, yet one is more convenient to patients, the extent to which CMA can be appropriately utilized depends largely on the perspective adopted by the analysis. Where equivalence is not demonstrated for all important outcomes, the analyst must provide explicit justification for using the cost-minimization approach in light of the study question and perspective. In large part, the interpretation of clinical equivalence will depend on the specific circumstances of the clinical trial, the range of outcomes being measured and the judgement of the analyst. In such cases it is difficult to provide specific guidance that would be appropriate in all cases.

6.3.3 WHOSE VIEWS OF CLINICAL EQUIVALENCE SHOULD BE PREEMINENT?

Definitions of clinical equivalence will depend on whose views we consider to be the most important (patients, clinicians, or society). Generally, lead investigators in clinical trials specify the primary and secondary health outcomes to be measured, with the identification of the primary outcome measure's being based on relevant clinical experience, published clinical evidence, and knowledge of patient needs. The crucial factor is to ensure that the choice of health outcome measures used to determine clinical equivalence is clinically meaningful to the patient.

6.3.4 OVER WHAT PERIOD SHOULD WE EVALUATE CLINICAL EQUIVALENCE?

The benefits of health care technologies will vary in relation to the time point at which they are measured. In a clinical trial the primary health outcome measure might exhibit statistically significant differences at 3 months but not at 6 or 12 months. In such circumstances, do we interpret the therapeutic interventions as being equivalent and, hence, appropriate for analysis in the context of a CMA? It is important to acknowledge that subsequent reanalysis is required to demonstrate continued clinical equivalence.

6.4 EFFECTIVELY TARGETING THE USE OF CMA

The current use of RCT evidence to support statements of clinical equivalence is inadequate, and clear and appropriate decision rules are required in the future to ensure that unambiguous evidence of clinical equivalence is a feature of future CMAs. In the absence of such evidence it would be potentially misleading to use flawed analyses as the basis for health care decision-making. While it is comparatively simple to identify circumstances in which the use of CMA as an economic methodology is clearly inappropriate, it is more difficult to specify unambiguous decision rules that identify circumstances in which clinical evidence clearly supports the use of CMA. The appropriateness of using CMA must be judged in the light of the totality of the clinical evidence supporting or refuting the hypothesis of therapeutic equivalence between two competing interventions, combined with the specialist knowledge and expertise required to place such evidence in context. However, certain limited guidance can be provided with regard to effectively targeting CMAs.

First, clinical evidence from a well-designed ET represents the gold standard in supporting claims of clinical equivalence in support of the use of CMA. However, even where data is available from an ET it still remains important to consider the extent to which the primary health outcome fully captures the benefits being derived from the health care treatments being compared. If other benefits are clinically meaningful to patients and clinicians, additional comparisons of clinical equivalence may be required.

Second, failure to prove clinical superiority should not be interpreted as providing evidence of clinical equivalence. In certain circumstances, and if planned into trial design, trial data may be re-analyzed to assess clinical equivalence, but such reinterpretation of the dataset requires further analysis if the use of CMA is to be justified. In particular, a non-inferiority statement should be stipulated in the clinical trial protocol to ensure that valuable information can still be derived even if superiority is not proven.

Third, the extent to which data from NIs can be used to justify CMAs is currently subject to a great amount of uncertainty. In particular, to what extent proof of non-inferiority represents an acceptable approximation of "therapeutic equivalence" and, hence, justifies the use of CMAs, is still open to debate.

Finally, where CMAs are based on valid claims of clinical equivalence derived from appropriate sources of RCT evidence, it represents an appropriate and powerful method of economic evaluation. However, it is crucial that in interpreting the results of CMAs, the informed decision-maker uses his or her clinical judgment to assess the quality and quantity of the evidence in support of therapeutic equivalence and, hence, identifies the theoretical justification for the use of CMA. In cases where the decision-maker does not accept claims of clinical equivalence, the results of the CMA should clearly not be used as the basis for decision-making.

6.5 CONCLUSIONS

The cost-minimization method of economic evaluation has always been employed in a more haphazard manner than other methods of economic evaluation. It is crucial to rectify this situation to ensure that only techniques that prove to be robust and reliable in improving health care decision-making are incorporated into the toolkit employed by the health economist. However, exactly how similar do outcomes have to be to support the application of this powerful economic methodology? The most appropriate design for a clinical trial to generate evidence that two health care technologies are identical or similar is the ET. Such trials are specifically designed for this purpose and, therefore, any differences that are identified between the health interventions being compared are neither clinically nor statistically significant.

It is essential that health economists and decision-makers are clear on what is meant by the concept of clinical equivalence and to acknowledge that, given the heterogeneous nature of patient populations and treatment outcomes, it is likely to prove impossible to achieve exact equivalence between competing health care interventions. Ultimately, it is up to the health economist to justify the use of CMA just as it is up to the decision-maker to judge the extent to which the results obtained should be influential in determining decision making.

REFERENCES

Alderson, P., Chalmers, I. (2003). Survey of claims of no effect in abstracts of Cochrane reviews. *British Medical Journal* **326**: 475.

Briggs, A. H., O'Brien, B. J. (2001). The death of cost-minimization analysis? *Health Economics* **10**(2): 179–84.

Donaldson, C., Hundley, V. et al. (1996). Using economics alongside clinical trials: Why we cannot choose the evaluation technique in advance. *Health Economics Letters* **5**: 267–269.

Gold, M., Siegel, J. et al. *Cost-effectiveness in health and medicine.* New York, Oxford University Press. (1996).

Greene, W., et al. (2000). Claims on equivalence in medical research: Are they supported by the evidence? *Annals of Internal Medicine* **132**: 715–722.

Hatala, R., Holbrook, A., Goldsmith, C.H. (1999). Therapeutic equivalence: All studies are not created equal. *Canadian Journal of Clinical Pharmacology* **6**: 9–11.

Huson, L. (2004). Statistical assessment of superiority, equivalence, and non-inferiority in clinical trials. *CR Focus* **12**(5): 1–4.

Jones, B., Jarvis, P., Lewis, A., Ebbutt, A.F. (1996). Trials to assess equivalence: The importance of rigorous methods. *British Medical Journal* **313**: 36–9.

Newby, D., Hill, S. (2003). Use of pharmacoeconomics in prescribing research. Part 2: cost-minimization analysis—when are two therapies equal?" *Journal of Clinical Pharmacy & Therapeutics* **28**(2): 145–50.

Pater, C. (2004). Equivalence and non-inferiority trials: Are they viable alternatives for the registration of new drugs? (III). *Current Controlled Trials in Cardiovascular Medicine* **5**(8).

Snappinn, S. (2000). Noninferiority trials. *Current Controlled Trials in Cardiovascular Medicine* **1**: 19–21.

Span, M., TenVergert, E. et al. (2006). Noninferiority testing in cost-minimization studies: Practical issues concerning power analysis. *International Journal of Technology Assessment in Healthcare* **22**(2): 261–266.

Tarnow-Mordi, W., Healy, M. (1999). Distinguishing between "no evidence of effect" and "evidence of no effect" in randomised controlled trials and other comparisons." *Archives of Disease in Childhood* **80**: 210–11.

Tramer, M., Reynolds, R. et al. (1998). When placebo controlled trials are essential and equivalence trials are inadequate. *British Medical Journal* **317**: 875–80.

Whitehurst, D., Lewis, M. et al. (2006). Retrospective equivalence analysis of superiority trials: What are the implications for trial-based economic evaluations? Health Economists' Study Group, York.

7 Cost-Effectiveness Analysis

Kenneth J. Smith and Mark S. Roberts

CONTENTS

7.1 THE RATIONALE FOR COST-EFFECTIVENESS ANALYSIS

As noted in prior chapters, the economic evaluation of pharmacotherapies and other health care interventions is growing in importance as the resources directed toward health care account for progressively larger portions of the budgets of governments, employers, and individuals. Making rational decisions under conditions of resource constraints requires a method for comparing alternatives across a range of outcomes, allowing a direct ranking of the costs and benefits of specific strategies for preventing or treating a particular illness.

Cost-effectiveness analysis (CEA) provides a framework to compare two or more decision options by examining the ratio of the differences in costs and the differences in health effectiveness between options. The overall goal of CEA is to provide a single measure, the incremental cost-effectiveness ratio (ICER), which relates the amount of benefit derived by making an alternative treatment choice to the differential cost of that option. When two options are being compared, the ICER is calculated by the formula:

$$\frac{C_{\text{Option 2}} - C_{\text{Option 1}}}{\text{Effectiveness}_{\text{Option 2}} - \text{Effectiveness}_{\text{Option 1}}}$$

In medical or pharmacoeconomic cost-effectiveness analysis, health resource costs (the numerator) are in monetary terms, representing the difference in costs between choosing option 1 or option 2. In cost-effectiveness analysis, the differential benefits of the various options (the denominator) are non-monetary and represent the change in health effectiveness values implied by choosing option 1 over option 2. Typically, these health outcomes are measured as lives saved, life years gained, illness events avoided, or a variety of other clinical or health outcomes. Unlike CEA, cost-benefit analysis values both the costs and benefits of interventions in monetary terms. Cost-utility analysis, a subset of CEA where intervention effectiveness is adjusted based on the desirability (or utility) of the resulting health states, is discussed in Chapter 9 as it relates to the cost-effectiveness of human papillomavirus (HPV) vaccine.

7.2   THE COST-EFFECTIVENESS PLANE

A pharmacoeconomic analysis is often interested in how much more of a health outcome can be obtained for a given financial expenditure. Limited resources may, many times, constrain choices between medical options. The cost-effectiveness plane serves to clarify when these choices may be easy or difficult.[1] The cost-effectiveness plane is typically drawn with the differences in cost (or the incremental cost) on the y-axis and the differences in effectiveness (or incremental effectiveness) between the two options on the x-axis (Figure 7.1). In this example we will compare an existing program with a new program. The existing program, acting as the comparator, will be at the origin of both the cost and effectiveness axes, depicting the current level of expenditure and benefit with which a new therapy is compared. The new therapy can be more expensive, less expensive, or equivalent in costs to the current option. Similarly, the new option can be more effective, less effective, or equivalent in clinical effectiveness as compared with the existing strategy or therapy.

This produces four possible options for the results of the analysis of a new strategy compared with an existing one. If the new program is less expensive and more effective than the existing program, then the point representing the new program falls into the southeast (SE) quadrant of the cost-effectiveness plane. Points in this quadrant are called *dominant*, and strategies that have such a characteristic should be chosen over the existing strategy due to their superior outcome at diminished costs. These strategies are "cheaper and better" than current therapy and should be adopted. Examples of strategies in this quadrant are laparoscopic cholecystectomy

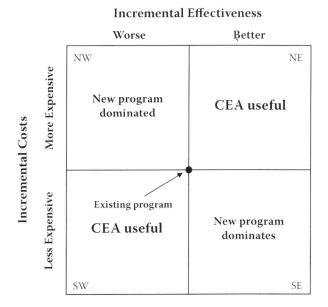

FIGURE 7.1   The cost-effectiveness plane.

compared with other therapies for symptomatic gallstones[2,3] or interventions to decrease cigarette smoking.[4,5]

If, on the other hand, the new program is more expensive and less effective than the existing one, then this program falls into the northwest (NW) quadrant of the plane. Strategies in this quadrant are considered to be *dominated* by the current strategy and should not be chosen due to poorer outcomes at greater cost. Although existing strategies in this quadrant are perhaps relatively rare, there are examples of strategies that do not appear to derive a benefit, yet incur substantially more health care costs than other options. Examples include amoxicillin prophylaxis compared with no antibiotic for dental procedures in patients at moderate risk for infective endocarditis[6] and magnetic resonance imaging vs. endocrinologic follow-up of patients with asymptomatic pituitary microadenomas.[7]

If the new program is either dominant or dominated (i.e., in the SE or NW quadrants), a formal CEA is not needed to assist the decision—the decision is (or should be) obvious. However, if the new program is both more effective and more costly, falling in the northeast (NE) quadrant, then a CEA would be useful to define the tradeoff between increases in costs and effectiveness and to calculate the cost per unit of effectiveness gained. Similarly, a CEA would also be useful if the new strategy fell into the SW quadrant as being both less costly and less effective than the existing program, once again to define the tradeoffs between programs and to ascertain the cost-effectiveness ratio. This graphical display emphasizes one of the most fundamental and important concepts of cost-effectiveness analysis; it is useful only when there is a tradeoff between the cost of a strategy and the benefit derived from that strategy.

TABLE 7.1
Basic Components of a Cost-Effectiveness Analysis

Component	Examples
Options/comparisons	Existing program compared with new program
Perspective of the analysis	Societal, health system, patient
Time horizon	1 month, 5 years, lifetime
Scope of the analysis	Population affected, inclusion (or not) of secondary or collateral effects
Measuring and valuing costs	Cost categories included in the analysis are determined by the perspective taken
Measuring and valuing outcomes	Life years saved, illnesses avoided, cases found
Time preference	Discounting future costs and effectiveness
Analytic models	Clinical trial data, decision analysis model
Accounting for uncertainty	Sensitivity analysis

7.3 BASIC COMPONENTS OF A COST-EFFECTIVENESS ANALYSIS

Several factors should be considered in the construction of a CEA (Table 7.1). A high-quality analysis will include and describe the relevant options, clearly state the perspective of the analysis, choose a relevant time horizon over which to track costs and effects, consider the appropriate population, accurately measure the costs and effectiveness of the competing options, account for the differential value of costs and outcomes that occur at different times in the future, and account for uncertainties of assumptions and values in the context of an appropriately constructed analytic model. Following is a description of these concepts in more detail.

7.3.1 ENUMERATION OF THE OPTIONS

A CEA requires a comparison between two or more options. A single option cannot be cost-effective in isolation—an option can be considered cost-effective or not cost-effective only in comparison with other options. Additionally, the cost-effectiveness of a strategy is highly dependent on the specific choice of comparators included in the analysis, and care must be taken to include all of the clinically reasonable options. At a minimum, the comparators include the current standard of care and a range of typically utilized options. A cost-effectiveness analysis of a new therapy compared with a strategy that is not typically used, or is used only in atypical circumstances, is not useful for clinicians or policy makers. It is often reasonable to include a "do nothing" option, especially if doing nothing is a legitimate clinical strategy, but also as a baseline comparator to assess the clinical realism of the model and analysis. In all cases, the strategies should be described in sufficient detail such that readers could replicate or implement the strategy in their own settings.

7.3.2 PERSPECTIVE OF THE ANALYSIS

Choosing the perspective or set of perspectives to be considered in a CEA is essential, as this choice determines the cost values to be contained in the analysis. For example, an analysis from the societal perspective considers all costs, while an analysis from the patient perspective would consider only costs borne by the patient. Other possible perspectives include the third-party payer (insurance) or health system perspective where costs for which these entities are responsible are considered in the analysis; the hospital or health agency perspective includes the costs of providing various health services. Whenever possible, the societal perspective should be included in the set of perspectives to be considered in analysis, because it is the broadest and is recommended for the reference case analysis by the Panel on Cost-Effectiveness in Health and Medicine.[8,9]

7.3.3 TIME HORIZON

The analyst must decide *a priori* how long the costs and effects of the various interventions in the analysis will be tracked. This is usually determined by the clinical features of the illness or its treatment. For example, a CEA of a new antibiotic for acute dysuria treatment in otherwise healthy women might appropriately have a very short time horizon of only a month, as there are virtually no long-term effects of either the disease or its treatments. On the other hand, cost-effectiveness analyses designed to value the effects of cardiovascular risk reduction need to assess the outcomes for much longer time periods; typically such an analysis would follow treatments and effects until death. In any case, all of the strategies must be followed or modeled for the same time horizon. Methods for modeling costs and effects, even in situations where this modeling extends beyond the existence of specific data, is provided in Chapters 2 and 4.

7.3.4 SCOPE OF THE ANALYSIS

An analysis might be relevant for an entire population or for only a relatively small population subgroup; the analyst will need to appropriately choose the cohort to be considered in the analysis. For example, if an intervention is to be directed toward elderly patients with diabetes in order to prevent diabetes complications, limiting the scope of the analysis to an elderly, diabetic population is a logical choice, while if the question is regarding diabetes prevention in adults, a broader population scope is required. The scope of outcomes to be considered is another important consideration. In the example above, a broad or narrow range of diabetes outcomes could be considered in an analysis of elderly diabetics. If a small number of complications are modeled, the data requirements of the model would be less but the conclusions might be limited compared with a model with a broader range of complications considered. However, a more comprehensive model would have greater data needs and require more complex model construction. Choosing the scope of an analysis often means finding a balance between simplicity and complexity, frequently determined by the clinical situation modeled and the question to be examined.

7.3.5 MEASURING AND VALUING COSTS

Data sources for costs must be found and incorporated into the analysis. Cost data can be obtained from clinical trials, but more often other sources will need to be utilized. In addition, the analyst will need to choose between micro-costing or macro-costing methodologies or some mix of the two, often based on the perspective taken in the analysis.[8,9] Micro-costing enumerates and identifies each item that is incorporated into a particular service, requiring detailed data on supplies used, personnel, room, and instrument costs, and often needing time-and-motion studies to accurately capture medical service costs. Macro-costing (or gross costing) uses data, often from large government databases, to estimate average costs for a care episode, for example the average cost of coronary artery bypass grafting or of a hospital stay for pneumonia. In the US, Medicare reimbursement data or the Healthcare Cost and Utilization Project (HCUP) database are often used for this purpose. Further detail on cost estimation can be found in Chapter 3.

7.3.6 MEASURING AND VALUING OUTCOMES

The effectiveness outcome for the analysis must be chosen and outcomes data found, often based on data availability. Randomized trials are excellent data sources on the effects of therapies, but study entrance criteria frequently limit applicability to a more general patient population (see Chapter 5 for more on this). Cohort studies are useful for risk factor determination and for determining the natural history of an illness. Administrative databases are excellent sources for broad population-based estimates of disease and for the effectiveness of therapies, unlike randomized trials which, in general, estimate efficacy. However, administrative databases often pose difficulties in accounting for possible confounding variables in the data set (see Chapter 5). Meta-analyses provide summary measures for parameters, but studies considered are generally limited to randomized trials, thus limiting generalizability. The perspective of the analysis may also influence the effectiveness outcome chosen. Life years or quality-adjusted life years (QALYs) gained are certainly relevant for analyses using the relatively broad-based societal or health system perspectives, but may not be as important when a narrower perspective is chosen, such as that of an individual hospital, when effectiveness measures such as bed day saved or drug administration error avoided might be more relevant.

7.3.7 TIME PREFERENCE

The differential timing of costs and outcomes should be considered in the analysis. This is typically accomplished through the use of discount rates, where costs and outcomes that occur in the present have higher values than those in the future (see Chapter 10).

7.3.8 CHOICE OF ANALYTIC MODELING METHOD

The analytic model must also be selected. Cost data from clinical trials can allow relatively straightforward calculation of incremental cost-effectiveness ratios between management options, often the intervention arms of the clinical trial. More often, data for the analysis must come from a variety of sources (see Chapter 5) and may require a decision analysis model as a framework for data synthesis.

7.3.9   ACCOUNTING FOR UNCERTAINTY

Finally, a sensitivity analysis to elucidate the effects of uncertainty on model results should be performed. There are many goals of sensitivity analysis, and methods for conducting such analyses are detailed in Chapter 12. During model construction and validation, sensitivity analysis is useful as a "debugging tool" to assure that the model behaves as it was designed to behave. After the model is finished, sensitivity analysis is useful to determine which variables have a large impact on the outcomes. Sensitivity analyses can be used to determine the cost-effectiveness ratio in specified subgroups of an analysis, as well as to determine how much a change in one variable will alter the cost-effectiveness ratio. Finally, probabilistic sensitivity analyses (described in Chapter 12) can be used to produce a version of a confidence limit or probability range around the cost-effectiveness ratio.

7.4   CALCULATION OF INCREMENTAL COST-EFFECTIVENESS RATIOS

The ICER requires a detailed enumeration of the costs and benefits of the strategies being compared. Methods for measuring and estimating the costs and benefits of strategies and interventions are often quite complicated, and are detailed in Chapters 3 and 10. In this section, we use the results of two existing pharmacoeconomic studies to illustrate the calculation and use of the ICER. Details of the enumeration of costs and outcomes in these studies are detailed in the studies themselves.[10,11]

The following example considers low molecular weight heparin (LMWH) compared with warfarin for the secondary prevention of venous thromboembolism in patients with cancer. Aujesky[10] used a decision analysis model and data from a variety of sources to estimate the incremental cost-effectiveness of two anticoagulant regimens. Analysis results, with effectiveness in life years, are outlined in Table 7.2.

Typically, the first step in calculation of ICERs among mutually exclusive options is to order the options by cost. LMWH is both more costly and more effective than warfarin, thus, neither strategy is dominant or dominated and a CEA would be useful. Subtracting the cost of the warfarin strategy from that of the LMWH strategy produces the incremental cost; the difference in life expectancy between strategies is the incremental effectiveness. Dividing the incremental cost by the incremental effectiveness produces the ICERs, $115,847 per life year gained, the unit cost of an additional life year occurring as a result of LMWH use rather than warfarin.

7.4.1   DOMINANCE AND EXTENDED DOMINANCE

Calculation of the ICER can be more complicated when more than two strategies are being considered. One of the complicating characteristics of the analysis of many

TABLE 7.2
Cost-Effectiveness of LMWH Compared with Warfarin for the Secondary Prevention of Venous Thromboembolism

Strategy	Cost	Life Expectancy (yrs)	Incremental Cost	Incremental Effectiveness	Incremental Cost-Effectiveness Ratio
Warfarin	$7720	1.377	–	–	–
LMWH	$15,329	1.442	$7609	0.066	$115,847

options is that some strategies may be dominated by others and should be removed from further analysis. As noted in the description of the cost-effectiveness plane, any strategy that is more expensive and less effective than an existing option for the same illness (e.g., is in the left upper quadrant compared with the existing strategy) is said to be strictly dominated; one would never choose such a strategy when an alternative would produce a better outcome at a cheaper price. Strict dominance is also termed strong dominance by some authors. A second type of dominance occurs when a particular strategy is more expensive and less effective than a linear *combination* of two other strategies. This is called *extended dominance*, and represents a situation where one could achieve a better outcome at less cost by treating a proportion of the population with a combination of two alternative strategies. Extended dominance can also be referred to as weak dominance. We illustrate both types of dominance in the following example.

Using a decision analysis model, we[11] performed a CEA of testing and antiviral treatment strategies for adult influenza, using days of influenza illness avoided as an effectiveness term in the analysis. Cost and effectiveness values estimated by this analysis are shown in Table 7.3. (Please note that in a separate analysis the other neuraminidase inhibitor, oseltamivir, was substituted for zanamivir, with similar cost-effectiveness results.) Once again, the first step in calculation of incremental

TABLE 7.3
Cost and Effectiveness Values for Influenza Management Strategies

Strategy	Cost	Illness Days Avoided
No testing or treatment	$92.70	0
Amantadine	$97.50	0.54
Rimantadine	$119.10	0.59
Zanamivir	$137.10	0.74
Testing then amantadine	$115.00	0.44
Testing then rimantadine	$125.50	0.48
Treating then zanamivir	$134.30	0.60

TABLE 7.4
Strategies Ordered by Cost

Strategy	Cost	Illness Days Avoided
No testing or treatment	$92.70	0
Amantadine	$97.50	0.54
Testing then amantadine	$115.00	0.44
Rimantadine	$119.10	0.59
Testing then rimantadine	$125.50	0.48
Testing then zanamivir	$134.30	0.60
Zanamivir	$137.10	0.74

cost-effectiveness ratios among mutually exclusive options is to order the options by cost. Doing so with these data results in Table 7.4. Next, options of lesser effectiveness and of equal or greater cost than another option are removed due to strict, or strong, dominance. These strictly dominated options, which are inferior both in terms of cost and effectiveness, do not need to be considered further in the analysis.[12] In this example, "Testing, then amantadine" costs more and is less effective than "Amantadine (without testing)." Thus, "Testing, then amantadine" is strictly dominated and can be removed from consideration. Similarly, "Testing, then rimantadine" also costs more and is less effective than the "Amantadine" strategy and the "Rimantadine (without testing)" strategy and, thus, can be eliminated due to strict dominance. Removal of these two strategies results in Table 7.5.

Then, starting with the second row, the differences in cost and effectiveness between that row and the preceding row are calculated. These results are the incremental cost and incremental effectiveness between the two adjacent strategies. The incremental cost divided by the incremental effectiveness produces the ICER, the cost per illness day prevented. This same procedure is then followed for the remaining rows in Table 7.6.

Next, the calculated ICERs are examined for extended, or weak, dominance of strategies.[13] This occurs when the ICER of a strategy is greater than the strategy below it, signifying that the subsequent strategy would be preferred. In this case

TABLE 7.5
Remaining Strategies when Strictly Dominated Strategies are Removed

Strategy	Cost	Illness Days Avoided
No testing or treatment	$92.70	0
Amantadine	$97.50	0.54
Rimantadine	$119.10	0.59
Testing then zanamivir	$134.30	0.60
Zanamivir	$137.10	0.74

TABLE 7.6
Calculation of the Incremental Cost-Effectiveness Ratio (ICER)

Strategy	Cost	Illness Days Avoided	Incremental Cost	Incremental Effectiveness	ICER
No testing or treatment	$92.70	0	–	–	–
Amantadine	$97.50	0.54	$4.90	0.54	$9.06
Rimantadine	$119.10	0.59	$21.50	0.05	$430.00
Test/Zanamivir	$134.30	0.60	$15.20	0.01	$1520.00
Zanamivir	$137.10	0.74	$2.80	0.14	$20.00

TABLE 7.7
Removal of Strategies Due to Extended Dominance

Strategy	Cost	Illness Days Avoided	Incremental Cost	Incremental Effectiveness	ICER
No testing or treatment	$92.70	0	–	–	–
Amantadine	$97.50	0.54	$4.90	0.54	$9.06
Zanamivir	$137.10	0.74	$39.60	0.20	$198.00

both "Rimantadine" and "Test/Zanamivir" have higher ICERs than Zanamivir; thus, these strategies would not be preferred over Zanamivir due to extended dominance and can be removed from consideration. Removing these strategies from the table and recalculating the ICER of Zanamivir compared with Amantadine results in Table 7.7.

This same procedure can be performed graphically using the cost-effectiveness plane.[8] Figure 7.2 depicts all the testing and treatment strategies on the cost-effectiveness plane. Starting with "No testing or treatment," the least costly option, a line is drawn to the strategy that produces the shallowest slope (i.e., the smallest ICER), which is "Amantadine." From Amantadine, the shallowest positive slope is to Zanamivir. The resulting line is the cost-effectiveness efficient frontier; any point not on this frontier is dominated, either by strict dominance or extended dominance, as illustrated by the "Testing" strategies and by the "Rimantadine" strategy.

All reasonable strategies should be included in cost-effectiveness analyses so that true ICERs can be calculated. For example, if the Amantadine strategy were omitted from the analysis above, the ICER of Zanamivir would be $60 per illness day avoided when compared with "No testing or treatment" rather than $198 when compared with Amantadine. Omitting Amantadine would not give a true picture of the incremental value of Zanamivir, i.e., it would not tell us how much more would be paid for the gains in effectiveness seen with Zanamivir compared with all other reasonable strategies.[8]

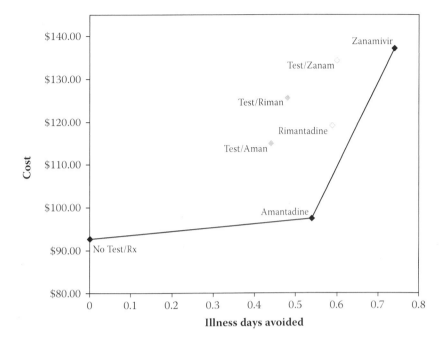

FIGURE 7.2   Cost and effectiveness values for influenza management strategies plotted on the cost-effectiveness plane. The line represents the cost-effectiveness efficient frontier, gray points denote strategies that are strictly dominated, and open points show strategies that are eliminated from consideration by extended dominance.

Similar considerations apply to the average cost-effectiveness ratio, here the cost divided by the illness days avoided; for example, the average cost-effectiveness ratio for Zanamivir is $137.1/0.74 or $185.27 per illness day avoided. When comparing mutually exclusive strategies, as we are in this example, the absence of incremental comparisons between strategies in the average cost-effectiveness calculation does not allow for elimination of dominated strategies or for calculation of incremental gains and costs between strategies.[8] The average cost-effectiveness ratio is useful in the evaluation of mutually compatible programs that are subject to a budget constraint, where programs are ranked, lowest to highest, by average cost-effectiveness ratio, then funded in that order until the budget is exhausted (see Chapter 1). Use of the average cost-effectiveness ratio in this fashion would maximize the health benefit for a given monetary expenditure; however, its use for this purpose has been largely theoretical to this point.

7.4.2   SENSITIVITY ANALYSIS

The next step in a CEA is the performance of sensitivity analyses. Typically, univariate, or one-way, sensitivity analyses are performed on parameter values, and further multiple parameter sensitivity analyses may also be performed. Further consideration of sensitivity analysis issues can be found in Chapter 12.

7.4.3 INTERPRETATION OF CEA RESULTS

To reiterate a prior point, CEA hinges on comparisons between strategies. A single option alone cannot be cost-effective; options can only be cost-effective compared with other options. The relative cost-effectiveness of one option compared with another is subject to interpretation and, perhaps as a result, the term "cost-effective" has been misused (although perhaps less so now than in the past, due to increasing familiarity with the true meaning of the term).[14] Cost-effective does not necessarily mean cost-saving. New health programs that are less costly and more effective than existing programs are clearly good buys, but a new program that costs more and is more effective than the existing program can be cost-effective without costs being saved, depending on how much is willing to be paid for a given health benefit. Cost-effective has also been incorrectly used to mean cost-saving when no determination of effectiveness differences between options has been performed; buying health insurance from one carrier that costs less than insurance from another carrier is not making a cost-effective decision when there is no comparison of health benefits between insurance plans; this would be a cost-minimization evaluation (see Chapter 6). Similarly, "cost-effective" has been misused to mean "effective" when there is no cost comparison. The correct meaning of "cost-effective" is that a program or strategy is worth the added cost because of the benefit it adds compared with other interventions. The application of the method requires a determination of the value of health care benefits as well as costs.

Returning to our influenza example, how can one interpret the incremental cost-effectiveness ratios of the amantadine and zanamivir strategies? One of the first steps in interpreting cost-effectiveness analyses is to understand what cost-effectiveness cannot do. It cannot make the "correct" choice; instead, it provides an analysis of the consequences of each choice. Cost-effectiveness analysis is not designed to address the social, political, or legal issues that might arise from a medical decision. Thus, if differing strategies involve questions of equity, social justice, legal responsibilities, or public opinion that need to be weighed in making a medical decision, consideration of more than strategy cost-effectiveness is necessary. Cost-effectiveness is one of many aspects of a decision to be considered and interpreted by decision-makers, be they physicians in the care of an individual patient or health policy makers in a broader population-based medical care context.[8]

Let us assume for now that sociopolitical issues are similar between our example strategies, allowing us to concentrate on the cost-effectiveness results as a major basis for the decision. In this case the question is: which strategy should we choose based on the ICERs calculated for each strategy? Or more bluntly, which strategy is the most "cost-effective"? The answer depends on the willingness-to-pay per unit health outcome (here, per illness day avoided). If the willingness-to-pay is less than $9 per illness day avoided, then "No testing or treatment" would be chosen, since the ICERs of the other strategies are ≥$9 per illness day. If willingness-to-pay thresholds are higher, other strategies would be chosen: Amantadine is chosen if the willingness-to-pay is $9 – $197, and Zanamivir is chosen if the willingness-to-pay is ≥$198 per illness day avoided.

How, then, is a reasonable cost-effectiveness willingness-to-pay threshold determined? This is a difficult question with no clear answer at this point, complicated by the many possible effectiveness values (life years gained, lives saved, illness days avoided, etc.) that could be considered. Cost-effectiveness comparisons between interventions using a common effectiveness measure can be useful in gaining a sense of an intervention's relative value. For example, if Treatment x for Disease X costs $100 per illness day prevented and is considered economically reasonable while Treatment y for Disease Y costs $500 per illness day avoided and is considered too expensive, then Treatment z for Disease Z costing $550 per illness day prevented might also be considered too expensive. However, the usefulness of this comparison depends on the similarity of illness days between Diseases X, Y, and Z. If Disease Z is worse than X or Y, then there might be a higher willingness-to-pay to avoid a more severe illness day from Disease Z than to avoid a more moderate illness day due to X or Y.

Sensitivity analysis may also be useful in the interpretation of results. If variation of analysis parameter values does not change the conclusion drawn from the base case analysis results, the analysis is said to be "robust," and increases the confidence in analysis results. Analyses that are not robust, where conclusions may change with variation of one or more parameter values, are termed "sensitive to variation," and their results are viewed with less confidence. Depending on the data used in the analysis, this confidence or uncertainty can be quantified through development of confidence intervals for cost-effectiveness ratios in empiric data sets or the use of probabilistic sensitivity analysis and acceptability curves when empiric data sets are not available. These issues are covered in greater detail in Chapter 12.

A number of other factors can make interpretation of CEAs challenging. Differences in analysis results can be due to methodologic differences between analyses. Cost-effectiveness analysis results are often dependent on the perspective, time horizon, and assumptions used in the analysis and, unless these factors are well-aligned between analyses, discordant results can arise based solely on these technical differences. Analyses using effectiveness values that are very specific to the medical scenario being examined, such as deep venous thrombosis prevented or lumbar discectomies avoided, may have few similar analyses available for comparison, making interpretation of their results challenging. Even if analyses with similar effectiveness values are available, their results could be difficult to compare with those of interventions for other disease processes using other effectiveness measures, thus limiting their comparability and interpretability. In these cases, a common effectiveness measure would facilitate cost-effectiveness comparisons over a broad spectrum of medical interventions. The use of quality-of-life utilities and QALYs in cost-utility analysis (as discussed in Chapter 9), along with methodologic recommendations to standardize analysis practices, such as those of the U.S. Panel on Cost-Effectiveness in Health and Medicine,[8] is largely motivated by the need to facilitate such comparisons, and has resulted in resources such as the online CEA Registry from Tufts University[15] to make direct comparisons possible.

7.5 SUMMARY

Cost-effectiveness analyses compare medical intervention strategies through the calculation of the incremental cost-effectiveness ratio, a measure of the cost of changes in health outcomes. These analyses can be performed on clinical trial data when information on both costs and effectiveness is available or, more commonly, through the use of decision analysis models to synthesize data from many sources. Interpretation of CEA results can be challenging due to the variety of health outcomes that can be used as the effectiveness term in these analyses and to the absence of a definitive criterion for "cost-effective." A subset of CEA, cost-utility analysis, attempts to make interpretation of results less difficult through the use of a common effectiveness term, the QALY.

REFERENCES

1. Black WC. 1990. The CE plane: A graphic representation of cost-effectiveness. *Med Decis Making* 10:212–214.
2. Bass EB, Pitt HA, Lillemoe KD. 1993. Cost-effectiveness of laparoscopic cholecystectomy versus open cholecystectomy. *Am J Surg* 165:466–71.
3. Cook J, Richardson J, Street A. 1994. A cost utility analysis of treatment options for gallstone disease: Methodological issues and results. *Health Econ* 3:157–68.
4. Ahmad S. 2005. The cost-effectiveness of raising the legal smoking age in California. *Med Decis Making* 25:330–40.
5. Johansson PM, Tillgren PE, Guldbrandsson KA, Lindholm LA. 2005. A model for cost-effectiveness analyses of smoking cessation interventions applied to a Quit-and-Win contest for mothers of small children. *Scand J Public Health* 33:343–52.
6. Agha Z, Lofgren RP, VanRuiswyk JV. 2005. Is antibiotic prophylaxis for bacterial endocarditis cost-effective? *Med Decis Making* 25:308–20.
7. King JT, Jr., Justice AC, Aron DC. 1997. Management of incidental pituitary microadenomas: A cost-effective analysis. *J Clin Endocrinol Metab* 82:3625–32.
8. Gold MR, Siegel JE, Russell LB, Weinstein MC, Eds. *Cost-effectiveness in health and medicine*. New York: Oxford University Press. 1996.
9. Drummond M, Sculpher M, Torrance G, O'Brien B, Stoddart G. *Methods for the economic evaluation of health care programmes*. Third edition. Oxford: Oxford University Press. 2005.
10. Aujesky D, Smith KJ, Cornuz J, Roberts MS. 2005. Cost-effectiveness of low-molecular-weight heparin for secondary prophylaxis of cancer-related venous thromboembolism. *Thromb Haemost* 93:592–9.
11. Smith KJ, Roberts MS. 2002. Cost-effectiveness of newer treatment strategies for influenza. *Am J Med* 113:300–7.
12. Weinstein MC. 1990. Principles of cost-effective resource allocation in health care organizations. *Int J Technol Assess Health Care* 6:93–103.
13. Cantor SB. 1994. Cost-effectiveness analysis, extended dominance, and ethics: A quantitative assessment. *Med Decis Making* 14:259–65.
14. Doubilet P, Weinstein MC, McNeil BJ. 1986. Use and misuse of the term "cost effective" in medicine. *N Engl J Med* 314:253–6.
15. Center for the Evaluation of Value and Risk in Health. The Cost-Effectiveness Analysis Registry [Internet]. (Boston), Institute for Clinical Research and Health Policy Studies, Tufts Medical Center. Available from: www.cearegistry.org.

8 Budget Impact Analysis

Lieven Annemans[*]

CONTENTS

8.1 INTRODUCTION

Every health economic evaluation must give rise to clear conclusions. Among other things, this means that it is reported for what indications, what patients, and in comparison with what alternatives a certain cost-effectiveness value was found. It is not acceptable to state in general terms that a medicine or a technology is cost-effective. This conclusion must always be accompanied by the indication, the target population, and the strategy with which comparisons were made. The conclusion must also indicate to what extent the results are robust (on the basis of the sensitivity analysis) and which variables should be subjected to further examination in the future.

It is also recommended that *the consequences of a decision on using a new medicine or technology should be represented at the level of the whole population.*

Birch and Gafni illustrate the point using the example of a purchase of cornflakes. Suppose you want to buy cornflakes and you compare the different products regarding their cost per 100g (some supermarkets give this information).[1] If you follow the rules of decision-making based on "value for money," you would choose the product with the lowest cost per 100g (assuming they all have the same quality). However, suppose you can buy only that product in a packet of 100 *kilograms* (a

---

[*] Copyright is retained by Dr. Lieven Annemans

slight exaggeration). In that case, you would certainly not opt for it because you do not have the budget for it. The same thing applies for medicines and technologies; a cost-effective result at the individual patient level can extrapolate to an immense budgetary impact at the population level, and this must at least be indicated to the policy maker. If no extra budgets are made available, the money must come from existing funds, and, therefore, other treatments will have to be sacrificed.

The same applies for medicines and technologies: a cost-effective result at the individual patient level may extrapolate to an immense budgetary impact at the population level and this plays a part in the policy decisions. The policy maker will certainly have to take this into account. This can be demonstrated by means of an admittedly abstract choice problem, as presented here below.[2]

8.1.1 A Choice Problem

Suppose you are the policy maker, and you have a budget of €1 billion available (or, if you prefer, £1 billion or $1 billion). There are eight new possible interventions, as shown in Table 8.1.[3]

TABLE 8.1
Summary of Eight New Interventions in a Choice Problem with Limited Budget

	Cost per Patient[1]	Number of Patients	Budget Impact[2]	% Success[3]	Gained QALYs in Case of Success[4]	Total QALYs[5]	ICER[6]
A*	€10000	60000	€600 M	25%	1.4	21000	€28571
B*	€4000	100000	€400 M	2%	9	18000	€22222
C*	€350000	1000	€350 M	90%	19	17100	€20468
D*	€500	500000	€250 M	1%	3.2	16000	€15625
E*	€10000	20000	€200 M	100%	0.6	12000	€16667
F*	€1000	200000	€200 M	50%	0.1	10000	€20000
G*	€500000	300	€150 M	100%	21	6300	€23810

(Handwritten annotations: A, B, C = A×B, D, E, Gained QALYs; F = ; B×D×E = Total QALYs; G = C/F)

[1] Incremental cost of the strategy. For example, A* is a new treatment for Alzheimer's disease and was compared with the current treatment A. The incremental cost per patient is €10,000.

[2] Product of the cost per patient and the number of patients. For A* this is €10000 x 60000 = €600 million.

[3] This is also incremental in relation to the current treatment. For instance, with A* the success rate is 85% while this was only 60% with current treatment A, a gain of 25%.

[4] This number applies only for successfully treated patients (in the case of A* this means 25% of 60000 = 15000 successfully treated patients.

[5] Product of the number of successfully treated patients and the number of QALYs per successfully treated patient: e.g., for A* this is 60000 x 25% x 1.4 = 15000 x 1.4 = 21000.

[6] Incremental Cost-Effectiveness Ratio. Ratio between the budget impact and the total number of QALYs, e.g., for A* this is €600M/21000 = €28571.

Every intervention has been examined for its cost-effectiveness at the level of the population. We see the cost per patient, the number of patients who are eligible, the total budgetary impact (the product of the number of patients and the cost per patient), the percentage of patients for whom the therapy works, the gain in quality-adjusted life years (QALYs) for each successfully treated patient, the total number of QALYs and, finally, the cost-effectiveness ratio.

The sum of the budgetary impact of the eight treatments is €2.15 billion, which is more than twice the available budget of €1 billion. Therefore, the policy maker must make choices and set priorities in order to generate the maximum number of QALYs with a limited budget.

The solution that results in the most QALYs for the set budget is that in which the interventions are ranked according to the last column, from the lowest (best) to the highest (worst) cost-effectiveness. This is done in Table 8.2. The interventions that are chosen are those at the top of the resultant list and a line is drawn where the budget is used up. With this solution, 55,100 QALYs are achieved (the sum of the first four lines in the total QALYs column). This number cannot be improved in any way.

An interesting observation is that the size of the budget (€1 billion) determines the maximum willingness to pay for a QALY. (In this example, this maximum willingness to pay is €20,468; see Table 8.2, 4th line, right-hand column.)

However, bearing in mind the considerations about equity, there are immediate doubts about whether the best choice has been made. It appears that therapy G is not chosen because its cost-effectiveness is not good enough. This is an admittedly expensive, but very effective, therapy for which only very few patients are eligible. These 300 patients would each gain 21 QALYs with this intervention. Clearly, this is a matter of the possibility of saving the lives of these people, who must be in a serious condition. Will these people simply be dropped while therapy F, which has a

TABLE 8.2
Solving the Choice Problem by Means of Cost-Effectiveness

	Cost per Patient[1]	Number of Patients	Budget Impact[2]	% Success[3]	Gained QALYs in Case of Success[4]	Total QALYs[5]	ICER[6]
D*	€500	500000	€250 M	1%	3.2	16000	€15625
E*	€10000	20000	€200 M	100%	0.6	12000	€16667
F*	€1000	200000	€200 M	50%	0.1	10000	€20000
C*	€350000	1000	€350 M	90%	19	17100	€20468
B*	€4000	100000	€400 M	2%	9	18000	€22222
G*	€500000	300	€150 M	100%	21	6300	€23810
A*	€10000	60000	€600 M	25%	1.4	21000	€28571

See notes for Table 8.1.

TABLE 8.3

Solving the Choice Problem with a Different Budgetary Impact

	Cost per Patient[1]	Number of Patients	Budget Impact[2]	% Success[3]	Gained QALYs in Case of Success[4]	*Total QALYs[5]*	*ICER[6]*
D*	€500	1500000	€750 M	1%	3.2	48000	€15625
E*	€10000	25000	€250 M	100%	0.6	15000	€16667
F*	€1000	200000	€200 M	50%	0.1	10000	€20000
C*	€350000	1000	€350 M	90%	19	17100	€20468
B*	€4000	100000	€400 M	2%	9	18000	€22222
G*	€500000	300	€150 M	100%	21	6300	€23810
A*	€10000	60000	€600 M	25%	1.4	21000	€28571

See notes for Table 8.1.

moderate success rate and limited gains in QALYs, will be reimbursed? It would not be surprising if policy makers were prepared to reimburse G and not F.

Let us go a step even further and suppose that there is a slight mistake with regard to the starting situation: it turns out that treatment D* does not apply to 500,000 patients but to 1,500,000; and treatment E* applies to 25,000 rather than 20,000 patients. Looking at the table again we find that the budget is used up after only these two interventions (Table 8.3). What policy maker could afford to reimburse only these two most cost-effective treatments, and not reimburse the rest? Logically, the policy maker will wish to limit the budget impact by putting downward pressure on the price of D*, or reimburse D* only for the highest risk category of patients in order to reduce the number of eligible patients.

This simple example shows the importance of budgetary impact. Cohen et al. state that the economic and equity rationale for carrying out budget impact analyses (BIA) is *opportunity cost*, or benefits forgone, measured in terms of utility or equitable distribution, by using resources in one way rather than another.[4] In other words, by choosing to use the budget in one way, decision-makers forgo other opportunities to use the same resources. The problem today is that there is not yet a clear insight into what is thought of as a large budgetary impact and what is a small one. This will depend to an important extent on the permitted growth of the budget.

8.2   GUIDELINES FOR BUDGET IMPACT ANALYSES

In 2007, Mauskopf et al. presented the first international guidelines for budget impact analyses (BIA).[5] Although these guidelines provide a very detailed insight into all issues related to the conduct and reporting of these analyses, the local implementation is not straightforward with regard to different aspects of BIA since the guidelines leave room for several interpretations and methodological options. We make an attempt here to make a set of clear standards for improving the consistency of analyses and results. The text aims to serve both those developing, as well as those reviewing, BIAs and making decisions.

A BIA is thereby defined as the best possible estimation of the financial consequences for the budget holder resulting from the adoption and diffusion of a new pharmaceutical drug or medical device over a well-defined time period. In the remainder of the text, we often refer to drugs but the same principles should count as well for devices.

8.2.1 PERSPECTIVE AND TARGET AUDIENCE

A budget impact of a new pharmaceutical drug or medical device should consider the perspective of the budget holder. This may be a national health insurance or a national health service, a private insurer, a hospital manager, etc. (see also Chapter 1).

8.2.2 OUTCOME

Given the perspective, all estimated expenses and savings must relate to the total health care impact. The narrower perspectives of the budget impact related to a drug only or related to the total pharmaceutical budget impact can also be shown, but the total health care budget impact is the primary outcome. It is also recommended to add information on the health impact on a population level, in line with a recommendation from Gafni and Birch. This may be in terms of complications avoided, cured patients, (quality-adjusted) life years saved, or other "hard" endpoints. As such, the decision-maker will not only receive an estimate of the financial impact but also about how many units of health, either disease-specific or generic, can be obtained on a population level.

8.2.3 HEALTH CONDITION AND TARGET POPULATION

The BIA addresses the impact of the use of a new drug in a well-defined health condition and target population. Therefore, a complete and detailed description of the health condition, its current treatment and related outcomes is essential. The potential target population must then include *all* patients who are eligible for the new drug and, hence, who might be given this new treatment in the time horizon of interest.

The target population must be defined starting from the approved indication, and—possibly—narrowed down to the population for which the reimbursement is requested. Of note, this target population may consist of new patients, but longstanding patients must also be considered for chronic diseases. Indeed, suppose a new treatment for patients with major depression, not only incident patients will be eligible, but also prevalent patients who have failed on previous treatments. Moreover, in some disease areas it may be that some prevalent patients currently have no adequate treatment option and that the introduction of a new drug enables them to be better treated (for instance, patients whose rheumatoid arthritis had been insufficiently controlled for several months or years). This is called induced demand, and means that the new drug may lead to market expansion, which, in such a case, must be taken into account in the analysis.

Regardless of induced demand, the target population may evolve over time organically because of diseases with an increasing incidence/prevalence over time, and this must be taken into account as well.

Within the target population, it is recommended that subpopulations be considered if there is evidence that such subpopulations are associated with different levels of effectiveness of the new drug or with different cost consequences. Importantly, the final estimated target population will depend on the market penetration of the new drug. This market penetration must be based on evidence, either from experience in other countries (if the drug was already launched there earlier) or from a similar drug in the same disease area that was launched earlier in the same setting, or based on market research studies. In the latter case, the report with methods and results of the market research study must be added to the appendix of the budget impact report.

Finally, possible off-label use of the new drug must also be discussed, its magnitude estimated and taken into account in the BIA.

8.2.4 The Intervention

The new drug must be fully described in terms of its efficacy, effectiveness, adverse events, and convenience of use. This description must focus on a comparison with the drugs and non-drug treatments that may be replaced by the new drug.

8.2.5 Time Horizon

The time horizon must meet the needs of the decision-maker. Therefore, it is recommended that a time horizon of 3 to 5 years be applied as a base case. It is, however, mandatory to show a flow of financial consequences on a yearly basis. Hence, instead of showing the total budget impact over only 3 to 5 years, the year-by-year impact must be shown. It is possible to show longer time horizons for BIAs related to chronic diseases, but it is suggested not to use a time horizon that does not allow validation of outcomes.

8.2.6 Comparators

A BIA must predict how a change in the current mix of drugs and other therapies used to treat a particular health condition will impact the flow of spending on that condition. Hence, the comparison must be made between a current intervention mix and a new intervention mix. The current intervention mix consists of those drugs (and possibly other treatments) that are currently used in the target population, and that may be replaced by the new drug. In case there are numerous current drugs and treatments that may be replaced by the new drug, it is possible to consider only the top three or top five of these drugs and treatments. Based on the above-mentioned market research, it must be estimated to which extent the new drug will replace each of those current drugs and treatments. Hence, the new intervention mix consists of the new drug plus the re-mix of the current drugs and treatments. It is important to account for the fact that the current intervention mix can also change over time, even without the introduction of the new drug. Finally, note that the abovementioned off-label use may occur within both the current mix and the new mix.

8.2.7 MODEL

A BIA requires a modeling approach for different reasons. For instance, if the available clinical trials do not describe the economic and health consequences of reaching an endpoint, other data sources must be consulted in order to obtain this type of information. The information from these different data sources must be combined in a model, in a similar way to that in cost-effectiveness studies (see Chapter 7). The model must be as simple as possible, but must be a correct reflection of the health condition, its natural history, and its consequences (as far as these consequences are affected by the new drug) for each year after the new drug is introduced into clinical practice. The model should be consistent with that used for the cost-effectiveness analysis (CEA), if there is one, with regard to clinical and economic assumptions.

It is important to note, however, that the complexity of the budget impact model and its alignment with the CEA model will depend on the type of health condition (acute health conditions and self-limiting health conditions may be associated with more simple models than chronic conditions or acute conditions with sequelae) and the type of intervention (preventive, curative, palliative, one-time, on-going, periodic). The final model structure must take into account these aspects and be justified accordingly. A budget impact model must be an open cohort model in the sense that individuals enter or leave the population.

The model must also be fully transparent. This means that all the data inputs must be clearly presented, together with their sources and their range of uncertainty (see 8.2.8, Data Sources) and that an electronic copy of the model should ideally be delivered to the decision maker.

The validity of the model must be assessed and the result of this assessment must be reported. The validation involves:

1. *Structure validation*: it is important to confirm that the framework that has been created is a good representation of the real situation.
2. *Content validation*: A peer reviewer should have the chance to examine the data input, sources, and the calculations of the model. This can be facilitated by providing the peer reviewer with an electronic version of the model.
3. *Outcomes validation*: The closer the model's clinical predictions approach reality, the greater the validity of the results. Obviously this cannot yet be examined for the branch with the new treatment, but can be done for the current mix.

8.2.8 DATA SOURCES

A BIA is meant to provide a range of predictions based on realistic estimates of the input parameter values in the model. To allow for the verification of the reliability of the data sources, each data input in the model must be documented by a clear reference to the data source from which the input was obtained. Moreover, the characteristics of each data source must also be described. This is essential, since the decision-maker must be able to verify whether the information in the data source is relevant to the considered target population.

The primary data sources should be published clinical trial estimates and comparator studies for efficacy and safety. Other data sources include population statistical information, health care databases, patient chart reviews, observational data, and—if data gaps are still present despite all the above sources—expert opinion (see Chapter 5). It is necessary that the data to which decision-makers have access also become accessible to the developers of the BIA. If assumptions will be needed (which is often the case), these must be realistic and justifiable, and their impact tested in the results section.

8.2.9 CALCULATIONS

The budget impact must be calculated on a yearly basis. For each year, the expenses associated with the current mix and the new mix, the medical resource use and costs associated with the consequences of the current mix and the new mix, the additional expenses due to the new intervention mix, the possible savings due to avoided medical resource use, and the net impact must be evaluated. This must be reported according to different scenarios as explained next.

As the BIA deals with financial streams over time, it is not necessary to discount the costs. Note that costs and savings need to be disease- and treatment-related, and must be calculated based on the product of resource use (induced or avoided) with the unit cost per resource item, from the perspective of the decision-maker, which often is noted as "charges" instead of real costs. The calculations should address the impact of compliance and persistence with therapy on the cost and outcomes of treatments. It may be, however, that the payer bears the cost anyway (e.g., even if poorly compliant, the patient still picks up the prescription).

8.2.10 REPORTING OF THE RESULTS

The main results of the BIA must not be presented as one base case estimate but, rather, as a range of plausible outcomes based on different scenarios (typical scenarios may be "best case" and "worst case"). Moreover, using a probabilistic sensitivity analysis (see Chapter 12) will enable the showing of the likelihood of different values in the range. Hence, descriptions such as, "according to our estimates, and based on the key assumptions, the budget impact of this drug will be with 80% of certainty below X million Euro in year 1, below Y million Euro in year 2, etc. ..." are recommended. Even when little is known about the degree of variability and the extent of correlation among parameters, an attempt should be made to produce such probabilistic results. Thus, all input data need to be described by a range and the BIA must show the impact of these ranges by means of one-way sensitivity analyses, as well as probabilistic sensitivity analysis. Moreover, the list of sensitivity analyses to be conducted must be established in agreement with the decision-maker. Last, the impact of all assumptions in the model must be clearly described, using alternative scenarios.

It is the intention that the quality and uniformity of budget impact analyses will improve based on these guidelines. The guidelines, however, do not inform the decision about what is or is not an acceptable budget impact. Further research with regard to the latter is required and is based on the unique characteristics of each situation.

REFERENCES

1. Birch, S., Gafni, A. 2006. Information created to evade reality (ICER): Things we should not look to for answers. *Pharmacoeconomics* 24(11):1121–31.
2. Eddy, D. 1992. Cost-effectiveness analysis. A conversation with my father. *JAMA* 267 (12).
3. Annemans, L. *Health economics for non-economists. An introduction to the concepts, methods and pitfalls of health economic evaluations.* Academia Press. XIV + 106 p. info@academiapress.be. 2008.
4. Cohen, J.P., Stolk, E., Niezen, M. 2008. Role of budget impact in drug reimbursement decisions. *J Health Polit Policy Law* 33(2):225–47.
5. Mauskopf, J.A. Sullivan, S.D., Annemans, L., Caro, J., Mullins, C.D., Nuijten, M., Orlewska, E., Watkins, J., Trueman, P. 2007. Principles of Good Practice for Budget Impact Analysis: Report of the ISPOR Task Force on Good Research Practices—Budget Impact Analysis. *Value in Health* 10 (5): 336–347.

9 Cost-Utility Analysis
A Case Study of a Quadrivalent Human Papillomavirus Vaccine

Erik J. Dasbach, Ralph P. Insinga, and Elamin H. Elbasha

CONTENTS

9.1 BACKGROUND AND INTRODUCTION

The purpose of this chapter is to introduce the reader to cost-utility analysis (CUA). We will do this by providing a brief background on CUA and reviewing a case study using it.

CUA is a special case of cost-effectiveness analysis (CEA), where the numerator of the incremental cost-effectiveness ratio (ICER) is a measure of cost (similar to other forms of CEA) and the denominator is measured typically using a metric called the *quality-adjusted life year* (QALY). A QALY accounts for both survival and quality of life (QoL) benefits associated with the use of a healthcare technology. The QoL component of the QALY is measured using a metric known as a *health utility*; hence, the term *cost-utility analysis* is used to describe this form of CEA. Background on the measurement of health utilities is discussed in Chapter 11.

Given that the QALY can be used to measure the survival and QoL benefits of a healthcare technology, the QALY can serve as a common metric from which to compare the benefits of very different healthcare technologies (e.g., migraine pharmacotherapy versus angioplasty). Thus, one of the primary advantages of conducting a CUA is that the ICER theoretically can be considered a common metric from which to compare the relative value of one health care technology (e.g., drug) with a completely different healthcare technology (e.g., vaccine).

This universal quality of a CUA is the primary reason many policy makers and reimbursement agencies prefer or require CUA when requesting a reimbursement dossier from a manufacturer. In fact, some reimbursement agencies have established ICER thresholds from which to determine whether a healthcare technology is cost effective. For example, the National Institute for Health and Clinical Excellence (NICE) has used the benchmark ICER of £30,000 per QALY gained as a threshold from which to judge whether a drug is cost effective for the National Health Service (NHS) in England.[1,2] In the United States, $50,000 per QALY gained has been frequently used in cost-effectiveness analyses as a threshold.[3,4] From a global perspective, the World Health Organization (WHO) has established a cost-effectiveness criterion indicating that a healthcare technology is cost effective if the ICER is less than three times the per capita gross domestic product (GDP) for a given country.[5]

Other decision-makers may use "league tables" of ICERs for commonly accepted healthcare technologies (e.g., renal dialysis) as a method for judging whether a healthcare technology is cost-effective or of good value. For example, the Center for the Evaluation of Value and Risk in Health at Tufts Medical Center maintains a Cost-Effectiveness Analysis Registry.[6] In particular, the Tufts-New England Medical Center Cost-Effectiveness Registry provides public electronic access to a comprehensive database of cost-effectiveness ratios in the published medical literature that can be used by decision-makers.

To summarize, CUA can serve as a general framework for conducting economic evaluations and a practical tool for decision-makers faced with making reimbursement decisions across widely different healthcare technologies. The role of CUA in drug development, reimbursement, and marketing are described in depth in Chapter 15. In the remainder of this section, we will focus on providing an example of the methodology undertaken in developing a CUA by reviewing a case study CUA of a vaccine developed to prevent four types of human papillomavirus (HPV) infection as well as associated diseases caused by HPV infection (e.g., cervical pre-cancers, cervical cancers, and genital warts). Results from this CUA as well as other economic evaluations[7] were used by policy makers in the United States in developing vaccine recommendations for a quadrivalent HPV vaccine in 2006.

9.2   CASE-STUDY: A COST-UTILITY ANALYSIS OF A QUADRIVALENT HUMAN PAPILLOMAVIRUS VACCINATION PROGRAM

9.2.1   BACKGROUND

Genital infections with HPV are among the most widespread sexually transmitted infections worldwide. Infection with HPV can cause cervical intraepithelial neoplasia (CIN); cervical, vaginal, vulvar, anal, penile, and head and neck cancers; anogenital warts; and recurrent respiratory papillomatoses (RRP). In 2006, the U.S. Food and Drug Administration approved the vaccine Gardasil® for use in girls and women 9 to 26 years of age for the prevention of the following diseases caused by HPV types 6, 11, 16, and 18:

* Cervical cancer
* Genital warts (condyloma acuminata)

and the following precancerous or dysplastic lesions:

* Cervical adenocarcinoma *in situ* (AIS)
* Cervical intraepithelial neoplasia (CIN) grades 2 and 3
* Vulvar intraepithelial neoplasia (VIN) grades 2 and 3
* Vaginal intraepithelial neoplasia (VaIN) grades 2 and 3
* Cervical intraepithelial neoplasia (CIN) grade 1

The Centers for Disease Control and Prevention's (CDC) Advisory Committee for Immunization Practices (ACIP) also recommended in 2006 that U.S. girls and women 11 to 26 years old be vaccinated with Gardasil (with a provision that females as young as 9 may also be vaccinated) to prevent cervical cancer, precancerous and low-grade lesions, and genital warts caused by HPV types 6, 11, 16, and 18. As part of the process for formulating this vaccine policy, CEAs of an HPV vaccine were required by the ACIP. Cost-effectiveness analyses conducted by the CDC, academia, and industry were thus presented to the ACIP. A summary of the clinical and health economic evidence considered by the ACIP, including various relevant CEAs conducted up to that time, has been reported elsewhere.[8] In this case study, we will review a cost-utility model that was developed by industry to support these deliberations. The analyses reviewed here are based on a previously published model.[9,10] For this case study, however, we will not focus on the myriad of analyses reported in these previous publications. Instead, this case study will present a few selected analyses that we develop here to specifically illustrate the value of CUA in reimbursement and policy decisions. In particular, we will highlight the role of QALYs in the analysis as this is a distinguishing feature from other forms of CEA.

9.2.2   Research Questions

The primary research questions this CUA answered were as follows:

1. In a setting of organized cervical cancer screening, what is the cost effectiveness of a quadrivalent HPV vaccination strategy that targets girls and women 12 to 24 years of age relative to a strategy of no vaccination in the United States from a healthcare system perspective over a 100-year analytic horizon?
2. In a setting of organized cervical cancer screening, is a quadrivalent HPV vaccination strategy that targets girls and women 12 to 24 years of age relative to a strategy of no vaccination in the United States cost effective?

9.2.3   Disease Model

To capture the indirect effects of vaccination on the entire population, we developed a dynamic disease transmission model.[11] Figure 9.1 depicts a simplified schematic of the health states tracked in the analysis. The model follows the U.S. population of persons greater than 12 years of age over an analytic horizon of 100 years. Persons enter the model into the susceptible state and, if vaccinated, the vaccinated state. Susceptible persons can become infected by different HPV types. Persons infected with HPV types 16 or 18 can become immune or progress to CIN 1, followed by CIN 2/3 and cervical cancer. Persons infected with HPV types 6 or 11 can become immune or progress to genital warts as well as low-grade CIN. Vaccinated persons can follow a path similar to that of susceptible individuals; however, the acquisition of infection and progression to disease is slowed through vaccination. At any point in time, persons can exit the model according to age, gender, and disease-specific mortality rates. The model consists of a system of ordinary differential equations

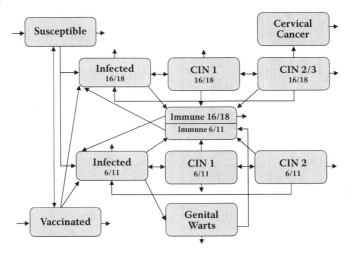

FIGURE 9.1   A simplified schematic of the HPV model.

(ODEs). We programmed all model equations and inputs in Mathematica® (Wolfram Research, Champaign, IL). We used the NDSolve subroutine in Mathematica version 5.2 to generate numerical solutions for ODEs making up the model.

9.2.4   SCREENING AND VACCINATION STRATEGIES AND PARAMETERS

Reference Strategy. The baseline reference strategy was routine cervical cancer screening as practiced in the United States. We used age-stratified data from the Kaiser Permanente Northwest health plan, the National Health Interview Survey (NHIS), and Behavioral Risk Factor Surveillance System (BRFSS)[12,13] to estimate rates for routine cytology screening. Estimates of cytology screening test characteristics were based on published studies.[14]

Comparator Strategy. The comparator strategy (i.e., quadrivalent HPV vaccination) was assumed to be routine quadrivalent (16/18/6/11) HPV vaccination of girls at age 12 combined with a temporary (i.e., 5-year) catch-up vaccination program for girls and women 12 to 24 years of age. We assumed this vaccination strategy would be combined with current cervical cancer screening practices. Moreover, we assumed that current cervical cancer screening practices would not change with the introduction of HPV vaccination.

The efficacy of the vaccine strategy in preventing incident HPV infection (HPV 6/11 or 16/18) was assumed to be 90%. We assumed the prophylactic efficacy of the vaccine in preventing HPV-related diseases (i.e., HPV 6-, 11-, 16-, and 18-related CIN and genital warts) was 95.2% and 98.9%, respectively.[15] The duration of protection provided by vaccination was assumed to be lifelong, as was done in previous models.[16–18] We assumed that the natural course of acquired infection and disease is unaltered following vaccine failure or loss of vaccine-induced immunity. Because this is a prophylactic vaccine, we did not assume any therapeutic benefits when administered to persons infected with HPV.

We assumed that 70% of adolescents would receive a three-dose vaccine before they turned 12, similar to the coverage rates used in previous models.[17,19,20] Coverage was also assumed to increase linearly from 0% up to 70% during the first 5 years of the program (i.e., 14% in year 1, 28% in year 2, etc.) and remain at 70% thereafter. We assumed that the annual vaccine coverage for three doses of vaccine for the catch-up program in girls and women 12 to 24 who were previously unvaccinated would increase linearly from 0% up to 50% during the first 5 years (i.e., 10% in year 1, 20% of unvaccinated in year 2, etc.) and then drop to 0% per year after 5 years.

9.2.5   ECONOMIC PARAMETERS

All costs were updated to 2005 U.S. dollars using the medical care component of the consumer price index. The direct medical costs for screening for and treatment of CIN, genital warts, and cervical cancer were based on administrative claims data and other sources.[21–23] We assumed the cost of the HPV vaccine for three doses and administration would be $360. All future costs and QALYs were discounted to present at a rate of 3% per year.

9.2.6 QoL Weight Parameters

One of the primary challenges with estimating QALYs in a CUA is estimating the QoL weights for the health states. When estimating a QoL weight, the range of potential values for a given health state are usually bounded by 0 and 1, where 1 corresponds to best imaginable health and 0 corresponds to death. Data for measuring the QoL weights (i.e., health utilities) can be obtained through a variety of approaches[24–26] and is discussed in detail in Chapter 11 on Patient Reported Outcomes.

For this CUA, we used estimates from studies reported in the literature. Table 9.1 summarizes the QoL weights used for the disease health states. We assumed females diagnosed with CIN1 and CIN2/3 would have quality weights of 0.91 and 0.87, respectively.[27,28] Males and females with genital warts were assumed to have a QoL weight of 0.91.[27] We assumed females with local and regional cervical cancer to have QoL weights of 0.76 and 0.67, respectively.[27] We derived a quality weight for invasive distant cancer of 0.48 from Gold et al.[29] using the 25th percentiles of female genital cancer weights. We assumed that the QoL weight for cervical cancer survivors after successful treatment would continue to be lower (i.e., 0.76) than that of healthy females.[30,31] The QoL weights for individuals harboring undiagnosed conditions of HPV, genital warts, CIN, and cervical cancer, and following successful treatment of CIN and genital warts, were assumed to be similar to those of individuals without HPV disease. We derived gender- and age-specific QoL weights from Gold et al.[29] to reflect the QoL impact of non-HPV related co-morbidities, which could potentially reduce the absolute gains in health utility achievable from preventing HPV disease.

9.2.7 Model Output: Epidemiologic

We used several measures to assess the epidemiologic impact of vaccination. Epidemiologic output included clinically diagnosed cases of CIN 1, CIN 2/3, invasive cervical cancer, and genital warts and cervical cancer-related deaths. These health states are shown in Figure 9.1.

TABLE 9.1
Health Utility Values

Health State	Estimate	Notation	Reference
Genital wart	0.91	QGW	28
CIN 1	0.91	$QCIN1$	27, 28
CIN 2	0.87	$QCIN2$	27, 28
CIN 3	0.87	$QCIN3$	27, 28
CIS	0.87	$QCIS$	27, 28
Localized cervical cancer treatment	0.76	$QLCC$	27
Regional cervical cancer treatment	0.67	$QRCC$	27
Distant cervical cancer treatment	0.48	$QDCC$	29
Cervical cancer survivor	0.76	$QCCS$	31
Healthy (age and gender specific)	0.70 to 0.93	QH	29

9.2.8   MODEL OUTPUT: QUALITY-ADJUSTED LIFE YEARS

As noted earlier, the QALY metric integrates all of the health benefits (i.e., quality and length of life) conferred by a healthcare technology into a single metric. To do this, the metric assigns QoL weights to each health state tracked in the model and integrates the sum of all of these adjusted health states over the planning horizon (0, 100). QoL weights for an individual experiencing a given condition were multiplied by the age and gender-specific QoL weight assigned to that individual. For example, if the life expectancy for a 55-year-old woman (age- and gender-specific QoL weight of 0.8) diagnosed with distant cervical cancer was 6 months (or 0.5 years), then the resulting number of undiscounted QALYs experienced would be valued at .19 (.5 x 0.48 x 0.8) QALYs. Hence, the QALY is calculated as the sum of the product of the expected time in the health state and the QoL experienced (i.e., QoL weight) over that time. The following equation shows the specific formula used to estimate QALYs.

$$QALY = \int_{0}^{100} \left[\sum_{i=1}^{17} QH_{fi} \begin{pmatrix} NH_{fi} - \left(1 - QGW_{f}\right)NGW_{fi} - \left(1 - QCIN1\right)NCIN1_{i} - \left(1 - QCIN2\right)NCIN2_{i} - \\ \left(1 - QCIN3\right)NCIN3_{i} - \left(1 - QCIS\right)NCIS_{i} - \left(1 - QLCC\right)NLCC_{i} - \\ \left(1 - QRCC\right)NRCC_{i} - \left(1 - QDCC\right)NDCC_{i} - \left(1 - QCCS\right)NCCS_{i} \end{pmatrix} \right. \\ \left. + \sum_{i=1}^{17} QH_{mi} \left(NH_{mi} - \left(1 - QGW_{m}\right)NGW_{mi} \right) \right] e^{0.03t} dt$$

Table 9.1 summarizes the health utilities assigned to each health state, the variable name for each health state represented in the equation, and the sources of the utility values. All variables in the equation beginning with N represent the total number of individuals with the associated conditions at time t. For example, NH represents the number of healthy individuals where f and m represent female and male respectively and i represents age. Hence, NHfi represents the number of females alive in age group i. NHmi represents the number of males alive in age group i. The model included 17 age groups.

It should be noted that we integrated the sum of quality-adjusted health states over the planning horizon (0, 100) because time is continuous. If time is treated as a discrete variable, as in many Markov models with fixed cycle length (e.g., 1 year), QALYs would be obtained as a sum of quality-adjusted health states from the present to 100 years.

Finally, we note that the age-specific QALY for females is reduced by time spent in diagnosed genital warts, CIN, and cancer states. Male age-specific QoL deteriorates by spending time with genital warts. All health states are multiplied by the age- and gender-specific weights to reflect the variation in QoL by age and gender groups.

9.2.9   Model Output: Economic

The economic output of interest from the model included total discounted costs and the incremental cost per QALY gained ratio. Both costs and QALYs were discounted at a 3% annual rate. We measured the cost-per-QALY ratio as the incremental cost difference between the two strategies divided by the incremental QALY difference between the two strategies.

9.2.10   Sensitivity Analyses

The focus of the sensitivity analyses reported here will be on the QoL weights and the influence changes in these weights have on the ICERs.

9.2.11   Epidemiologic Results

Table 9.2 summarizes some of the public health benefits of the vaccination strategy (i.e., vaccination of girls and women 12 to 24 years of age) relative to no vaccination in the United States. Specifically, Table 9.2 shows the cumulative additional cases of HPV-16/18/6/11-disease prevented in the United States with vaccination relative to no vaccination at years 10, 20, 50, 70, and 100 following the introduction of vaccination. For example, in row 2, column 4 of Table 9.2, the vaccination strategy compared with the no vaccination strategy is projected to reduce the number of cases of HPV 16/18-related cervical cancer by over 100,000 cases 50 years following the introduction of the HPV vaccine program in the U.S. population.

9.2.12   QALY Results

To estimate QALYs, we multiplied the amount of time spent in each of the disease states shown in Table 9.2 by the quality life weights in Table 9.1. Figure 9.2 shows

TABLE 9.2
Cumulative Additional Cases of HPV-16/18/6/11—Disease Prevented in the United States with Vaccination Relative to No Vaccination

	Years Since Vaccination Program Started				
	10	20	50	70	100
Cervical Cancer Deaths	0	479	19,701	41,458	76,544
Cervical Cancer	20	6,140	103,578	189,947	324,426
CIN 2/3	26,531	570,853	3,145,945	4,961,776	7,711,992
CIN1	8,533	189,860	900,595	1,378,583	2,097,669
Genital Warts	250,336	2,955,871	11,024,892	16,365,481	24,403,341

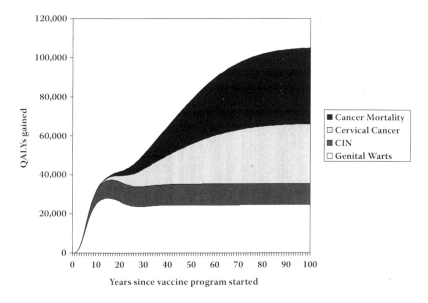

FIGURE 9.2   Undiscounted QALYs gained with vaccination over time.

the net QALYs gained (undiscounted) over time with vaccination relative to no vaccination by disease (health) state. The total QALY gained for the vaccination strategy would be estimated by calculating the area under the curve. Overall, prevention of genital warts accounted for 33% of the total QALYs gained over 100 years. In addition, prevention of cervical cancer deaths, cervical cancer cases, and CIN cases accounted for 29%, 25%, and 14% of the total QALYs gained over 100 years, respectively. Figure 9.3 shows the net discounted QALYs gained over time with vaccination relative to no vaccination by disease state. The total QALYs gained for the vaccination strategy would again be estimated by calculating the area under the curve. Overall, preventing genital warts accounted for 45% of the total QALYs gained over 100 years, which is higher than in the undiscounted analysis. This was because the discounted value of preventing the other HPV diseases was reduced in relative magnitude as these diseases increased their relative proportion of the total QALYs gained further out in time when compounded discounting had a greater impact in reducing their contribution to total QALYs gained. Cervical cancer deaths, cervical cancer cases, and CIN cases thus accounted for only 20%, 19%, and 17% of the total discounted QALYs gained over 100 years, respectively.

9.2.13   Cost-Effectiveness Results

To assess the cost-effectiveness of the vaccination strategy, we estimated the total discounted costs and effects (i.e., QALYs) accrued over a 100-year period for each strategy. These total costs and QALYs are shown in columns 2 and 3, respectively, in Table 9.3. Next, we calculated the incremental cost incurred to achieve an incremental gain in benefit with vaccination relative to no vaccination. These incremental

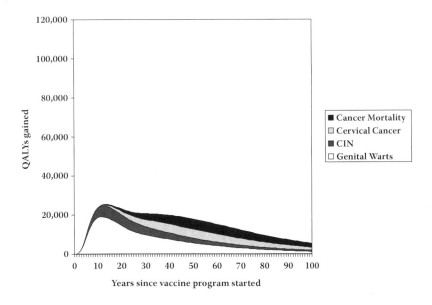

FIGURE 9.3   Discounted QALYs gained with vaccination over time.

TABLE 9.3

Cost-Effectiveness Analysis of an HPV Vaccination Program that Targets Girls and Women under the Age of 25 Relative to No Vaccination in the United States

Strategy	Total Costs (1,000s)	Total QALYs (1,000s)	ΔCosts (1,000s)	ΔQALYs (1,000s)	ΔCosts / ΔQALYs (ICER)
No Vaccine (screening only)	$174,340,679	6,476,910			
Quadrivalent Vaccine (12 to 24 girls and women)	$179,818,630	6,478,399	$5,477,951	1,489	$3,680

Note: Δ = the incremental difference between strategies.

---

costs and effects are shown in columns 4 and 5. Note that the total discounted QALYs gained over 100 years in the U.S. population (i.e., 1,489,000) were calculated by estimating the area under the curve in Figure 9.3. The final column shows the ratio of the incremental costs to incremental QALYs gained (i.e., the ICER). The ICER for vaccination was $3,680 per QALY gained.

We also explored a variety of sensitivity analyses where we varied the QoL weights assigned to the health states. We have summarized the results of these sensitivity analyses in Table 9.4. For example, in row 1, column 3, of Table 9.4, we

TABLE 9.4
Summary of Incremental Cost-Effectiveness Ratios for Sensitivity Analyses

Input Variable	ΔQALYs (1,000s)	ICER
Increase quality of life weight decrement by 50%	2,084	$2,629
Reference case	1,489	$3,680
Decrease quality of life weight decrement by 50%	893	$6,132
No protection against HPV types 6/11 (e.g., no genital wart benefit)	895	$10,103
No quality of life weight decrement (i.e., life years gained)	298	$18,387

show the ICER decreases to $2,629 per QALY gained when we assumed the decrement in the QoL weights for the disease states were 50% greater. The reason for the decrease in the ICER is evident from column 2, which shows that an additional 595,000 QALYs would be gained relative to the reference case if we assumed the decrement in the QoL weights for the disease states was 50% greater. However, when we assumed the decrement in the QoL weights for the disease states was 50% less, the ICER increased to $6,132 per QALY gained (row 3). Again, column 2 shows fewer QALYs would be gained relative to the reference case if the QoL weights for the disease states were 50% less.

We also examined two other scenarios where we partially or completely eliminated the QoL benefits of the vaccine. In one scenario, we eliminated any benefits associated with protecting against HPV 6/11 infection and disease. The resulting ICER under this scenario increased to $10,103 per QALY gained. This increase in the ICER was attributable to two factors. First, the number of QALYs gained relative to the reference case was less. Second, the total cost of the vaccination strategy was significantly higher than the total cost of the vaccination strategy in the reference case because the reduction in the costs of preventing genital warts was eliminated from this scenario. Finally, we examined a scenario where no QoL benefits would be realized by preventing CIN, genital warts, and cancer (i.e., all of the benefits were due to life extension only, with no improvement in QoL). The resulting ICER increased to $18,387 per QALY gained. Again, the QALY benefits gained in this scenario (i.e., 298,000) were significantly less than the reference case. In fact, these QALYs gained represent only survival gains (i.e., life years gained).

9.3   COMMENTARY

The primary research question this case study aimed to answer was, "What is the cost-effectiveness of a quadrivalent HPV vaccination strategy that targets girls and women 12 to 24 years of age relative to a strategy of no vaccination in the United States from a healthcare system perspective over a 100-year analytic horizon?" We found that for the reference case analysis the ICER was $3,680 per QALY gained.

The second research question this case study aimed to answer was, "Is a quadrivalent HPV vaccination strategy that targets girls and women 12 to 24 years of age relative to a strategy of no vaccination in the United States cost effective?" Based on thresholds used by cost-effectiveness analyses in the United States, a quadrivalent HPV vaccine would be considered cost-effective as the ICER is less than $50,000 per QALY gained.[3,4] Similarly, based on threshold ICERs set by NICE in the UK and the WHO, quadrivalent HPV vaccination would also be considered cost-effective from these perspectives. Finally, if one were to compare the ICER to ICERs of other commonly accepted medical technologies using the Cost-Effectiveness Analysis Registry at Tufts Medical Center, quadrivalent HPV vaccination would be considered cost effective.[6] For example, the ICER for dialysis in end-state renal disease (ESRD) in the United States ranges from $50,000 to $100,000 per QALY gained.[32] Given that Medicare reimburses for dialysis for ESRD in the United States, HPV vaccination would represent a good value relative to dialysis for ESRD. Similar conclusions to these have been reached within U.S. policy-making contexts. For instance, the ACIP at the CDC concluded that, based on CEA models from industry, academia, and the government, vaccination of 9 to 26-year-old females with the quadrivalent vaccine was a solid investment, with ICERs within an acceptable range of cost effectiveness.[7] All of the cost-effectiveness models reviewed by the ACIP in this deliberation reported incremental cost per QALY gained ratios.[9,18,–20,33]

Thus, one of the primary benefits of using CUA is the ability to provide decision-makers with a common yardstick from which to assess the relative value of a healthcare technology. If we had examined cost per cervical cancer case avoided in this CUA, we would not have been able to compare the ICER with the ICER of healthcare technologies that do not prevent or treat cervical cancer. In fact, this very issue was subsequently raised at the ACIP when evaluating the cost-effectiveness of a rotavirus vaccine.[34] The cost-effectiveness analysis presented to the ACIP only reported ICERs that used cases of rotavirus avoided and life years gained in the denominator because QoL weights were not available to account for the childhood morbidity associated with rotavirus. The ACIP noted that these metrics limited their ability to assess the value of the rotavirus vaccine relative to other vaccines they had deemed as being cost effective. As a result, the ACIP recommended that QALYs be incorporated into the cost-effectiveness analysis in order to better assess the acceptability of the cost-effectiveness of rotavirus vaccination.[34]

Another benefit of CUA is that it allows for all the benefits of a healthcare technology to be considered. For example, we showed the impact of not accounting for QoL benefits in the sensitivity analyses. In particular, the ICER increased almost fivefold to $18,387 per QALY gained when we eliminated the QoL benefits of preventing genital warts, CIN, and cervical cancer. As shown in Figure 9.2 and Figure 9.3, these quality benefits exceeded the mortality benefits. In addition, these QoL benefits were realized sooner in the population than were the survival benefits. Hence, using survival gains as a metric for evaluating HPV vaccines significantly undervalues the benefits of the vaccine. For other disease areas such as arthritis and migraine, QoL decrements would account for virtually the entire health benefits associated with any intervention and an analysis of life-years gained would be inappropriate.

Given the ability of CUA to facilitate comparing the relative value of differing healthcare technologies, CUA has enjoyed significant growth as a preferred method of CEA in the field. The CUA is not without its limitations. In particular, many over the years have been critical of using the QALY as the denominator in the ICER because either the metric is too complex and not pragmatic or not complex enough to accurately characterize how individuals value the QoL weights.[35] As a result, others have proposed alternative metrics. However few CEAs have adopted these other metrics. Hence, the literature on CUA with QALYs continues to grow and facilitate a language from which to compare the relative value of different healthcare technologies.

REFERENCES

1. NICE. NHS. National Institute for Clinical Excellence. Guide to the methods of technology appraisal Issue date: June 2008. http://www.nice.org.uk/media/B52/A7/TAMethodsGuideUpdatedJune2008.pdf accessed July 23, 2008.
2. Devlin N, Parkin D. 2004. Does NICE have a cost-effectiveness threshold and what other factors influence its decisions? A binary choice analysis. *Health Econ* 13(5):437–52.
3. Eichler HG, Kong SX, Gerth WC, Mavros P, Jonsson B. 2004. Use of cost-effectiveness analysis in health-care resource allocation decision-making: How are cost-effectiveness thresholds expected to emerge? *Value in Health* 7(5):518–28.
4. Grosse SD. 2008. Assessing cost-effectiveness in healthcare: History of the $50,000 per QALY threshold. Expert Rev. *Pharmacoeconomics Res* 8:165–178. 2008.
5. WHO. World Health Organization. Choosing Interventions that are Cost Effective (WHO-CHOICE) Tables of costs and prices used in WHO-CHOICE analysis. http://www.who.int/choice/costs/CER_levels/en/index.html: accessed July 28, 2008.
6. Center on the Evaluation of Value and Risk in Health (2008). The cost-effectiveness analysis registry, Tufts-New England Medical Center, ICRHPS. http://www.tufts-nemc.org/cearegistry/data/docs/PhaseIIIACompleteLeagueTable.pdf accessed July 28, 2008.
7. ACIP. ACIP Record of the Proceedings June 29–30, 2006. http://www.cdc.gov/vaccines/recs/acip/downloads/min-jun06.pdf: accessed July 30, 2008.
8. Markowitz LE, Dunne EF, Saraiya M et al. Quadrivalent human papillomavirus vaccine: Recommendations of the Advisory Committee on Immunization Practices (ACIP). *MMWR* 2007. 56:1–24. 2007.
9. Elbasha EH, Dasbach EJ, Insinga RP. 2007. Model for assessing human papillomavirus vaccination strategies. *Emerg Infect Dis* 13(1):28–41.
10. Elbasha EH, Dasbach EJ, Insinga RP. 2008. A multi-type HPV transmission model: Assessing the epidemiologic and economic impact of a quadrivalent HPV vaccine. *Bull Math Biol* 70:2126–2176.
11. Brisson M, Edmunds WJ. 2003. Economic evaluation of vaccination programs: The impact of herd-immunity. *Med Decis Making* 23(1):76–82.
12. Hewitt M et al. 2004. Cervical cancer screening among U.S. women: Analyses of the 2000 National Health Interview Survey. *Prev Med* 39(2):270–8.
13. Insinga RP et al. 2004. Pap screening in a U.S. health plan. *Cancer Epidem Biomarkers Prev* 13(3):355–60.
14. Bigras G, de Marval F. 2005. The probability for a Pap test to be abnormal is directly proportional to HPV viral load: Results from a Swiss study comparing HPV testing and liquid-based cytology to detect cervical cancer precursors in 13,842 women. *Br J Cancer* 93(5):575–81.
15. Merck & Co., Inc. GARDASIL Prescribing Information. www.gardasil.com/downloads/gardasil_pi.pdf: accessed July 30, 2008. 2007.

16. Stratton K. Committee to Study Priorities for Vaccine Development. Institute of Medicine. *Vaccines for the 21st century: A tool for decisionmaking. Appendix 11. Human Papillomavirus* pp. 213–222. Washington DC: National Academy Press. 2000. http://www.iom.edu/report.asp?id=5648 accessed July 30, 2008.
17. Goldie S, Grima D, Kohli M, Weinstein M, Wright T, Franco E. 2003. A comprehensive natural history model of human papillomavirus (HPV) infection and cervical cancer: Potential impact of an HPV 16/18 vaccine. *Value in Health* 5(6):576.
18. Goldie SJ, Kohli M, Grima D, Weinstein MC, Wright TC, Bosch FX, Franco E. 2004. Projected clinical benefits and cost-effectiveness of a human papillomavirus 16/18 vaccine. *J Natl Cancer Inst* 96(8):604–15.
19. Sanders GD, Taira AV. 2003. Cost effectiveness of a potential vaccine for Human papillomavirus. *Emerg Infect Dis* 9(1):37–48.
20. Chesson HW, Ekwueme DU, Saraiya M, Markowitz LE. 2008. Cost-effectiveness of human papillomavirus vaccination in the United States. *Emerg Infect Dis* 14(2):244–51.
21. Medstat 2. MarketScan R database, Thomsom Medstat. Ann Arbor, MI. Rockville, MD: Agency for Health Care Policy and Research. http://www.ahrq.gov/clinic/epcsums/cervsumm.htm: accessed July 30, 2008. 1999.
22. Kim JJ, Wright TC, Goldie SJ. 2002. Cost-effectiveness of alternative triage strategies for atypical squamous cells of undetermined significance. *JAMA* 287(18):2382–90.
23. Insinga RP, Dasbach EJ, Myers E. 2003. The health and economic burden of genital warts in a set of private health plans in the United States. *Clin Infect Dis* 36(11):1397–403.
24. Froberg DG, Kane RL. 1989. Methodology for measuring health-state preferences. 2. Scaling methods. *J Clin Epidemiol* 42(5):459–71.
25. Neumann PJ, Goldie SJ, Weinstein MC. 2000. Preference-based measures in economic evaluation in health care. *Annu Rev Public Health* 21:587–611.
26. Dasbach EJ, Teusch, SM. Quality of life. In Dasbach EJ, Haddix, AC, Corso, PS, Eds. *Prevention effectiveness: A guide to decision analysis and economic evaluation.* Second Edition. 2003. NYC, Oxford University Press, 2003.
27. Myers ER, Green S, Lipkus I. Patient preferences for health states related to HPV infection: Visual analogue scales vs. time trade-off elicitation. Proceedings of the 21st International Papillomavirus Conference, Abstract No. 390.2 2004. Mexico City, Mexico. 2004.
28. Insinga RP, Glass AG, Myers ER, Rush BB. 2007. Abnormal outcomes following cervical cancer screening: Event duration and health utility loss. *Med Decis Making* 27(4):414–22.
29. Gold MR, Franks P, McCoy KI, Fryback DG. 1998. Toward consistency in cost-utility analyses: Using national measures to create condition-specific values. *Med Care* 36(6):778–92.
30. Andersen BL. 1996. Stress and quality of life following cervical cancer. *J Nat Cancer Inst Monographs* [21], 65–70.
31. Wenzel L, DeAlba I, Habbal R, Kluhsman BC, Fairclough D, Krebs LU, Anton-Culver H, Berkowitz R, Aziz N. 2005. Quality of life in long-term cervical cancer survivors. *Gynecol Oncol* 97(2):310–7.
32. Neumann PJ, Rosen AB, Weinstein MC. 2005. Medicare and cost-effectiveness analysis. *N Engl J Med* 353(14):1516–22.
33. Kulasingam SL, Myers ER. 2003. Potential health and economic impact of adding a human papillomavirus vaccine to screening programs. *JAMA* 290(6):781–9.
34. ACIP. ACIP Record of the Proceedings June 25–26, 2008. http://www.cdc.gov/vaccines/recs/acip/meetings.htm: accessed September 5, 2008.
35. Gold MR, Patrick DL, Torrance GW, et al., Identifying and valuing outcomes. In Gold MR, Patrick DL, Torrance GW, et al., Eds. *Cost-effectiveness in health and medicine* Ch. 4, Oxford University Press. 1996.

10 Some Problems/ Assumptions in Pharmacoeconomic Analysis

Stuart Birks

CONTENTS

10.1 INTRODUCTION

Previous chapters have outlined three commonly used evaluation techniques, cost-benefit analysis (CBA), cost-effectiveness analysis (CEA), and cost-utility analysis (CUA). They are all used to assist in decision-making. It might be thought that this involves only undertaking the calculations and then applying a decision rule. For example, the simplest rule in CBA is to proceed in all cases where CBA gives a positive net present value. According to the criterion, this means that in each approved case benefits exceed costs, so a net gain to society is achieved. However, it may not be desirable to rely solely on such a decision rule. The rule can result in poor decisions when there are mutually exclusive alternatives.* In addition, there may be reservations about the distributional effects of the approach. These arise because gains and losses are simply added up to get a net present value. Some people may gain a lot, while others may lose. We may be concerned about the actual allocation of costs and benefits, rather than just their totals.†

Briefly, then, a purely mechanical approach may not be satisfactory. The technique and the decision rule may not always give the best answer. Also, in a democracy it might be considered important that the final decision be left to elected representatives. In other words, the actual process of policy making/decision-making may be important.‡ In recent decades an emphasis on "evidence-based policy" would suggest a mix of analysis and political input, with the former serving to inform the latter. While noting this point, this chapter will focus on some problems in analysis.

10.2   STEPS IN THE ANALYSIS

If intended for practical purposes, the role of analysis is generally to improve decision-making. For any resource allocation decision there may be many factors to consider. A decision rule approach requires that the mass of relevant information be somehow condensed into one number. Three steps are involved. First, the components in relation to the specific problem have to be identified and measured. This can be difficult, and will involve expertise beyond that commonly possessed by an economist. In other words, a cross-disciplinary approach is required. A health specialist may be aware of the relevant clinical dimensions associated with a treatment, and an economist should have an understanding of the economic dimensions. However, perhaps neither is well informed on the psychological and social factors

---

* Mutually exclusive alternatives occur when there is a specific resource that, if used on one project, is no longer available for others (hence there is an *opportunity cost* in terms of alternative options forgone). For example, a piece of land could be used for a hospital or a rest home, but not both. Even if both give positive net present value, only one of them can be undertaken. In this situation, it is suggested that the one with the highest net present value be chosen so as to achieve the greatest benefit for society.

† This is just one of several criticisms that can be raised about the approach. For a broadly based critical perspective on the application of neoclassical microeconomics to policy decisions see Chapter 14 of Hunt.[1] A more fundamental concern is the allocation of decision-making responsibility. At one extreme, decisions could be made according to a mechanical decision rule, either as above, or in a more involved form. At the other extreme, decision-makers could have full discretion in their choices. In a democracy, there are elected representatives entrusted to make decisions on people's behalf. It is to be hoped there is some reasoned basis for the decisions that they make, but they may be able to add insights that are not incorporated into mechanical approaches. They may be able to consider preferences, as with distributional aspects, or there may be specific local considerations not covered in general evaluations, for example. In practice, small, routine decisions are likely to be made according to established rules, whereas larger, one-off decisions are more commonly made by appointed/elected decision-makers.

‡ The current move by some academic economists into the growing area of "happiness research" indicates both recognition of our lack of understanding of this issue and acknowledgment of its possible importance.[3]

that may affect preferences and perceived costs and benefits.[*] The need for a mix of health and economic information is clearly described from the introduction to Dasbach, Elbasha, and Insinga,[4] and Goldie et al.[5] beginning with a reference to health, economic, and national policy perspectives.

Second, some or all of the selected components of costs and benefits will have to be valued. To the extent that the analysis is based on dollar values, market or other prices ("shadow prices") must be determined. Shadow prices are needed if there is no market for the item, or if it is considered that the market prices are misleading. Moreover, as some costs and benefits occur in the future, estimates will have to be made as to future prices, along with a mechanism for comparing values over time. Goldie et al. refer to the quality adjustment of life expectancy as a form of valuation.[5] For this to be the case, the basic unit of "currency" is a healthy year of life.

Third, some form of analysis will have to be undertaken to convert the information into the measures to which the decision rule can be applied. These might be net benefits, benefit:cost ratios, or cost per quality-adjusted life year (QALY), for example.

10.3   POTENTIAL PROBLEM AREAS

Techniques are applied at each step in the analysis. How useful are these techniques? Do we know that they will address the issues in such a way as to give the "right" answers, or are they simply commonly accepted methods? In other words, are they based on logic and proof, or rhetoric and persuasion? Ideas change over time. Methods applied and accepted in the past may be considered unsatisfactory now. Present approaches will almost certainly be thought questionable at some time in the future. To some degree, we are simply faced with a problem of having to make difficult decisions, so we rely on approaches that will hopefully give reasonable results most of the time. At worst, the techniques simply legitimize the decisions taken. A technique removes some of the responsibility from the decision-makers on the basis that they followed "best practice," rather than acting subjectively or according to personal prejudice. In this section, two broad aspects of analysis are considered. First we look at discounting, then consider the identification of preferences as a basis for measuring or valuing costs and benefits.

10.3.1   DISCOUNTING

Aggregation is the process of grouping together items and treating them as if they were the same. We aggregate diverse expenditures by using dollar values as a common measure. We give figures for the number of patients treated, even though individual treatments may vary. There is an assumption that all patients are the same.[†] Aggregation is central to the process of reaching one number on which to apply a decision rule.

---

[*] Tyler[2] describes the importance of **procedural justice**, suggesting that people are more willing to accept decisions, even those that are against their interests, if they believe that the processes followed were fair.

[†] Similarly, in Goldie's model, it is assumed that all persons residing in a particular health state are indistinguishable from one another.[5]

Frequently, we have to aggregate over time. When dollar values are used, it is commonly accepted that a dollar today is not equivalent to a dollar next year. At the very least, a dollar today could be set aside to earn interest, thereby having a value greater than one dollar by next year. For this and other reasons, it is widely accepted that, when aggregating monetary values over time, we should adjust for timing. Hence, we could compound the values to give some value in the future, taking into account the interest that could be earned. More commonly, we would follow this process in reverse, by discounting future values to give a measure of "present value."

At its simplest interpretation, given a sequence of payments over time, the present value of the sequence is the sum of money that, if held today, could be invested at the specified interest rate so as to allow the holder to just recreate the payments.* If I could earn 10% interest, then $100 today could turn into $110 in 1 year and $121 in 2 years. If I wanted to spend $100 this year, $110 next year and $121 the year after, then it would not matter if I were paid those sums at those times, or if I received $300 now. With $300 now, I could spend $100 now, while investing $100 for 1 year and $100 for 2 years. Alternatively, if I could also borrow at 10% interest and I wanted to spend $300 now, then it would not matter whether I received all $300 now, or three yearly payments of $100, $110, and $121. The nature of the required calculations is described in the appendix to this chapter.

In summary, *if it is possible to borrow or lend at the same rate of interest*, then it is possible to convert any pattern of payments and receipts over time into any other pattern so long as they both have the same present value (calculated by discounting at that rate of interest). The present value figure gives us all the information we need. Aggregation over time is acceptable because timing is not important.

10.3.1.1 What Discount Rate?

It is well recognized that streams of monetary values over time can be combined through discounting. The discussion above indicates one possible justification for this approach, subject to the assumption that borrowing and lending is possible at a rate of interest equal to the discount rate. It is an approximation for several reasons:

1. Borrowing and lending rates commonly differ.
2. There may be further distortions due to differing tax treatments of interest earned and paid. Interest income may be taxed, but it may be possible to offset against losses elsewhere. Interest payments may be made from after-tax income (as with home mortgages), or be considered as a deductible expense, as with mortgage interest on investment properties, thereby coming out of before-tax income.
3. Interest payments and receipts will be measured differently if considered from the point of view of individuals (concerned about the effect on them, and hence looking at the net-of-tax sums), or the government, or society, concerned about the overall effect from their perspectives.

---

* Other interpretations can apply when other discount rates are used. These are based on other reasons for having positive "time preference," whereby the present is valued more highly than the future.

4. Interest rates are also sensitive to inflation. Lenders commonly want higher interest when inflation is high. The extra interest is really a response to the falling purchasing power of the money they have lent. There is therefore a capital repayment component in the interest payment. Economists talk of nominal and real interest rates. Nominal rates are those actually charged or paid. Real rates are the percentages paid after adjusting for the distorting effects of inflation. As a simple example, if the nominal interest rate is 10% and inflation is 10%, then $100 lent for a year would give the lender $110 at the end of the year. This is just enough to buy what could have been bought with $100 at the start of the year, so the lender is no better off. The $10 interest is nothing more than a part of the repayment of capital, and the real interest rate is zero. Moreover, if tax on interest has to be considered, this means that inflation is causing a portion of the real capital to be taxed on repayment.

Prevailing interest rates are set through financial markets and are influenced by market demand and supply. It could be considered that this process fails to reflect society's preferences. For example, it is sometimes suggested that individuals, thinking of themselves, may have a shorter time horizon than society as a whole, which may be considering future generations. Placing a lower value on the future equates to discounting at a higher rate. It is therefore widely thought that the individual/private discount rate is too high, and that the social discount rate should be lower.

Goldie et al. adopt a societal perspective, discounting future costs and life years at an annual rate of 3%.[5] If we use a discount rate other than that at which we can borrow or lend, then our interpretation of discounting breaks down. It would not be possible to switch between any two payment streams of the same present value. Some other justification for ignoring timing would then be required.

An alternative interpretation might be that we are indifferent between the two streams, so timing is not important. This does cause a problem, however. If we are indifferent at the chosen discount rate, and we can borrow and lend at another rate, then we have an incentive to actively borrow or lend. Consider a social discount rate of 5% and a prevailing interest rate of 10%. Society would be indifferent between $100 now and $105 next year, but $100 now could earn interest and become $110 in a year's time. Society (or the government on society's behalf) has an incentive to defer $100 of spending now, so as to be able to spend $110 next year. If the rates are constant, it has an incentive to defer every $100 of spending now, and it could also defer every $110 of spending next year so as to be able to spend $121 the following year, and so on. In fact, if the social rate is lower than the market rate, it would make sense to defer all spending indefinitely.

More probably, the more current spending is curtailed, the greater the value that would be placed on an additional dollar of current spending, and the more future potential spending is increased, the lower the value seen in an additional dollar spent in the future.* The social and private rates would therefore move closer together. As we do not see major spending deferral, perhaps the difference in rates is very small. Alternatively, if the decision is political, then public decisions (including the choice of discount rate) may be shaped by the expression of individual preferences through the political process, or through politicians' placing emphasis on short-term political considerations.

10.3.1.2 First-Best and Second-Best Solutions

Economic analysis frequently aims to describe a "best" solution based on structures assumed in economic theory under conditions of perfect competition. These solutions have been referred to as "first-best" solutions. Perfect competition is seldom if ever observed in real world markets. First-best solutions may therefore not be the best for the real world. The optimal decision for the real world, recognizing the inevitable distortions from perfect competition, is called the second best. A classic article on the Theory of Second Best is Lipsey and Lancaster.[6] The points they raise are relevant here. The argument that future benefits would be undervalued in evaluations using standard discount rates should be considered in the context of the operation of the economy as a whole. Note that a common approach in economic theory is to make an implicit assumption that other parts of the economy are functioning properly. The undervaluing of future benefits is then the only distortion to consider. In other words, we could aim for a "first-best" solution. However, if there are distortions elsewhere that cannot be removed, then a first-best solution is not attainable. The problem then becomes far more complex.

In making the case for lower or zero discount rates for health benefits, it has been suggested that there would be underinvestment in health care if standard discount rates are used. However, a case could also be made that there is underinvestment in numerous private-sector areas. The argument goes as follows. Private-sector investors are aware that outcomes are uncertain. If an investment turns out badly, the costs to them can be severe. They are therefore likely to want a higher expected return to compensate them for the risks they face. This is called risk aversion. The outcome of numerous private investments from the perspective of society as a whole is far less uncertain. Some projects succeed, others fail, and there is some averaging out overall. From a social perspective, therefore, it is desirable for many individual risks to be ignored. Therefore, there are potential private-sector investments that are socially desirable, but are not undertaken due to risk aversion. The private sector is underinvesting. Health care investments and private-sector non-health care investments are competing against each other for limited funds. If lower requirements are set for health investments, more of them will be approved, further reducing (or "crowding out") other investment.

---

* This is an example of marginal analysis, which is widespread in economics. Additional costs and benefits are unlikely to be constant as quantities increase. This indicates a limitation of cost-effectiveness measures or cost:benefit ratios that, being ratios, conceal the scale of activity at which they were calculated. There is no reason to assume the same cost-effectiveness for a screening program reaching 70% of a target population and the same program reaching 90% of the population. As Goldie states, "screening is not equally accessible to all groups of women,"[5] and Dasbach describes Taira's finding of cost-effectiveness varying with coverage.[4]

This is a major problem in the application of theory. The world assumed by the theory is a simplification. There may be systematic distortions, such as the one above. These limit the practical value of the theory. At the same time, decisions have to be made on some basis. The term used to describe simplified approaches to decision-making is "heuristics." Perhaps, then, theory could be considered as giving an analytic basis for some heuristic approaches that we can and do use as a loose guide to our decision-making. They may be helpful, but they are approximations, and will not always give us the most appropriate answers.

10.3.2   DISCOUNTING NON-MONETARY UNITS

A clear distinction separating CEA and CUA from CBA is that the latter requires dollar values to be placed on all the costs and benefits that are considered. In contrast, CEA and CUA include non-monetary measures. As mentioned previously, one popular non-monetary measure in health economics is the QALY. Hence, CEA is often applied in terms of cost per QALY gained from treatments. For the purposes of illustration of non-monetary measures, the following discussion will consider just life years.[*]

The problem of discounting non-monetary units can be considered in two steps. First, is it meaningful to add up quantities and then undertake analyses in relation to the totals? Second, if the answer to the first question is yes, should we then adjust for the timing of the quantities by discounting (i.e., discounting at a non-zero rate)? The first question is important because it asks what meaning can be given to the units used. Discussion on discounting such units commonly focuses only on the second question, as if the question were solely one of deciding whether to discount at a non-zero rate, and, if so, what rate should be chosen.

10.3.2.1   Is it Meaningful to Add Up Quantities?

Consider the outcome of a treatment's being measured in terms of increased life expectancy, or life years gained. Is it meaningful to talk of total life years? It might be helpful to think of some other item, such as motor vehicles. Would we find it helpful to consider the number of motor vehicles produced in a year, or in a decade? Motor vehicles include motorcycles, cars, buses, trucks, and even motor boats. Even taking cars alone, there are numerous makes and models. The differences may be unimportant, but an annual data series showing motor vehicles by volume could look very different from a series by value, which can be affected by the types of vehicles produced. Nevertheless, volume figures are sometimes presented as an indication of output. What about volume figures for a decade? It would be rare for economists to refer to numbers such as these. They may be used for descriptive purposes, but are unlikely to be used for analysis, especially in relation to costs. Timing of production might be considered important, and costs over a decade would almost certainly be discounted. If we find it misleading with cars, would it not be equally misleading with life years?

---

[*] For a novel (and fictional) approach to placing a monetary value on life, see Johnson.[7]

There is a fundamental process involved when we are adding up in this way. Whenever we group items, whether quantities or values, we are aggregating, and are therefore at risk of encountering aggregation problems. These arise because aggregation can involve the loss of information, or misleading simplifications. The key requirement for aggregation is homogeneity of the components of the aggregate. When an aggregate variable (such as total output) is used in a specific analysis, a context is defined. This includes the variable's relationships with other variables (such as total cost). There is no loss of information if the relationships are identical for each component of the aggregate (such as each motor vehicle). Conversely, if the relationships differ, we are approximating (as with using an estimate of average cost).* Similarly, if we are using aggregate output when our real concern is with benefits, there is an implicit assumption that all units provide equal benefit.†

Hence, there are problems at the first stage. We are making implicit homogeneity assumptions as soon as we group life years in the context of a cost-effectiveness analysis.

10.3.2.2   What Do Discounted Quantities Mean?

Consider now the concept of discounting motor vehicle production as we might discount dollar values. With annual value of production figures, we could calculate their present value through discounting at an appropriate rate. So, instead of simply adding up motor vehicles, a volume measure, can we make some equivalent adjustment for the actual year in which the vehicles are produced? The result would not be in the same units as the undiscounted total. Just as we talk of present value, which is different from the sum of annual dollar values, we would have to talk of some unit such as "present motor vehicles." The production of 100,000 motor vehicles a year for 10 years would not give us one million motor vehicles. At a 10% discount rate it would equate to the production of 675,904 "present motor vehicles." Can we be comfortable with this concept? We do not use it when considering motor vehicles. Should we use it when considering life years? Instead of referring to a life expectancy at birth of 75 years, should we discount at 10% per annum and talk of a life expectancy of 11 "present years"?

There is a way this approach can be explained. It is not that we are avoiding valuing life years. Rather, without open acknowledgment, we are implicitly valuing them, but in another currency. The prices of all life years at the same time are assumed equal. This, in relation to quality-adjusted life years, has been encapsulated in the expression that a QALY is a QALY is a QALY (see, for example,[10]). If we think of it, this may not be something we are willing to accept. The position runs counter to that expressed in the "fair innings" viewpoint, which is based on the idea

---

* Birch (8) gives an example of the Simpson paradox, where one treatment appears better than another when considering a sample from a population as a whole, but the results are reversed when considering the population divided into two sub-groups, rich and poor, for which the effects differ.

† Aggregation of health state values is discussed in Brazier, Ratcliffe, Salomon, and Tsuchiya.[9] They assume that some form of aggregation is acceptable. Their focus is on the method of aggregation, questioning whether the mean or median response should be used. This indicates a further set of options to consider when constructing an aggregate.

that people who have already lived a certain amount of time have had fair innings, whereas younger people deserve more.[11*]

If life years are then discounted to calculate present life years, it is assumed that the implicit values of a life year change in a systematic way according to the timing. All that is missing from this approach for us to be able to go from present life years to dollars is an exchange rate.

The length-of-life issue raises another possible complication. What if the effects of a treatment for an individual can be felt over several years? The effects may well differ according to the age, and hence the life expectancy, of the patient. Consider, for example, a treatment with the simple effect that it prevents instant death, after which the individual can live as normal. This might give 10 years of life to a 75 year old, but closer to 60 years of life to a 25 year old. In other words, the effects of a treatment could depend not only on the treatment itself, but also on the types (or age groups) of individuals treated. Should treatments then be assessed in relation to each type separately? Even when assessed for one group, results may vary. For the analysis to produce a single figure, this uncertainty will have to be ignored.

10.3.2.3 What Discount Rate Should Be Used?[†,‡]

Much controversy exists about the choice of discount rates, and whether costs and benefits should be discounted at the same or different rates. In recognition of this, Drummond and Jefferson[13] suggest that sensitivity analyses be done using alternative discount rates, including zero. One reason that zero discount rates have been suggested in both the health and the environmental area is that the benefits are likely to be felt some time in the future, whereas many costs are incurred now. It has been argued that discounting at a positive rate counts against activities with more distant benefits. Discounting at a zero rate results in these benefits' being more prominent, and is therefore thought by some to be more desirable. The argument is flawed. It is claiming that the approach should be taken not because of some inherent validity in the reasoning, but because the results more closely reflect the advocates' wishes. However, a discount rate should not be chosen simply because it gives the result we want. There should be some stronger rationale. If the results are considered unacceptable when using an economically justified discount rate, then perhaps the problem lies elsewhere in the analysis. For example, perhaps we should consider the (explicit or implicit) values placed on the future benefits.

Those who want a lower or zero discount rate are really saying that the analysis is based on prices of future life years that are too low. A zero discount rate means that we should be prepared to set aside as much now to gain a future life year as we

---

* Considering fair innings, it may be paradoxical that people's preferences are used to estimate specific QALYs, but they are ignored when aggregating QALYs.

† This issue is discussed in detail in Chapter 7 of Gold, Siegel, Russell, and Weinstein.[12]

‡ Note that the question of choice of discount rate is generally posed in terms of a search for some constant rate to apply. Hence there is an implicit assumption that the rate does not vary over time.

are willing to spend for an extra life year this year. That same sum would grow over time, so more is effectively being allocated per life year in the future.*

If we treat discounting (including at a zero rate) as a means of condensing a series of life years over time into one number, we could apply the same test as for present value. If two series equate to the same total number of present life years, is it possible to convert from either series into the other? If so, then we could consider them equivalent, and the actual timing unimportant. Can we forego current life years in exchange for future life years, or vice versa? For individuals, this may be difficult, although there could be some scope for shifting quality of life from one year to another. For society as a whole, there is more flexibility. Nevertheless, the ability to shift may not match the discount rate being used for financial transactions.

Failing the ability to shift, would we be comfortable with an assumption that we (or society) are indifferent between the two series? One interpretation of discounting is based on "time preference," with the view that people value the present more highly than the future. For a person to be indifferent between two sums of money, one now and the other at some time in the future, it would generally be expected that the future sum would be larger (and, if discounted to the present, the discounted value would equal the sum available now). It is not clear that we would view years of life in the same way. First, mainstream economics assumes that people get utility from the consumption of goods and services. The more they consume overall, the greater their utility. Were it possible to simply suspend a year of life, so as to live it some time in the future, then it would also be possible to leave wealth to accumulate, enjoying the much larger sum at the later date. Given that possibility, a year of life in the future would be far preferable to a year of life now. Put more simply, if life will be so much better in the future, it is preferable to increase future life rather than life in the present (for individuals or for society as a whole).† This is the reverse of the monetary evaluation, one argument of which states that people will be better off in the future, so an additional dollar then would be valued less than an additional dollar now.‡ As a curiosity, Jeremy Bentham, the most prominent name associated with utilitarianism, is reported to have said that he would rather live the rest of his life 1 year per century.[16]

---

* When applied to the environment, the argument could be that future consequences of environmental damage are greater than currently commonly believed, and the costs of repairing the damage will rise if the problem is not addressed soon. However, logic aside, it may be politically easier and more persuasive to use the argument that discounting shows a lack of concern for the future, hence the call for a zero discount rate for environmental issues.

† This raises a fundamental issue. While there are attempts to limit world population growth, large sums are being spent on health care, including health care of the elderly. Analyses such as CBA and CEA are concerned with efficient use of resources, given specified objectives, focusing on costs and benefits for people who are alive. Future generations have only an indirect say in these decisions, to the extent that they are a factor influencing the preferences of the current population. Besides efficiency, we are also concerned about equity issues and perhaps broader aspects of an implicit social contract. For these, the distribution of costs and benefits is important. People's perceptions of the decision-making processes may also be important, as can be seen in literature on procedural justice (see third footnote).

‡ This is based on the concept of diminishing marginal utility. Note that the link between utility and wellbeing is more complex than assumed in current mainstream microeconomics. Earlier thinking on utility was not restricted to its being a function of goods and services (see [14]), and recent developments in the area of happiness research are also based on a broader view.[15]

In summary, there is no clear answer as to what discount rate should be chosen, or even if the aggregation and discounting process has any validity. At best, it could perhaps be argued by analogy that, if an approach is valid for monetary measures, then a similar method may suit non-monetary measures. A deeper investigation of the assumptions required for this raises serious concerns. An alternative approach could be to forgo the attempt to find a single number, presenting instead a broader range of information to assist decision-makers.*

10.3.3 MEASURING PREFERENCES

Mainstream economic theory includes the assumption that people's preferences are exogenous. In other words, they are taken as given, determined outside the theory. This is understandable, given the emphasis on static analysis and *ceteris paribus* assumptions in this body of theory. Static analysis does not consider adjustments over time, and at any one time, preferences are fixed. In addition, under the economic "ideal" of perfect competition, people are assumed to be perfectly informed. Even where imperfect information is assumed, it is interpreted as the information's being incomplete, rather than actually false, or misleading. This does not reflect the real world. In practice, issues are highlighted, opinions are shaped, people are persuaded to see things from particular perspectives, and understanding is influenced by experience, the media, and the attitudes of others.

10.3.3.1 Whose Preferences?

QALYs or other measures, including monetary valuations, are required for assessing outcomes or benefits, and sometimes costs, associated with interventions. Goldie et al. considered costs and clinical benefits, but recognized the need for data on patient and parent preferences.[5] There are not well-functioning markets for all the aspects that should be considered. Preferences must be deduced by other means. One approach is by asking people, as with stated-preference techniques.† Who should be asked, and how?

When considering the effects of a health care intervention, some studies ask health care professionals, others ask patients, and yet others ask the general public. These may give different answers. They have differing levels of understanding, their emotional commitments to the issues may differ, and they are taking different perspectives. Moreover, people's preferences may change according to their circumstances.‡,§

---

* This point has been made in Bos, Postma, and Annemans.[17]
† For a brief overview of stated preference techniques in health care evaluations, including discussion of problems and limitations, see Bridges.[18]
‡ A specific problem has been identified with patients' preferences, namely "peak" effects and "end" effects.[19] People's remembered perceptions are heavily influenced by the extremes (peaks) and by the situation at the end, as with pain that suddenly stops, compared with an equivalent pain that then gradually eases, with the former being considered worse.
§ An additional dimension is the extent to which findings from a study can be applied. Do they relate to that study sample alone, or are they more useful than that? In other words, there are issues of transferability and generalizability (Reference 20, Chapter 10).

When obtaining survey results, information is passed on to the participants. The results can depend on people's prior knowledge and the information given. In addition, views can change when people are responding in a communal situation where there has been some general discussion. It is not clear whether these changes are due to people's refining their views or adapting so as to appear to conform to the general view. This has been discussed in a health context,[21] also raising the point that individuals' valuations may differ depending on whether they are considering a personal or societal perspective. A similar point has been made in Richardson and Smith[22] on willingness to pay for a QALY. Group influence on expressed views has also been discussed in the broader context of deliberative democracy.[23]

Whereas markets provide a price (hopefully the equilibrium price), surveys give individual preferences. These must then be combined to get an overall figure. Utility theory and welfare economics stress that a person may be able to indicate a preference ordering, stating if A is preferred over B, but this is an ordinal measure. As such, it does not say by how much A is preferred, nor is it possible to compare the degree of one person's preference to that of someone else. For that, cardinal measures are required. Nevertheless, some method of aggregation is needed so as to combine individual preferences to obtain a measure for the evaluation. Wiseman[24] uses two alternative methods to show that the choice of method can affect the result. It is therefore not enough to know that preferences have been elicited.

These issues have been discussed in the health economics literature. Wider problems with preferences have been largely ignored by most of today's economists, but afforded a lot of attention in the literature on policy process, on the media, and on sociolinguistics and discourse analysis. It is to these that we now turn.

10.3.3.2 The Role of Process and Persuasion

While the following comments are raised in the context of pharmacoeconomics, they have a wider relevance in terms of economic approaches more generally, and in relation to public deliberation on policy issues.

Techniques are applied, and their results may have an impact on decisions that are made. Are the techniques legitimate? How much weight should be placed on the results? If they are accepted, is this because of the inherent merit of the studies, or is there just some tacit agreement to be persuaded by these analyses?

Adam Smith, sometimes referred to as the "father" of modern economics, gave a series of lectures on rhetoric in 1762 and 1763.[25] This was not remarkable at the time. Smith reflected a long tradition (dating back to classical Greece) where both logic and rhetoric were considered central to a good education. Briefly, we could consider logic to be concerned with proof, whereas rhetoric is concerned with persuasion. When describing the rhetoric of political debate, whereby policy decisions are made, Smith used the term "deliberative eloquence." People are not necessarily swayed by detailed, technical, logical arguments. It is more likely that they would be persuaded by simple points and rhetorical techniques such as humor, the use of analogy, or appeals to authority or to emotion.

While this perspective could be used to consider political debate, it has also been suggested that the same techniques may influence our understanding of economics. This point is discussed at length in a book called *The Rhetoric of Economics*.[26]

McCloskey considers the extent to which accepted economic findings do not have a firm basis in logic. There are numerous examples. Economic theory might conclude, within a narrowly defined theoretical framework, that competition is desirable. We cannot logically claim that this result applies in the real world without showing that the theory reflects the real world. Failing that, an acceptance of the view requires a leap of faith. We are persuaded, but not on the basis of logic.

Literature on the processes of policy making can also be seen to draw on the scholarship of rhetoric. Dunn,[27] for example, lists eleven "modes of argumentation." These are ways in which positions can be presented so as to persuade people to a particular viewpoint. Logic is not mentioned, and the presentation of logical arguments may not be very effective in comparison with other approaches—advertising and celebrity endorsement immediately come to mind. The results of studies may be convincing, although this is not necessarily related to the quality of the studies themselves.* Persuasive methods include "authority," the use of a source or personality that people trust, and "analogy," applying an approach in one context that people already accept in another (even though it may not, in fact, be suitable). Some of the techniques that analysts apply may have achieved acceptance on such grounds as well.

Literature on critical discourse analysis focuses on the use of selected words to emphasize a particular perspective, and on broader approaches to "frame" issues in desirable ways. Fairclough[29] refers to "ideological-discursive formations" that groups may use to define debate in a way that favors their perspective. Attitudes to health conditions may differ according to whether they are seen as resulting from individual behavior or as a consequence of social circumstances, for example.

Such analyses could be considered as "macro" approaches to rhetoric, as compared with traditional rhetoric, which is "micro" in focus, looking at individuals in debate.† Public perceptions and media presentation of issues will be heavily influenced by dominant terminology and frames. Considine[30] describes policy as the result of competition between groups, each trying to create the dominant perspective. In a similar vein, other literature emphasizes the setting of agendas.[31–33]

Public perceptions are shaped by the information that is transmitted in these processes. It might be hoped that debate in the media would result in an informed public. Bourdieu doubts this. He suggests that television favors people he terms "fast thinkers."[34] He does not mean that they actually think quickly. Rather, they are able to give quick answers that will be accepted. Far from thinking, they are simply tapping in to currently held beliefs, thereby getting instant audience acceptance and giving the appearance of being knowledgeable. His point could apply to much of the mass media. Consequently, dominant frames are emphasized, prior beliefs reinforced, and false perceptions perpetuated. This can have a significant impact on people's understanding of issues and priorities, at least those with which they have little or no direct personal experience.

---

* McCloskey[26] devotes much attention, in her book and elsewhere, to the distinction between statistical significance and economic or policy significance. She stresses that many refereed studies fail to note the difference, resulting in questionable policy conclusions. See also chapter 6 of Donaldson et al.[28]

† This is drawing on the economic distinction between microeconomics, looking at individual units or markets, and macroeconomics, which considers a broad-brush approach to the economy as a whole.

10.4   CONCLUDING COMMENTS

The title of this book indicates that the aim is to go from theory to practice. Terms used in several texts on economic evaluation in health are best practice, or the current convention. This is no mistake. Theory is not conclusive on the methods to be used. In fact, it could be argued that any approach taken is subject to valid criticisms. There is often a conflict between theory and practice. Analysts are charged with undertaking assessments and making policy recommendations. They cannot avoid the issues by saying that the data do not exist or the theories are deficient. In many cases, ad hoc or pragmatic approaches may be used, while theories are being developed in parallel or subsequently. In some areas of economics, theories have been developed in an attempt to find a rationale for existing analytical practices.[*]

Where theories are used, they could be questioned in terms of their own validity (given their assumptions), and in terms of their applicability in a particular situation. In relation to the latter, assumptions may be made as a basis for an approach, after which the conclusions could be treated as if they apply regardless of the assumption. This is a particular problem when assumptions are not explicitly stated, as with exogenous preferences. Debates on approaches also indicate that methods are sometimes chosen not on the basis of their legitimacy, but because they give the desired results. More generally, approaches may be chosen less on the basis of logic, and more on the basis of rhetoric or persuasion. They are plausible, or appealing.

This does not mean that analyses are necessarily giving wrong results. Rather, we cannot be sure that they will give the right results, or at least better answers than by some other means. However, we should at least acknowledge the limitations of our understanding.

APPENDIX

A.1   DISCOUNTING

Mathematically, discounting can be considered as follows:

Imagine investing \$X at a rate of interest, r, for one year, with the interest to be paid at the end of the year. You would get back your \$X, plus \$rX in interest, or \$(1+r)X in total. It has grown by a factor (1+r). In other words, on this basis \$1 now is equivalent to \$(1+r) next year and \$(1+r)^n in n years time. Consider this process in reverse. \$1 next year can be obtained by investing \$1/(1+r) now. We would say that the present value of \$1 next year, discounted at a rate, r, is \$1/(1+r).

If you were to invest \$X for additional years, the sum would increase by a factor of (1+r) each year. After 2 years you would have \$(1+r)^2 X, and after n years you would have \$(1+r)^n X. Considering this in reverse, \$1 in n years' time is equivalent to \$1/(1+r)^n now.

---

[*] Indicative planning is one example.[35]

We can apply this to a stream of dollar sums, X_0 to X_n, for years 0 (the present) to n. This would give us the present value (PV) of the sums of money. The formula would be:

$$PV = X_0 + (1/(1+r))X_1 + (1/(1+r)^2)X_2 + (1/(1+r)^3)X_3 + \ldots + (1/(1+r)^n)X_n$$

REFERENCES

1. Hunt EK. *History of economic thought: A critical perspective.* 2nd ed New York: HarperCollins. 1992.
2. Tyler T. 2000. Social justice: Outcome and procedure. *Int. J. Psychol.* 35(2):117–125.
3. Veenhoven R. World Database of Happiness, Erasmus University Rotterdam. http://worlddatabaseofhappiness.eur.nl/. Accessed May 28, 2009.
4. Dasbach EJ, Elbasha EH, Insinga RP. 2006. Mathematical models for predicting the epidemiologic and economic impact of vaccination against human papillomavirus infection and disease. *Epidemiol. Rev.* 28(1):88–100.
5. Goldie SJ, Kohli M, Grima D, et al. 2004. Projected clinical benefits and cost–effectiveness of a human papillomavirus 16/18 Vaccine. *J. Natl. Cancer Inst.* 96(8):604–615.
6. Lipsey RG, Lancaster K. 1956. The General Theory of Second Best. *Rev. Econ. Studies.* 24(1):11–32.
7. Johnson BS. *Christie Malry's own double-entry.* London: Picador. 2001.
8. Birch S. Making the problem fit the solution: Evidence-based decision-making and "Dolly" economics. In: Donaldson C, Mugford M, Vale L, Eds. *Evidence-based health economics: From effectiveness to efficiency in systematic review.* London: WileyBlackwell. 2002:133–147.
9. Brazier J, Ratcliffe J, Salomon JA, Tsuchiya A. *Measuring and valuing health benefits for economic evaluation.* Oxford: Oxford University Press. 2007.
10. National Institute for Clinical Excellence. (2004) Scientific and Social Value Judgements. Retrieved May 23, 2008, from http://www.nice.org.uk/nicemedia/pdf/boardmeeting/brdmay04item6.pdf.
11. Nord E. 2006. Severity of illness and priority setting: Worrisome lack of discussion of surprising finding. *J. Health Econ.* 25(1):170–172.
12. Gold MR, Siegel JE, Russell LB, Weinstein MC, Eds. *Cost-effectiveness in health and medicine.* New York: Oxford University Press. 1996.
13. Drummond MF, Jefferson TO. 1996. Guidelines for authors and peer reviewers of economic submissions to the BMJ. *British Medical Journal.* 313(7052):275–283.
14. Bentham J. *An introduction to the principles of morals and legislation* New York: Hafner. 1973.
15. Layard PRG. *Happiness: Lessons from a new science.* New York: Penguin Press. 2005.
16. Hazlitt W. *The spirit of the age, or, Contemporary portraits.* London: Oxford University Press. 1904.
17. Bos JM, Postma MJ, Annemans L. 2005. Discounting health effects in pharmacoeconomic evaluations: Current controversies. *Pharmacoeconomics.* 23(7):639–649.
18. Bridges JFP. 2003. Stated preference methods in health care evaluation: An emerging methodological paradigm in health economics. *Appl. Health Econ. Health Pol.* 2(4):213–224.
19. Oliver A. 2004. Should we maximise QALYs?: A debate with respect to peak-end evaluation. *Appl. Health Econ. Health Pol.* 3(2):61–66.

20. Glick HA, Doshi JA, Sonnad SS, Polsky D. *Economic evaluation in clinical trials.* Oxford: Oxford University Press. 2007. (Gray A, Briggs A, Eds. Handbooks in Health Economic Evaluation).

21. Akunne AF, Bridges JFP, Sanon M, Sauerborn R. 2006. Comparison of individual and group valuation of health state scenarios across communities in West Africa. *Appl. Health Econ. Health Pol.* 5(4):261–268.

22. Richardson J, Smith RD. 2004. Calculating society's willingness to pay for a QALY: Key questions for discussion. *Appl. Health Econ. Health Pol.* 3(3):125–126.

23. Ryfe DM. 2005. Does deliberative democracy work? *Ann. Rev. Polit. Sci.* 8(1):49–71.

24. Wiseman V. 2004. Aggregating public preferences for healthcare: Putting theory into practice. *Appl. Health Econ. Health Pol.* 3(3):171–179.

25. Smith A. *Lectures on rhetoric and belles lettres: Delivered in the University of Glasgow by Adam Smith, reported by a student in 1762–63.* London: Nelson. 1963.

26. McCloskey DN. *The rhetoric of economics.* 2nd ed Madison, WI: University of Wisconsin Press. 1998.

27. Dunn WN. *Public policy analysis: An introduction.* 3rd ed Upper Saddle River, NJ: Pearson Prentice Hall. 2004.

28. Donaldson C, Mugford M, Vale L, Eds. *Evidence-based health economics: From effectiveness to efficiency in systematic review.* London: WileyBlackwell. 2002.

29. Fairclough N. *Critical discourse analysis: The critical study of language.* London: Longman. 1995.

30. Considine M. *Making public policy: Institutions, actors, strategies.* Cambridge: Polity Press. 2005.

31. Cobb RW, Ross MH, Eds. *Cultural strategies of agenda denial: Avoidance, attack, and redefinition.* Lawrence, KS: University Press of Kansas. 1997.

32. Rochefort DA, Cobb RW, Eds. *The politics of problem definition: Shaping the policy agenda.* Lawrence, KS: University Press of Kansas. 1994.

33. Hilgartner S, Bosk CL. 1988. The rise and fall of social problems: A public arenas model. *Am. J. Sociol.* 94(1):53–78.

34. Bourdieu P. *On television.* Ferguson PP, Trans. New York: New Press. 1998.

35. Masse P. 1962. French Methods of Planning. *J. Indust. Econ.* 11(1):1–17.

11 Patient-Reported Outcome Measures

Dianne Bryant, Gordon Guyatt,
and Renée J.G. Arnold

CONTENTS

11.1 PATIENT-REPORTED OUTCOME MEASURES

A patient-reported outcome (PRO) is a direct subjective assessment by patients about aspects of their health, including symptoms, function, emotional well-being, quality of life, utility, and satisfaction with treatment. PROs ask patients to evaluate the impact and functional implications of the disease or treatment to reflect their interpretation of the experience, which is influenced by their internal standards, intrinsic values, and expectations. As such, PROs provide unique information that is unavailable from other sources.[1]

Direct measurement of health from the patient's perspective is an increasingly used outcome measure in clinical trial research. This phenomenon reflects a shift away from an exclusive emphasis on safety and efficacy, and from research that in the past focused narrowly on laboratory and clinical indicators of morbidity. Measuring patients' experience and the extent to which they can function in their daily activities is crucial when the primary objective of treatment is to improve how the patient is feeling. In fact, even when the goal of treatment is to reduce the incidence of seemingly straightforward outcomes like stroke or myocardial infarction, capturing the variability in patients' function and feelings will provide important complementary information if variability in the adverse morbid outcome varies in severity (e.g., a mild versus severe stroke).

11.2 HEALTH AND HEALTH MEASUREMENT

11.2.1 THE WORLD HEALTH ORGANIZATION

The World Health Organization (WHO) defines health as a state of complete physical, mental, and social well-being.[2] The WHO's International Classification of Functioning, Disability, and Health (ICF)[3] was developed to provide a standard language and framework to describe and measure health and health-related states. Within the ICF system, health outcomes are classified according to the effect upon body function, body structure, limitations in activities, and limitations in participation. Health outcomes that measure body function include measures of physiological functions of body systems (e.g., ejection fraction, glucose level, depression, pain, etc). Outcomes that measure body structures include measures of anatomical parts and their components (e.g., x-ray to measure fracture healing, computed tomography to measure tumor size, etc). Activity is defined as the performance of an action, whereas participation, more broadly, is defined as involvement in meaningful activities and fulfillment of roles that are socially or culturally expected of that person. Impairments are problems with body functions or structures. Having an impairment of a body structure (e.g., disc hernia) or function (e.g., reduced range of motion) may contribute to limitations in activities, including activities of daily living, walking, or driving a car, that might also contribute to restrictions in participation. Comprehensive assessment of an individual's health will include measures of body systems and function, as well as limitations in activities and participation.

11.2.2 HEALTH-RELATED QUALITY OF LIFE

Health-related quality of life (HRQoL) instruments measure the broad concept of health (physical, mental, and social well-being) by inquiring into the extent of difficulty with activities of daily living (including work, recreation, and household management) and how difficulties affect relationships with family, friends, and social groups, capturing not only the ability to function within these roles, but also the degree of satisfaction derived from doing them. HRQoL instruments often contain items that measure body function (e.g., pain, depression, anxiety) and limitations with activities and participation.

Within the construct of HRQoL, it is common to come across the terms *disease-specific* and *generic*. A disease-specific measure is tailored to inquire about specific aspects of health that are affected by the disease of interest (for example, specific to acne). In contrast, a generic instrument measures general health status, including physical symptoms, function, and emotional dimensions of health relevant to all health states, including healthy individuals.[4]

Disease-specific instruments are more responsive to small but important changes in health than are generic measures.[5] Because the items on a disease-specific HRQoL instrument are so focused on a particular disease, however, they cannot be used to compare the impact of one disease with another. In fact, in some cases, disease-specific measures are so specific that comparisons between different populations within the same disease are not possible (e.g., pediatric versus adult populations). On the other hand, generic HRQoL instruments are useful when measuring the impact of a specific illness or injury across different diseases, severities, and interventions.[4]

A number of previously widely used health profiles such as the Sickness Impact Profile (SIP)[6-11] and the Nottingham Health Profile (NHP)[12-16] are now of largely historical interest; health profiles developed from the Medical Outcomes Study, including the 36-Item Short-Form Health Survey (SF-36)[17-19] and 12-Item Short-Form Health Survey (SF-12)[20] have come to dominate the field of generic health status measurement.

11.2.3 ECONOMIC EVALUATION OF HEALTH

When making decisions on behalf of patient groups, decision-makers must weigh the benefits and risks of treatment, but must also consider whether the benefits are sufficient to merit the health care resources that must be spent to provide them. Limited societal resources necessitate that in order to add a program, society must forgo some other benefit—if the envelope for health spending is fixed, than another health program must be reduced. An economic analysis can inform these decisions. The primary distinction between this paradigm and HRQoL is the inclusion of explicit valuation of both resource consumption and patient-important benefit and harm.

Economic analyses include methods to evaluate different effects (death, effects of stroke on HRQoL, effect of reduction in acne on HRQoL) in the same metric. One way to create the same units is through the concept of preferences. Utilities and values are different types of preferences. Whether you are dealing with utilities or values depends on how questions on measurement instruments are framed; are participants being asked to consider outcomes that are certain (values) or uncertain (utilities)?

The Standard Gamble is the classical method of measuring utility, based directly on the axioms first presented by von Neumann and Morgenstern (utility theory) that describes how a rational individual "ought" to make decisions when faced with uncertainty.[21] During administration of the Standard Gamble, the participant suffering from a health problem, such as severe hip osteoarthritis (in reality or hypothetically), imagines that there is an intervention that will result in a return to perfect health but that there is a risk of death associated with the intervention. Participants are asked to specify the largest probability of death they would be willing to accept before declining the intervention and choosing to remain in their current (suboptimal) health state. The larger the probability of death that the subject is willing to accept, the lower value they place on their current health state. The utility of the present health state—as in all utility measures—is placed on a continuum between death (typically give a value of 0) and full health (typically given a value of 1.0).

For instance, let us assume an individual suffering from severe hip osteoarthritis would be indifferent between his or her current health state and the gamble when the probability of dying is 50%. This would mean that the utility the individual places on a year in this health state is 0.5, in contrast to a year in perfect health, which would be worth 1.0—hence the concept of the QALY (quality-adjusted life year).

The Time Trade-Off[22] is a measure of values. It asks participants to imagine living their lives in their current health states and to contrast this with the alternative of perfect health in exchange for a shorter lifespan (preference-based measured). The administrator provides alternatives of years of life in the present health state versus years of life in perfect health. The more years a subject is willing to sacrifice in exchange for a return to perfect health, the worse the subjects perceive their current health state (see Figure 11.1 for an example with human immunodeficiency virus [HIV]). Utility is calculated by subtracting the number of years sacrificed from the number of years of life remaining divided by the number of years remaining. The number of years remaining is estimated using actuarial tables. So, for instance, if an individual with 30 years of life remaining with severe hip osteoarthritis was ready to trade off 15 of those years to achieve 15 years in full health, the QALYs allocated to 1 year with arthritis would be 0.5.

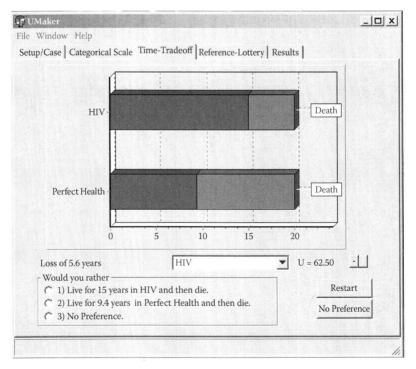

FIGURE 11.1 Time trade-off with HIV health states. Participants are asked to express their preference for living with HIV for 15 years and then dying or living in perfect health for an increasing number of years (less than 15 years) and then dying, until the point of indifference (no preference). Reproduced with permission from U–Maker (Sonnenberg).

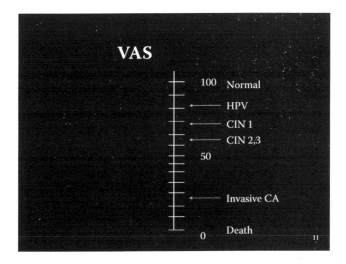

FIGURE 11.2   Visual analog scale.

Another common value-based measure is the Feeling Thermometer (FT). When completing the FT, participants rate their health status using a visual analog scale presented in the form of a thermometer from 0 (worst) to 100 (best)[23–25] (see Figure 11.2 for an example of a visual analog scale for human papillomavirus [HPV] health states).

Measuring preferences for health states using the Standard Gamble or Time Trade-Off is time consuming and can be complex. An alternative method is to use a pre-scored multi-attribute health status classification system. Some common systems include the Quality of Well-Being Scale,[26] Health Utilities Index (HUI),[27–30] European Quality of Life Scale (EQ-5D),[31] and Short Form 6D (SF-6D).[32–35] In general, patients are asked to rate their ability to function in physical, emotional, and social aspects of life, reporting on their health state rather than on their preference for different health states. The patient's preference is assigned on the basis of a mathematical model using preference ratings of health states that have been derived from a random sample of the general population.

11.3   MEASURING PATIENT SATISFACTION

Measurement of patient satisfaction is commonly used to evaluate treatment outcomes. Studies document that satisfied patients are more likely to comply with treatment protocols,[36,37] to use medical care services,[38,39] and to maintain a relationship with a specific provider.[40] Lack of clarity concerning the meaning of satisfaction has, however, been identified as a major weakness.[41–47] Patient ratings of satisfaction are generally directed at either the process of care or treatment outcome,[48] the latter of which is of most interest to clinicians.

Satisfaction may be best thought of as a construct, like health, that cannot be measured directly. Those who have investigated items that are important to patients in determining satisfaction have recommended going beyond inquiry about physical symptoms and function of the diseased body part to include items that probe satisfaction with resolution of social effects of the disease.[49,50] Some have suggested that patient expectations and experiences play a role in defining satisfaction, though the evidence is inconsistent.[51,52]

Experts in the field of measurement of patient satisfaction with treatment outcomes suggest that researchers should develop satisfaction instruments in much the same way they would approach the development of a new measure of quality of life, including the use of qualitative methods for item generation.[48,53] In consulting with the patients, the main objective should be to identify particular contexts in which the affected body part has different meanings, and tailor questions about satisfaction accordingly.

As with HRQoL, the challenge in developing an instrument to measure satisfaction is capturing the necessary content to appropriately measure the construct. In fact, several authors who have compared satisfaction ratings between measures on the same patients have found substantial differences.[54,55] To date, most existing instruments were developed from the perspective of the provider or institution and not the patient.

Like HRQoL, several types of satisfaction measures exist. For example, there are global ratings that contain one or two general questions about overall satisfaction, or multidimensional indexes that probe different aspects of satisfaction, including such things as emotions, desires, perceptions, and expectations.

One disadvantage of global ratings is that they do not capture what patients are considering when reporting their satisfaction. Because of this, global instruments are generally found to be unreliable and tend to be highly skewed.[43,55-57] As with HRQoL, there are also generic and disease-specific instruments to measure satisfaction. Generic instruments can be used to assess satisfaction in any population, whereas disease-specific scales are designed for use in specific patient populations. The pros and cons of generic versus disease-specific instruments are similar to those outlined in Section 11.2.2.

11.4 WHAT ARE THE PROPERTIES OF A GOOD MEASUREMENT INSTRUMENT?

The choice of instrument should align itself with the objectives of the clinician, researcher, or policy-maker. The intent may be to (1) discriminate between patients with different disease severity at a point in time (e.g., whose asthma is impairing function to a greater degree and who to a lesser degree), (2) to predict patient outcome (e.g., functional status may predict mortality in heart failure patients), or (3) to evaluate change following an intervention (e.g., which stroke patients have improved and which have not). To be useful for application in a research and clinical setting for the first two intentions, instruments must be valid (measure what they are supposed to measure—discriminative validity) and reliable (provide consistent ratings between repeated measures in a stable population). If the intention is to evaluate change following treatment, the instrument must be valid (longitudinal validity) and responsive (able to detect important change, even if the magnitude of the change is small).

11.4.1 Validity

An assessment of the validity of a new instrument is an evaluation of whether the instrument measures what was intended. Instruments with the greatest potential for validity will have, in choosing items, consulted with patients, and perhaps clinician experts or patients' family members who have experience with the disease to ask how the disease affects their lives.

One of the first steps in selecting an instrument is to review the items that make up the questionnaire. In some cases, the authors of an instrument will describe its content or include the instrument in an appendix (more common in online publications than in hard copy) so that clinicians can use their own experiences to decide whether what is being measured reflects what is important to patients (*face validity*) in a comprehensive way (*content validity*).

Readers or researchers can use several strategies to provide empirical evidence of the validity of the outcome measure. For example, they can investigate the *criterion validity* of the instrument, which is an assessment of whether the instrument behaves the way it should when compared with a gold standard measurement of the construct (e.g., the gold standard for virtual colonoscopy using imaging approaches is standard colonoscopy). Although measures of body function and structure are likely to have a gold standard reference, there is no gold standard for quality of life.

Construct validity assesses the extent to which the instrument relates to other measures of theoretical concepts (constructs) in the way that it should. Types of construct validity include convergent and discriminant validity. *Convergent validity* examines the degree to which interpretations of scores on the instrument being tested are similar to the interpretation of scores on other instruments that theoretically measure similar constructs. For example, we would expect that patients with poorer performance on a 6-minute walk test will have more dyspnea in daily life than those with better walk test scores, and we would expect to see substantial correlations between a new measure of emotional function and existing emotional function questionnaires.

Discriminant validity predicts weaker correlations with less closely related measures. For instance, one might expect a lower correlation between spirometry and daily dyspnea than between the walk test and daily function. To improve the strength of the inference, investigators pre-specify the magnitude of the correlation that is expected (e.g., no correlation $r<0.20$; weak $r>0.20$—0.35; moderate $r>0.35$—0.50; strong $r>0.50$). They would then administer multiple instruments (spirometry, walk test, other dyspnea questionnaires, global ratings of function) to a group of patients suffering from chronic obstructive pulmonary disease (COPD) to determine the agreement between predicted and observed correlations. The better the agreement between predicted and observed correlations, the stronger is the evidence for construct validity.

The appropriate way to design a study to investigate these types of validity for a discriminative instrument is by looking at the correlations between measures at a single point in time. Such correlations reflect an instrument's *cross-sectional construct validity*.

Conversely, the appropriate way to measure validity for evaluative instruments is by looking at the correlations in change over time between measures. For example, COPD patients who deteriorate in their six-minute walk test score should, in general, show increases in dyspnea, whereas those whose exercise capacity improves should experience less dyspnea; a new emotional function measure should show improvement in patients who improve on existing measures of emotional function. Such correlations reflect an instrument's *longitudinal construct validity*.

11.4.2 RELIABILITY

Reliability is defined as the extent to which an instrument is free from measurement (random) error. In practice, reliability refers to the extent to which an instrument discriminates between individuals in a population in a consistent manner when respondents are in stable health.

The mathematical relationship that defines reliability can be explained by the ratio of the variability in scores between patients to the total variability (i.e., between and within patient variability). Scores obtained on a reliable instrument will demonstrate relatively small differences between scores upon repeated administrations in patients who are stable in their condition (i.e., small within-person variability). Reliability will always appear to be greater when measured in a heterogeneous population with greater variability in scores between patients (e.g., includes patients with no limitations to those with severe limitations) than in a homogeneous population.

An instrument free of random error will have a reliability of 1.0 as long as there is some between-patient variability. As the amount of random error increases in relation to the between-patient variability, the measure of reliability will approach 0. Common expressions of the magnitude of reliability are *Kappa*, when the scale is categorical and *intraclass correlation coefficient* (ICC) when the scale is continuous. Several potential influences may affect the reliability of an instrument, including learning effects, regression to the mean, alterations in mood, circumstance and conditions of administration, and the length of time between assessments. It is also possible that real changes have occurred between consecutive assessments. The most important frequently neglected determinant of reliability is the variability in patient's status on the underlying attribute.

Different techniques to measure the reliability of an instrument include test-retest and inter-rater. *Test-retest reliability* is a measure of the magnitude of the agreement between ratings in repeated administrations of the instrument in a population with a stable health condition. There is no gold standard timeframe between subsequent administrations of the instrument; repeated administrations too close together face criticisms that high levels of agreement reflect patients' ability to remember previous responses, whereas administrations at large intervals run the risk of real changes having occurred within the sample of patients. In general, convention would suggest that any time from 1 to 4 weeks is appropriate, but this will be largely determined by the length of time that patients are expected to remain stable in their condition.

Inter-rater reliability is a measure of the magnitude of the agreement between ratings given by different raters administering the same instrument in a population with a stable health condition. The literature contains some discussion around study design for inter- and intra-rater reliability that suggests that the timing of ratings (e.g., time of day), by different raters, location, and patient position may influence agreement between raters.[58] Depending on the instrument, raters may be able to assess the same patient at fairly tight intervals whereas other outcomes may need to be measured on different days (e.g., measuring maximum strength that requires recovery time).

Internal consistency reliability is quite different from test-retest and inter-rater reliability, and measures the extent to which items in an instrument yield similar scores in the same patients on a single administration. The internal consistency reliability coefficient (R) is used to calculate the standard error of measurement (SEM), which provides an easily defined estimate of the reproducibility of individual measurements (SEM = $\sigma(1 - R)^{1/2}$) and can be used to determine whether true change has occurred within an individual ($\sqrt{2}$ x SEM).[59] Internal consistency is very limited as a measure of reliability because it relates only to the correlation between items on a single administration, and makes no attempt to assess the degree of variability on repeated administration of a measure.

11.4.3 SENSITIVITY TO CHANGE, RESPONSIVENESS, AND MINIMALLY IMPORTANT DIFFERENCE

Many people use the terms "sensitivity to change" and "responsiveness" interchangeably, but by some definitions there are important differences. Sensitivity to change has been defined as the ability of an instrument to measure true change in the state being measured regardless of whether it is relevant or meaningful to the patient or clinician.[60] In contrast, responsiveness has been defined as the ability of the instrument to detect change that is important to the patient in the state being measured even if that difference is small.[60,61] It follows that the minimally important difference (MID) is defined as the smallest difference in score in the outcome of interest that informed patients or informed proxies perceive as important, either beneficial or harmful, and that would lead the patient or clinician to consider a change in management.[62,63]

The magnitude of change that constitutes an MID for many objective outcomes may be intuitive to the clinician (changes in platelet count or serum creatinine). For most PRO measures however, the magnitude of change that constitutes an MID is not self-evident, creating difficulties with interpreting the results of studies that report changes in PRO. In studies that show no difference in HRQoL when patients receive a treatment versus a control intervention, clinicians should look for evidence that the instrument has been shown to be responsive to small or moderate-sized effects in a similar population in previous investigations. In the absence of this evidence, it is unknown whether the intervention was ineffective or whether the instrument was not responsive.

11.5 INTERPRETING THE RESULTS OF A STUDY THAT REPORTS PATIENT-REPORTED OUTCOMES

Physicians often have limited familiarity with methods of measuring how patients feel or their ability to do the things they need or want to do. At the same time, published articles recommend administering or withholding treatment on the basis of its impact on patients' well-being. Thus, if a measure is to be clinically useful, its scores must be interpretable. Interpretability is greatly enhanced if we know the magnitude of the change in score that is important—the MID.

Strategies to define important change have included distribution-based approaches and anchor-based approaches. In general, distribution-based approaches relate the magnitude of the effect to some measure of variability. For example, in a simple before–after comparison, one could calculate the difference between scores before and after treatment divided by the standard deviation of scores at baseline; the resultant statistic is coined the "effect size." In a parallel groups design, the effect size is generated by calculating the difference in scores between the treatment and control group divided by the standard deviation of the change that patients experienced during the study.

A rough rule of thumb for interpreting effects sizes is that changes of a magnitude of 0.2 represent small changes, 0.5 moderate changes, and 0.8 large changes.[64] Interpretation using effect sizes remains problematic because it is sensitive to the homogeneity of the distribution of the sample of patients who participated in the study (i.e., estimates of variability will vary from study to study). In other words, the same difference between treatment and control will appear as a large effect size if the sample is homogenous (patients are similar and thus there is a small between-patient variability, which defines the standard deviation) and as a small effect size if the sample is heterogeneous (patients are dissimilar and thus there is large between-patient variability).

On the other hand, anchor-based approaches involve comparing the magnitude of the change observed on a PRO to an anchor or independent standard that is itself interpretable. The anchor may be defined by achieving change on some external criteria, for example, changing category increasing on a well-known classification system for disease or functional severity (e.g., moving from New York Heart Association Functional Classification III to II) or moving in or out of a diagnostic category (e.g., from depressed to non-depressed, or the reverse).

Another common anchor-based approach, the global rating of change, follows patients longitudinally and asks them to report whether they got better, stayed the same, or got worse. If better or worse, patients rate how much change has occurred—for example, they may rate the degree of change from 1 (minimal change) to 7 (a very large change), where 1 to 3 indicates a small but important change. In the most common way of using this approach, the investigators estimate the MID as the average of the change scores on the PRO that corresponds to a small but important change (that is, the average change in patients who have rated themselves as 1 to 3 on the degree of change rating).

11.6   EXAMPLE OF USE OF HRQOL IN HPV
DECISION-ANALYTIC MODELING

Goldie and colleagues[65] used age-specific quality weights for non-cancer states (range from 0.92 in women aged 25–34 years to 0.74 in women older than 85 years) based on data from the Health Utilities Index (Mark II Scoring System) and quality weights for the time spent in cancer health states (range 0.65 for Stage I to 0.48 for Stage IV invasive cervical cancer) from utility estimates by the Institute of Medicine's Committee to Study Priorities for Vaccine Development. These weights were then multiplied by the time spent in the health state and then summed to calculate the number of QALYs in the cost-effectiveness model (see Chapter 9 on use of utilities in HPV modeling).

11.7   SUMMARY

Patient-reported outcome measures provide information gathered directly from the patients about their experiences with the disease and its treatment. Because of the unique perspective offered by patient-reported instruments, direct measurement of health from the patient's perspective is popular and has replaced more objective measures as the primary outcome of interest for a broad spectrum of clinical conditions. For the purpose of evaluating studies that include patient-reported outcomes, it is important to understand the fundamentals of reliability, validity, and responsiveness of the outcome measure being used in addition to appraising the validity of the study. To make wise management decisions, patients and clinicians need to know the magnitude of the effect of treatments on a variety of outcomes, including patient-reported outcomes. Investigators must choose an informative method to present their findings to enhance the interpretability and applicability of their results in a clinical setting.

REFERENCES

1. Rothman ML, Beltran P, Cappelleri JC, Lipscomb J, Teschendorf B. 2007. Mayo/FDA Patient-Reported Outcomes Consensus Meeting Group. Patient-reported outcomes: Conceptual issues. *Value in Health* 10 (Nov–Dec)(Suppl 2):S66–75.
2. Preamble to the Constitution of the World Health Organization as adopted by the International Health Conference. Official Records of the World Health Organization, no. 2, p. 100 and entered into force on 7 April 1948 19–22 June, 1946. signed on 22 July 1946 by the representatives of 61 States. New York.
3. World Health Organization. Towards a common language for functioning, disability, and health: ICF The International Classification of Impairment, Disability, and Health. Geneva: World Health Organization. 2002. Report No: WHO/EIP/GPE/CAS/01.3.
4. Jackowski D, Guyatt G. 2003. A guide to health measurement. *Clin Ortho Related Res* 413:80–9.
5. Wiebe S, Guyatt G, Weaver B, Matijevic S, Sidwell C. 2003. Comparative responsiveness of generic and specific quality-of-life instruments. *J Clin Epidemiol* 56 (1):52–60.
6. Bergner M, Bobbitt RA, Carter WB, Gilson BS. 1981. The sickness impact profile: Development and final revision of a health status measure. *Med Care* 19(8):787–805.

7. Bergner M, Bobbitt RA, Kressel S, Pollard WE, Gilson BS, Morris JR. 1976. The sickness impact profile: Conceptual formulation and methodology for the development of a health status measure. *Int J Health Serv* 6(3):393–415.

8. Bergner M, Bobbitt RA, Pollard WE, Martin DP, Gilson BS. 1976. The sickness impact profile: Validation of a health status measure. *Med Care* 14(1):57–67.

9. de Bruin AF, Buys M, de Witte LP, Diederiks JP. 1994. The sickness impact profile: SIP68, a short generic version. First evaluation of the reliability and reproducibility. *J Clin Epidemiol* 47(8):863–71.

10. de Bruin AF, Diederiks JP, de Witte LP, Stevens FC, Philipsen H. 1997. Assessing the responsiveness of a functional status measure: The sickness impact profile versus the SIP68. [Review] [38 refs]. *J Clin Epidemiol* 50(5):529–40.

11. de Bruin AF, Diederiks JP, de Witte LP, Stevens FC, Philipsen H. 1994. The development of a short generic version of the sickness impact profile. *J Clin Epidemiol* 47(4):407–18.

12. Hunt SM, McEwen J. 1980. The development of a subjective health indicator. [Review] [62 refs]. *Sociol Health Illn* 2(3):231–46.

13. Hunt SM, McKenna SP, McEwen J, Backett EM, Williams J, Papp E. 1980. A quantitative approach to perceived health status: A validation study. *J Epidemiol Commun Health* 34(4):281–6.

14. Hunt SM, McEwen J, McKenna SP. 1985. Measuring health status: A new tool for clinicians and epidemiologists. *J R Coll Gen Pract* 35(273):185–8.

15. Hunt SM, McKenna SP, McEwen J, Williams J, Papp E. 1981. The Nottingham health profile: Subjective health status and medical consultations. *Soc Sci Med [A]* 15(3 Pt 1):221–9.

16. Hunt SM, McKenna SP, Williams J. 1981. Reliability of a population survey tool for measuring perceived health problems: A study of patients with osteoarthrosis. *J Epidemiol Commun Health* 35(4):297–300.

17. McHorney CA, Ware JE, Jr, Raczek AE. 1993. The MOS 36-item short-form health survey (SF-36): II. Psychometric and clinical tests of validity in measuring physical and mental health constructs. *Med Care* 31(3):247–63.

18. McHorney CA, Ware JE, Jr, Lu JF, Sherbourne CD. 1994. The MOS 36-item short-form health survey (SF-36): III. Tests of data quality, scaling assumptions, and reliability across diverse patient groups. *Med Care* 32(1):40–66.

19. Ware JE, Jr, Sherbourne CD. 1992. The MOS 36-item short-form health survey (SF-36). I. Conceptual framework and item selection. *Med Care* 30(6):473–83.

20. Ware J, Jr, Kosinski M, Keller SD. 1996. A 12-item short-form health survey: Construction of scales and preliminary tests of reliability and validity. *Med Care* 34(3):220–33.

21. Von Neumann J, Morgenstern O. *Theory of Games and Economic Behaviour.* Princeton, NJ: Princeton University Press. 1944.

22. Torrance GW, Thomas WH, Sackett DL. 1972. A utility maximization model for evaluation of health care programs. *Health Serv Res* 7(2):118–33.

23. Schunemann HJ, Griffith L, Jaeschke R, Goldstein R, Stubbing D, Guyatt GH. 2003. Evaluation of the minimal important difference for the feeling thermometer and the St. George's respiratory questionnaire in patients with chronic airflow obstruction. *J Clin Epidemiol* 56(12):1170–6.

24. Schunemann HJ, Griffith L, Stubbing D, Goldstein R, Guyatt GH. 2003. A clinical trial to evaluate the measurement properties of 2 direct preference instruments administered with and without hypothetical marker states. *Med Decision Making* 23(2):140–9.

25. Puhan MA, Guyatt GH, Montori VM, Bhandari M, Devereaux PJ, Griffith L, et al. 2005. The standard gamble demonstrated lower reliability than the feeling thermometer. *J Clin Epidemiol* 58(5):458–65.

26. Kaplan RM, Anderson JP. The quality of well–being scale! Rationale for a single quality of life index. In: Walkee SR, Rosser R, Eds. *Quality of Life: Assessment and Application.* London: MTP Press. 1988. p. 51–77.

27. Torrance GW, Feeny DH, Furlong WJ, Barr RD, Zhang Y, Wang Q. 1996. Multiattribute utility function for a comprehensive health status classification system. Health utilities index mark 2. *Med Care* 34(7):702–22.

28. Boyle MH, Furlong W, Feeny D, Torrance GW, Hatcher J. 1995. Reliability of the health utilities index—mark III used in the 1991 cycle 6 Canadian general social survey health questionnaire. *Qual Life Res* 4(3):249–57.

29. Feeny D, Furlong W, Boyle M, Torrance GW. 1995. Multi-attribute health status classification systems. Health Utilities Index. [Review] [58 refs]. *Pharmacoeconomics* 7(6):490–502.

30. Torrance GW, Furlong W, Feeny D, Boyle M. 1995. Multi-attribute preference functions. Health utilities index. [Review] [83 refs]. *Pharmacoeconomics* 7(6):503–20.

31. EuroQol—a new facility for the measurement of health-related quality of life. The EuroQol Group. *Health Policy* 16(3) 1990: 199–208.

32. Brazier J, Roberts J, Deverill M. 2002. The estimation of a preference-based measure of health from the SF–36. *J Health Econ* 21(2):271–92.

33. Brazier J, Roberts J, Tsuchiya A, Busschbach J. 2004. A comparison of the EQ-5D and SF-6D across seven patient groups. *Health Econ* 13(9):873–84.

34. Tsuchiya A, Brazier J, Roberts J. 2006. Comparison of valuation methods used to generate the EQ-5D and the SF-6D value sets. *J Health Econ* 25(2):334–46.

35. Kharroubi SA, Brazier JE, Roberts J, O'Hagan A. 2007. Modeling SF-6D health state preference data using a nonparametric Bayesian method. *J Health Econ* 26(3):597–612.

36. Raper J, Davis BA, Scott L. 1999. Patient satisfaction with emergency department triage nursing care: A multicenter study. *J Nurs Care Qual* 13(6):11–24.

37. Thomas JW, Penchansky R. 1984. Relating satisfaction with access to utilization of services. *Med Care* 22(6):553–68.

38. Lee Y, Kasper JD. 1998. Assessment of medical care by elderly people: General satisfaction and physician quality. *Health Serv Res* 32(6):741–58.

39. Marquis MS, Davies AR, Ware JE, Jr. 1983. Patient satisfaction and change in medical care provider: A longitudinal study. *Med Care* 21(8):821–9.

40. Wartman SA, Morlock LL, Malitz FE, Palm EA. 1983. Patient understanding and satisfaction as predictors of compliance. *Med Care* 21(9):886–91.

41. Abramowitz S, Cote AA, Berry E. 1987. Analyzing patient satisfaction: A multianalytic approach. *Qrb Qual Rev Bull* 13(4):122–30.

42. Fitzpatrick R, Hopkins A. 1983. Problems in the conceptual framework of patient satisfaction research: An empirical exploration. *Sociol Health Illn* 5(3):297–311.

43. Locker D, Dunt D. 1978. Theoretical and methodological issues in sociological studies of consumer satisfaction with medical care. *Soc Sci Med* 12(4A):283–92.

44. Sitzia J, Wood N. 1997. Patient satisfaction: A review of issues and concepts. *Soc Sci Med* 45(12):1829–43.

45. Williams B. 1994.Patient satisfaction: A valid concept?. *Soc Sci Med* 38(4):509–16.

46. Williams B, Coyle J, Healy D. 1998. The meaning of patient satisfaction: An explanation of high reported levels. *Soc Sci Med* 47(9):1351–9.

47. Hudak PL, McKeever PD, Wright JG. 2004. Understanding the meaning of satisfaction with treatment outcome. *Med Care* 42(8):718–25.

48. Hudak PL, Wright JG. 2000. The characteristics of patient satisfaction measures. *Spine* 25(24):3167–77.

49. Hudak PL, McKeever P, Wright JG. 2007. Unstable embodiments: A phenomenological interpretation of patient satisfaction with treatment outcome. *J Med Humanit* 28(1):31–44.

50. Hudak PL, Hogg-Johnson S, Bombardier C, McKeever PD, Wright JG. 2004. Testing a new theory of patient satisfaction with treatment outcome. *Med Care* 42(8):726–39.
51. Linder-Pelz S. 1982. Social psychological determinants of patient satisfaction: A test of five hypothesis. *Soc Sci Med* 16(5):583–9.
52. Kane RL, Maciejewski M, Finch M. 1997. The relationship of patient satisfaction with care and clinical outcomes. *Med Care* 35(7):714–30.
53. Lynn MR, McMillen BJ. 2004. The scale product technique as a means of enhancing the measurement of patient satisfaction. *Can J Nursing Res* 36(3):66–81.
54. Ross CK, Steward CA, Sinacore JM. 1995. A comparative study of seven measures of patient satisfaction. *Med Care* 33(4):392–406.
55. Ware JE, Jr. 1978. Effects of acquiescent response set on patient satisfaction ratings. *Med Care* 16(4):327–36.
56. Blais R. 1990. Assessing patient satisfaction with health care: Did you drop something? *Can J Prog Eval* 5:1–13.
57. A guide to direct measures of patient satisfaction in clinical practice. Health services research group. *CMAJ* 146(10) 1992:1727–31.
58. Hays RD, Anderson RT, Revicki D. Assessing the reliability and validity of measurement in clinical trials. In: Staquet MJ, Hays RD, Fayers PM, Eds. *Quality of life assessment in clinical trials: Methods and practice*. Oxford: Oxford University Press. 1998. p. 169.
59. Stratford PW, Goldsmith CH. 1997. Use of the standard error as a reliability index of interest: An applied example using elbow flexor strength data. *Phys Ther* 77:745–50.
60. Liang MH. 2000. Longitudinal construct validity: Establishment of clinical meaning in patient evaluative instruments. [see comment]. [Review] [37 refs]. *Med Care* 38(9 Suppl):84–90.
61. Kirshner B, Guyatt G. 1985. A methodological framework for assessing health indices. *J Chronic Dis* 38(1):27–36.
62. Schunemann HJ, Puhan M, Goldstein R, Jaeschke R, Guyatt GH. 2005. Measurement properties and interpretability of the chronic respiratory disease questionnaire (CRQ). *COPD: J Chronic Obstruct Pulmon Dis* 2(1):81–9.
63. Schunemann HJ, Guyatt GH. 2005. Commentary—goodbye M(C)ID! Hello MID, where do you come from? comment. *Health Serv Res* 40(2):593–7.
64. Cohen J. *Statistical power analysis for the behavioral sciences*. 2nd ed. Hillsdale, NJ.: Lawrence Erlbaum Associates. 1988.
65. Goldie SJ, Kohli M, Grima D, et al. 2004. Projected clinical benefits and cost-effectiveness of a human papillomavirus 16/18 vaccine. *J Natl Cancer Inst* 96(8):604–15.

12 Sensitivity Analysis

Maarten J. Postma

CONTENTS

12.1 INTRODUCTION

With the widespread use of modeling in pharmacoeconomics, sensitivity analysis has become an important tool for investigating the models being developed and used. In this respect, modeling is conceived as the simulation of complex systems in reality. In particular, a model can be defined as a simplification of such complex relationships, as simple as possible, yet reflecting all relevant aspects of reality. We know that such a model has to be both internally and externally valid, but, in addition, it is important to know its properties regarding the changes in the outcomes in relation to changes in the inputs or parameters. The set of parameters reflects those characteristics of reality that were deemed relevant for simulating the specific realities of interest. The latter may be the costs, savings, and health gains of a specific therapeutic treatment. The parameters may be concerning epidemiology, progression of disease, and unit costs. The generic investigation of these changes in the outcomes in relation to changes in the input parameters is generally labeled sensitivity analysis (SA).

This chapter deals with SA of models in all of its dimensions. The role envisaged for SA will be discussed by considering the pharmacoeconomic (PE) guidelines throughout the world. Most country-specific guidelines do specify a particular role of SA for judging the appropriateness of models and for selecting those analyses that reflect state-of-the-art PE analysis. Relevance of such PE guidelines is high as, often, reimbursement filings for new drugs must adhere to these and might be denied if this is not the case. Indeed, in the Netherlands, Gardasil® (4-valent human papillomavirus vaccine) has been denied reimbursement within the reference pricing system for individual use due to an inadequate PE reimbursement file (www.cvz.nl). In particular, absence of full and adequate SA on all parameters considered relevant was the primary critique.

After discussing the PE guidelines around the world, this chapter will focus on the terminology surrounding SA. All types will be formally defined and illustrated, often using recent work on the human papillomavirus (HPV) vaccine. Next to the different types of SA, scenario analysis will be discussed as yet another technique that is sometimes seen as part of SA, that, however, does exhibit its own specific features, warranting separate consideration and explicit distinguishing from SA.

12.2   PE GUIDELINES AROUND THE WORLD

Various countries around the world have now specified PE guidelines on how to perform a state-of-the-art and good-practice PE analysis. Often, these PE guidelines are formally required for drug reimbursement files submitted by manufacturers to local and national authorities—for example, to have a new drug admitted to reference pricing systems. The International Society for Pharmacoeconomics & Outcomes Research (ISPOR) has summarized the PE guidelines for those countries that have them available. Table 12.1 shows country-specific guidelines referring to SA, both regarding ranges and values for parameters to be investigated and regarding exact methods to be used (Table 12.1 is directly taken from the website www.ispor.org, by selecting countries and individual guidelines). Notably, some countries that do have PE guidelines lack specific ones for SA. In particular, this was the case for Australia, Denmark, Israel, Russia, Taiwan, and South Korea. All other countries included in ISPOR's overview do specify formal requirements for SA.

From Table 12.1 it follows that PE guidelines often require that SA be undertaken "for key (uncertain) variables over plausible ranges or 95% confidence intervals for parameter values if available." Regarding the techniques, all types are generally advised:

- One-way or univariate SA, in which one (key/uncertain) parameter is varied at a time
- Two-way or bivariate SA, if two parameters are both varied at the same time
- Multivariate SA, if multiple parameters (notably more than two) are varied at the same time
- Best-case analysis, reflecting a specific type of multivariate SA in which all parameters are set at those values in the pre-specified ranges to render the most favorable cost-effectiveness ratio
- Worst-case analysis, reflecting a specific type of multivariate SA in which all parameters are set at those values in the pre-specified ranges to render the most unfavorable cost-effectiveness ratio
- Probabilistic SA, also referred to as Monte Carlo analysis, reflecting the most comprehensive type of analysis in which, for all key and uncertain parameters, probability distributions are specified and multiple simulations are performed

Now that we have noted its importance, illustrated by the inclusion of specific requirements for SA in PE guidelines, the different types of SA will be discussed in the next sections, in many cases illustrated by recent work on the HPV vaccine published in a supplement of the journal *Vaccine*.[1]

TABLE 12.1
Country-Specific Pharmacoeconomic Guidelines on Sensitivity Analysis: Parameters and Value Ranges to be Investigated and Methods to be Used (Univariate or One-Way, Bivariate or Two-Way, Multivariate and Probabilistic Sensitivity Analysis)

Country	Sensitivity Analysis—Parameters and Range	Sensitivity Analysis—Methods
Austria	All key uncertain parameters, within a defined area, or probabilistic	One-way, multi-way, may be probabilistic analysis
Baltic	Main assumption variables, confidence interval	Details of the statistical tests performed
Belgium	Interval estimates should be presented for each parameter in the economic evaluation. All different aspects of uncertainty in the evaluation should be addressed. Confidence interval around the ICER; Cost-effectiveness plane; cost-effectiveness acceptability curve; Tornado diagrams.	Probabilistic sensitivity analyses should be performed on all uncertain parameters in a model.
Brazil and Cuba	For all uncertain parameters, a plausible range must be defined for each parameter	One-way, multi-way, probabilistic analysis when adequate
Canada	Capture the full range of variability or uncertainty that is relevant for each model input.	One-way, two-way, multi-way, scenario analysis, Monte Carlo simulation
China	All key uncertain parameters, within a defined area, or best/worst case scenario	One-way, multi-way, may be probabilistic analysis Details be given of the statistical tests performed
Finland	On uncertain parameters at credible range	Not specific
France	Maintain uncertain variables.	A distinction is made between univariate and multivariate analysis, and also between first order and second order analysis.
Germany	The individual input parameters are varied within a range, which may be based on realistic considerations or a schematic variation. Details are given in the guideline.	A probabilistic analysis or a different multivariate approach. Details are given in the guideline.
Hungary	On uncertain parameters.	One-way, two–way.
Ireland	Justify the choice of variables and ranges used.	Details be given of the statistical tests performed
Italy	Those parameters which have the most influence on the final results. Effectiveness use CI, range of cost decided by author.	Better showing simultaneous effect of the variations for the more important parameters

Continued

TABLE 12.1 (Continued)
Country-Specific Pharmacoeconomic Guidelines on Sensitivity Analysis: Parameters and Value Ranges to be Investigated and Methods to be Used (Univariate or One-Way, Bivariate or Two-Way, Multivariate and Probabilistic Sensitivity Analysis)

Country	Sensitivity Analysis—Parameters and Range	Sensitivity Analysis—Methods
New Zealand	All assumptions should be subject to SA.	Univariate, Multivariate (best and worst case estimate),
Norway	All key uncertain parameters, within a defined area, or best/worst case scenario	One-way, multi-way, probabilistic SA.
Poland	On uncertain parameters at credible range.	One-way, multi-way, may be probabilistic analysis
Portugal	Key uncertain parameters. For population data, use CI; others, justified intervals used in detail on the basis of empirical evidence.	Not specific
Scotland	Present the associated 95%CI.	Prefer probabilistic SA (Monte Carlo simulation or Bayesian approach)
Spain	Uncertain parameters, using ± 2 SD, or favorable and unfavorable extreme values	Not specific
Sweden	At central assumptions and parameters	Not specific
Switzerland	The variation range accepted for key parameters should be plausible	The sensitivity of study conclusions should be examined in detail.
The Netherlands	All key uncertain parameters, within a defined area and best/worst case scenario	One-way, multi-way and probabilistic analysis
UK (England and Wales)	All inputs used in the analysis will be estimated with a degree of impression. The most appropriate ways of presenting uncertainty are confidence ellipses and scatter plots on the cost-effectiveness plane and cost-effectiveness acceptability curves.	Probabilistic SA.
United States	All uncertain parameters, high/low value, best/worst scenario, 95% CI, variable distribution.	At a minimum, univariate SA should be undertaken and for important parameters, multivariate SA. Where parameter uncertainty is a major concern, simulation should be undertaken.

12.3   SENSITIVITY ANALYSIS

SA is often explicitly differentiated from the so-called "base-case analysis."[2] In the base case, parameter values are all set at their most likely values. Base-case parameter values result in the base-case estimate for the ratio, typically representing a point estimate. For example, in their analysis on multiregional health-economic outcomes of HPV vaccination, Rogoza et al. estimated base-case cost-effectiveness of HPV vaccination at 12 years of age at €22,672 per life-year gained (€18,472 per QALY) and £21,962 per life-year gained (£18,037 per QALY) for the Netherlands and the United Kingdom, respectively (Table 12.2).[3]

Also, it is often argued that parameter values should be set conservatively in the base case if uncertainty is high and specification of most-likely values is difficult. For example, for the HPV vaccine, exact full duration of protection is obviously not yet known, given the current maximum length of clinical trials at around 6 years. It could, thus, be argued that base-case analyses on the cost-effectiveness of the HPV vaccine should not use durations of protection beyond 6 years, let alone lifelong protection, despite the knowledge that protection is still high after 6 years and is not likely to wane within the next few years. Alternatively, a most likely and probably still conservative period of 10 years could be used.

Table 12.2 classically presents point estimates for cost-effectiveness. Obviously, this is not the only information that we want; base-case numbers alone do not provide us with all of the information required for full insight into decision-making regarding, for example, reimbursement of the HPV vaccine. SA typically adds crucial information to the base-case analysis: it shows (1) how a plausible range for uncertain key parameters translates into ranges for cost-effectiveness rather than point estimates only; and (2) how changes in the input parameters affect the cost-effectiveness outcomes.

12.3.1   DETERMINISTIC SA

All SA, except for probabilistic SA, is sometimes labeled as deterministic. In uni-, bi-, and multivariate SA, generally, probabilities, rather than full density functions (often represented as histograms of probability distributions of continuous random variables), are applied. In fact, predefined inputs for parameter values are entered into the PE model and outcomes for these inputs are listed. If all key parameters are varied one-by-one using such predefined ranges (for example, plus and minus 20% of base-case values) the SA is univariate or one-way. One-way SA is often represented using Tornado diagrams. Figure 12.1 shows an example of a Tornado diagram for an analysis of HPV vaccination—again of teenage girls—in this case for Ireland. The figure is taken from Suárez et al. in a specific multiregional analysis on HPV vaccine cost-effectiveness, with specific focus on vaccine characteristics and alternative vaccination assumptions and scenarios.[4] As such, the paper uses SA as an instrument to investigate impacts of alternative characteristics and assumptions. It clearly shows that the price of the vaccine is an important and influential parameter; however, cost-effectiveness in this analysis is most sensitive to the discount rate.

TABLE 12.2
Per Woman Discounted Total Lifetime Costs, QALYs, and Life Years (LYs), with Discounted and Non-Discounted[a] Cost-Effectiveness Ratios for Current Screening and Vaccination Compared With Current Screening in Five Regions.[b]

	Canada	Netherlands	Taiwan	United Kingdom	United States
Costs					
No vaccine	CA$ 906	€123	NT$ 4112	£ 216	US$2144
Vaccine	CA$ 1163	€403	NT$ 14,911	£ 409	US$2232
Incremental	CA$ 258	€280	NT$10,879	£ 193	US$87
QALYs					
No vaccine	28.689	42.344	27.759	25.518	28.359
Vaccine	28.700	42.359	27.776	25.529	28.370
Incremental	0.011	0.015	0.017	0.011	0.011
LYs					
No vaccine	28.696	42.348	27.763	25.521	28.365
Vaccine	28.704	42.360	27.777	25.530	28.372
Incremental	0.008	0.012	0.015	0.009	0.008
Incremental Cost-Effectiveness					
Discounted, per QALY	CA$ 22,532	€18,472	NT$ 632,559	£ 18,037	US$7828
Discounted, per LY	CA$ 31,817	€ 22,672	NT$ 738,972	£ 21,962	Dominates[c]
Undiscounted, per QALY	CA$ 1249	€ 5679	NT$ 93,508	£ 1449	US$ 11,156
Undiscounted, per LY	CA$ 1554	€ 6785	NT$ 105,267	£ 1627	Dominates[c]

[a] Costs, LYs, and QALYs are discounted according to region-specific guidelines (www.ispor.org); [b]Results are expressed in country- or region-specific currencies; [c]Vaccination and screening is cost saving and more effective compared to screening alone.

Source: adapted from Rogoza et al.,[3] reproduced with permission.

Figure 12.2 shows an example of a bivariate, or two-way, sensitivity analysis, also taken from Suárez et al.[4] In this particular case, the percentage of cross-protection for some non-vaccine serotypes was investigated in conjunction with discounting outcomes against Polish PE guideline values versus undiscounted outcomes. It can be seen from the lines that the undiscounted results are quite insensitive to inclusion of assumed cross-protection, whereas the discounted results do show some relevant sensitivity. Two-way sensitivity analysis is typically represented by different lines, as in Figure 12.2. Alternatively, a 3-dimensional graph can be constructed, as was done, for example, by Hubben et al. to depict the dependencies on discount rates for

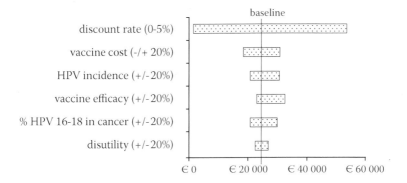

FIGURE 12.1 One-way sensitivity analysis on the incremental cost-effectiveness (€/QALY) for vaccinating teenage girls against HPV in Ireland: sensitivity analysis on parameter uncertainty and variability by varying each parameter ±20% and the discount rate between 0% and 5% (adapted from Suárez et al.,[4] reproduced with permission).

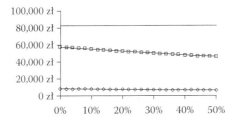

FIGURE 12.2 Two-way sensitivity analysis on the incremental cost-effectiveness (Zloty/QALY) for vaccinating teenage girls against HPV in Poland: discounting (squares) or nondiscounting (diamonds) versus percentage cross-protection against some non-vaccine serotypes at efficacies from 0 to 50%, line represents the potential threshold for favorable cost-effectiveness at 3 times GDP per capita (adapted from Suárez et al.,[4] reproduced with permission).

health and costs separately for infant pneumococcal vaccination in the Netherlands (Figure 12.3).[5,6]

Rozenbaum et al. typically present a best-case and a worst-case cost-effectiveness for their analysis on antenatal HIV testing in the Netherlands.[7] Taxonomy in best- and worst-case analyses can sometimes be a bit counter-intuitive as, for example, in this specific publication, a higher prevalence of HIV among pregnant women contributes to an improved cost-effectiveness. Yet, a higher prevalence is difficult to be envisaged as "best" in many other respects. In particular, the authors estimated that antenatal HIV testing would cost €6495 per life-year gained in the best case (maximum cost-effectiveness ratio), whereas antenatal testing would be cost saving in the worst case.

12.3.2 PROBABILISTIC SA

Probabilistic SA concerns the assignment of formal probability distributions or density functions to specific parameters in the model. Probabilistic SA is sometimes

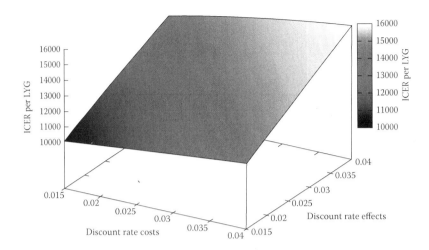

FIGURE 12.3 Two-way SA on the incremental cost-effectiveness in € per life-year gained (LYG) for vaccinating infants with the 7-valent pneumococcal conjugate vaccine in the Netherlands: discounting of costs (one x-axis) versus discounting of health (effects) (Adapted from Hubben et al.[5] & Postma,[6] reproduced with permission).

referred to as stochastic SA. This type of analysis was first suggested by Doubilet et al.[8] Generally, these probability distributions are designed for the mean values of the selected parameters (second-order SA), rather than for the sample data from which the estimated mean is derived (first-order). Using these distributions, typically 1000 or more simulations are done using random draws from the defined distributions in each simulation. Each individual one (often referred to as "replicate") from these multiple simulations translates into an estimate of the incremental cost-effectiveness ratio. Again from the Suárez et al. paper,[4] Figure 12.4 shows a scatter plot of 10,000 replicates around the base-case estimate of cost-effectiveness for vaccinating teenage girls against HPV in Ireland. Both nondiscounted, as well as discounted, outcomes using a 3.5% discount rate (according to the UK PE guideline), are shown.

Probabilistic SA (or PSA) is often further represented in a cost-effectiveness acceptability curve (CEAC). The CEAC shows, for a range of acceptability or willingness-to-pay (often denoted with λ), the proportions in the scatter plot that are below each individual λ. Figure 12.5 shows the corresponding CEAC to the scatter plot in Figure 12.4. Additionally, a CEAC with 2% discounting is included in the figure, possibly better reflecting the Irish underlying time preference (see Chapter 10 on discounting). For example, it can be read that with a discount rate of 3.5%, approximately 80% of replicates correspond to a cost-effectiveness ratio below €50,000 per QALY. Also, 95% of replicates, or more, provides an acceptable cost-effectiveness if λ is chosen at €40,000 or more, using a discount rate of 2%.

Of course, the major issue in probabilistic SA concerns the exact choice and specification of the probability distributions for the mean parameter values. In the absence of adequate information, often uniform or triangle distributions are taken over plausible ranges with the base-case parameter values as midpoints or expected values. In particular, for both of these types of distributions, a minimum

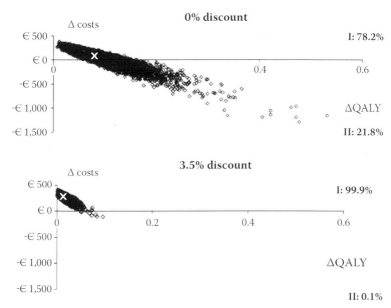

Replicates in the bottom right hand quadrant indicate QALYs gained at a reduced cost; replicates in the top right hand quadrant indicate QALYs gained at an increased cost.

FIGURE 12.4 Scatter plot from the probabilistic sensitivity analysis on the incremental cost-effectiveness (€/QALY) for vaccinating teenage girls against HPV in Ireland: non-discounted (0%) and discounted (3.5%) results being shown for the base case (x) and for 10,000 replicates (diamonds), I and II represent the first two quadrants from the cost-effectiveness plane, no replicates in the other two quadrants (adapted from Suárez et al.,[4] reproduced with permission).

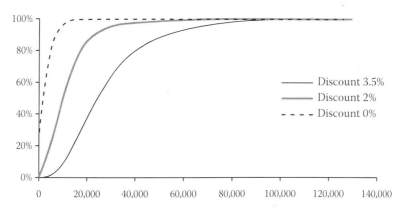

FIGURE 12.5 Cost-effectiveness acceptability curve on the incremental cost-effectiveness (€/QALY) for vaccinating teenage girls against HPV in Ireland for three levels of discounting with willingness-to-pay (λ) on the x-axis, represented by €/QALY, and the proportion of replicates below the λ threshold on the y-axis; corresponding to the scatter plot in Figure 12.4 (adapted from Suárez et al.,[4] reproduced with permission).

and maximum are defined, with equal probabilities for each value in between for the uniform distribution and increasing probabilities from the minimum or maximum if moving to the predefined top of the triangle. Also, referring to the central limit theorem, normal distributions are often considered. Indeed, Suárez et al.[4] used uniform distributions for parameters such as unit costs and screening coverage, and normal distributions for vaccine effectiveness and sensitivity of screening. De Vries et al.[9] used normal and triangle distributions for transition probabilities in the decision tree reflecting progression to aspergillosis and candidosis underlying their analysis of cost-effectiveness of itraconazole prophylaxis against invasive infections for neutropenic cancer patients. Also, Postma et al.[10] used normal and uniform distributions for average length of stay, antibiotic prescriptions, and indirect costs of production losses in their analysis of the cost-effectiveness of treatment with oseltamivir for influenza patients. Additionally, in line with theories underlying the formal estimation of relative risks (RR), they used lognormal distributions for RRs regarding advantages of oseltamivir treatment on antibiotic prescriptions, hospitalizations, deaths, and production losses.

Briggs advocates the use of beta distributions for specific parameters.[11] Beta distributions model events that take place within minimum and maximum values. Given their natural limitation between 0 and 1, these distributions are particularly suitable for risks (for example, of dying or hospitalization). In particular, in an analysis on beta-blocker therapy for chronic heart failure, beta distributions were used for risks of initial, second, third, and fourth or more hospitalizations and for risks of dying at home or in hospital, next to lognormal distributions for RRs and normal distributions for unit costs.[11]

With the majority of pharmacoeconomic models being defined in MS Excel™ and DATA (TreeAge Software Inc.), it is relevant to briefly consider how both packages facilitate PSA. In particular, PSA is a built-in feature of DATA, with a function of Monte Carlo analysis as an explicit analytic option. For Excel, several add-ons that allow PSA exist. For example, @Risk (Palisade) has been explicitly developed and often used for this purpose.[10]

12.3.3 Scenario Analysis

Not always formally distinguished as such, it does make sense to briefly consider scenario analysis as a specific type of SA. Scenario analysis is sometimes defined as exploring possible future paths given specific decisions and actions taken in the present. Pharmacoeconomic modeling, in a sense, also involves present decisions— for example, on which social time preference to choose, which price to set for a new drug —with impacts on cost-effectiveness in (near) future years. Some of the parameters in the model merely reflect decisions by policy makers (which discount rate to choose), manufacturers (pricing), and other stakeholders. These parameters can thus be seen as reflecting instrumental variables, i.e., instruments with which cost-effectiveness can be guided, rather than chance variables impacting probabilistically on the cost-effectiveness outcome. Varying these instrumental variables and parameters, therefore, also reflects the results of choices more than the results of uncertainty.

For those parameters reflecting instrumental variables in the pharmacoeconomic model, it wouldn't make sense to include them in PSA. The effects on the outcomes of varying this set of parameters could be labeled scenario analysis and would typically closely resemble a univariate SA on these parameters. The discount rate and prices of the new product investigated (for example, of the HPV vaccine) are typical examples of parameters not to be included in PSA, but in scenario analysis. As scenario analysis obviously closely resembles univariate SA, it is indeed often done as part of univariate SA and not formally distinguished as such.

12.4 SUMMARY

This chapter reviewed methods currently used in sensitivity analysis for pharmacoeconomic models. In particular, it considered deterministic versus probabilistic sensitivity analysis, univariate versus multivariate analysis, and scenario analysis as a specific form of sensitivity analysis.

REFERENCES

1. Franco EL, Drummond MF (Eds.). 2008. Health economics of HPV vaccination for cervical cancer prevention: Historical developments and practical applications. *Vaccine* 26: Suppl 5.
2. Gold MR, Siegel JE, Russel LB, Weinstein MC (Eds.). Cost-effectiveness in health and medicine. New York: Oxford University Press, 1996.
3. Rogoza RM, Ferko N, Bentley J, Meijer CJLM, Berkhof J, Wang K-L, Downs L, Smith JS, Franco EL. 2008. Optimization of primary and secondary cervical cancer prevention strategies in an era of cervical cancer vaccination: A multi-regional health economic analysis. *Vaccine* 26S:F46–F58.
4. Suárez E, Smith JS, Bosch FX, Nieminen P, Chen C-J, Torvinen S, Demarteau N, Standaert B. 2008. Cost-effectiveness of vaccination against cervical cancer: A multi-regional analysis assessing the impact of vaccine characteristics and alternative vaccination scenarios. *Vaccine* 26S:F29–F45.
5. Hubben GAA E, Bos JM, Glynn DM, Van der Ende A, Van Alphen L, Postma MJ. 2007. Enhanced decision support for policy makers using a web interface to health-economic models: Illustrated with a cost-effectiveness analysis of nationwide infant vaccination with the 7-valent pneumococcal conjugate vaccine in the Netherlands. *Vaccine* 25:3669.
6. Postma MJ. 2008. Public health economics of vaccines in the Netherlands: Methodological issues and applications. *J Public Health* 16:267–73.
7. Rozenbaum MH, Verweel G, Folkerts DKF, Dronkers F, Van den Hoek JAR, Hartwig NG, De Groot R, Postma MJ. 2008. Cost-effectiveness estimates for antenatal HIV testing in the Netherlands. *Int J STD & AIDS* 19:668–75.
8. Doubilet P, Begg CB, Weinstein MC, Braun P, McNeil BJ. 1985. Probabilistic sensitivity analysis using Monte Carlo simulation. A practical approach. *Medical Decision Making* 5:157–77.
9. De Vries R, Daenen S, Tolley K, Glasmacher A, Prentice A, Howells S, Christopherson H, de Jong-van den Berg LTW, Postma MJ. 2008. Cost effectiveness of Itraconazole in the prophylaxis of invasive fungal Infections. *PharmacoEconomics* 26:75–90.
10. Postma MJ, Novak A, Scheijbeler HWKFH, Gyldmark M, Van Genugten MLL, Wilschut JC. 2007. Cost effectiveness of Oseltamivir treatment for patients with influenza-like illness who are at increased risk for serious complications of influenza. *PharmacoEconomics* 25:497–509.

11. Briggs AH. Handling uncertainty in economic evaluation and presenting the results. In Drummond M and McGuire A (Eds.) *Economic Evaluation in Health Care*. New York: Oxford University Press 2001. 172–214.

13 Use of Pharmacoeconomics in Drug Reimbursement in Australia, Canada, and the United Kingdom
What Can We Learn from International Experience?

Michael Drummond and Corinna Sorenson

CONTENTS

13.1   INTRODUCTION

Several countries around the world have been using pharmacoeconomics as part
of their formal decision-making process for the pricing or reimbursement of pharmaceuticals. Australia was the first jurisdiction to adopt such a policy in 1993 and
was quickly followed by New Zealand and several Canadian provinces. In addition, several European countries request economic submissions for some, or all, new
medicines, including Belgium, Finland, Ireland, Norway, The Netherlands, Portugal,
Sweden, and the United Kingdom. Similar policies have also been recently adopted
by some Eastern European countries, plus jurisdictions in Asia (e.g., South Korea)
and Latin America (e.g., Brazil).

   Now that there is growing international experience with the use of pharmacoeconomics, the question arises as to whether jurisdictions that do not currently use
this approach can learn from previous attempts. This is of particular interest in the
United States at present, given the debate about the use of "comparative effectiveness research" and the possibility of federal government interest in this, and related,
approaches. Over the last couple of years, there has been growing interest and discussion in the United States around establishing a more formalized process or system
for conducting comparative-effectiveness research (CER).[*] Based on these discussions, various proposals have been put forward around the call for a centralized comparative research entity, each with different configurations regarding its governance,
remit, methods, and role in decision-making. While none of the proposals has yet to
be adopted on the congressional level, with continued debate over the nuances of a
CER entity, a wide range of stakeholders (e.g., U.S. government, business, insurers,
providers, consumers, and coalitions) support such initiatives and it appears highly
likely that some CER organizational form will be introduced in the United States.

   Until a new CER entity is introduced, the use of pharmacoeconomics in the
United States is largely decentralized, with several jointly operating health technology assessment (HTA) entities. For example, the Effective Health Care (EHC)
program at the Agency for Healthcare Research and Quality (AHRQ) includes a
collection of research centers that review existing evidence or generate new evidence
and analytic tools. Additionally, the Centers for Medicare and Medicaid Services
(CMS) has the Medicare Coverage Advisory Committee (MCAC); each of the 50
state Medicaid programs has some form of HTA procedure for drugs (the state of

---

[*] While definitions differ, comparative effectiveness research entails the evaluation of alternative treatment
options to treat the same condition, primarily via clinical studies.

Washington recently extended its HTA program to also cover devices, diagnostics, and procedures); and 13 states participate in the Drug Effectiveness Review Project (DERP). Many private health plans and pharmacy benefit managers (PBMs) also operate HTA programs, and pharmacoeconomic analyses are frequently conducted by manufacturers, consulting firms, and academic departments.

The focus of this chapter is to review experience overseas and to assess whether any lessons can be learned from international use of pharmacoeconomics. The discussion will concentrate on experience in Australia, Canada, and the United Kingdom, as these are the three countries with the most extensive use of pharmacoeconomics to date. The introduction of the human papilloma virus (HPV) vaccine in Australia, Canada, the United Kingdom, and the United States will then be explored to highlight the different approaches to pharmacoeconomics in these countries. Finally, the focus will be on potential implications for the United States, given the current policy debate, drawing on the strengths and weaknesses of other jurisdictions.

13.2 USE OF PHARMACOECONOMICS OVERSEAS

13.2.1 AUSTRALIA

Since 1993, pharmacoeconomic studies have formed part of submissions made by manufacturers to the Pharmaceutical Benefits Advisory Committee (PBAC). The PBAC makes recommendations to government ministers on the listing of drugs on the Pharmaceutical Benefits Schedule (PBS). This is the list of drugs given outside of public hospitals that receive a public subsidy. Therefore, PBS listing is usually essential if a new drug is to secure a substantial market share.

Manufacturers' submissions have to be produced in accordance with a set of guidelines set forth by the PBAC (Commonwealth of Australia 2007) and are then assessed by an independent review group. The activities are also supported by an economics subcommittee of the PBAC that contains several well-known Australian health economists. Based on the evidence and subsequent discussion, the PBAC will recommend that the drug be listed, either at the price proposed by the manufacturer or at a lower price. The committee can also reject or defer applications. The final price of the drug, if listed, is agreed upon by another government committee, after a consideration of several other factors (e.g., overseas prices, expected expenditure).

Australia has the greatest experience in the use of pharmacoeconomics and much has been written about the PBAC. One of the most interesting papers is that by George et al. (2001), who reviewed the outcome of several submissions to the PBAC and discussed why particular drugs had been approved or rejected by the committee. They found that the PBAC was unlikely to list a drug if the incremental cost per life-year gained exceeded 76,000 Australian dollars and unlikely to reject a drug for which the additional cost per life-year gained was less than 42,000 Australian dollars. However, the cost-effectiveness ratio was not the only factor determining the reimbursement decision. Other factors included the scientific rigor and relevance of the evidence for comparative safety, efficacy, and cost-effectiveness of the drug; the lack, or inadequacy, of alternative treatments currently available; the perceived need in the community; whether the drug is likely to be used only in a hospital setting; and the seriousness of the health condition for which the drug was indicated.

13.2.2 CANADA

The use of pharmacoeconomics in Canada began at the provincial level, most notably in Ontario and British Columbia (Ontario Ministry of Health 2004; Anis et al. 1998). However, in 2002 the Common Drug Review (CDR) was established, involving all provinces with the exception of Quebec.

The CDR is administered by the Canadian Agency for Drugs and Technologies in Health (CADTH). CADTH, formerly the Canadian Coordinating Office for Health Technology Assessment, or CCOHTA, is the central agency for the coordination of HTA activities in Canada. In addition to administering the CDR, CADTH undertakes some of its own HTAs of drugs and other health technologies. It also developed the Canadian Guidelines for Economic Evaluation (CADTH 2006), which lay out key methodological standards and serve as the template for submissions to the CDR.

The CDR was established in the hope of securing standardized access to new drugs across the whole of Canada. However, its recommendations still need to be adopted by individual provinces because the provision of health care is a provincial, rather than federal, responsibility in Canada. Some provinces still retain their own drug review committees and may occasionally come to a different view from that of the CDR. In addition, there are other activities involving the use of pharmacoeconomics, such as the Joint Oncology Drug Review, which seeks to establish guidelines for the use of cancer drugs both within, and outside, hospitals.

The main challenges facing the CDR have been set out in a recent paper by Laupacis (2006), who was the founding chair of its expert committee (CEDAC). These challenges include the variable quality of manufacturer submissions and the problems of dealing with drugs for rare diseases, which are often expensive and for which the clinical evidence is often sparse.

13.2.3 UNITED KINGDOM

Activities in HTA in the U.K. are coordinated by the National Coordinating Centre for Health Technology Assessment (NCCHTA). The NCCHTA manages the National Health Service (NHS) research program in HTA and also administers contracts for the National Institute for Health and Clinical Excellence (NICE).

Established in 1999, NICE is the most well-known HTA entity in the U.K. It issues guidance on the use of health technologies and healthcare interventions to the NHS in England and Wales. It has four major programs of work, in investigational procedures, technology appraisal, clinical guidelines, and the evaluation of public health interventions.

The work program on technology appraisal has attracted the most discussion and debate owing to several high-profile decisions to recommend against the use of some technologies, especially expensive new cancer drugs. NICE does not control the reimbursement or pricing of drugs; the latter is a matter for the manufacturer.

However, a negative recommendation from NICE usually results in highly restricted use of a given product.

As in Australia and Canada, NICE's technology appraisal process involves a submission from the manufacturer, undertaken in accordance with the institute's methodological guidelines (NICE 2008). The manufacturer's submission is then assessed by an independent review group, which may provide just a critique or may undertake its own study, depending on the precise nature and complexity of the appraisal being conducted. NICE distinguishes between single technology appraisals, which are simpler and consider only one drug, and multiple technology appraisals, which are longer, more complex, and typically consider three or more drugs for treating the same condition.

The role of pharmacoeconomics in NICE's technology appraisals is quite extensive and assessments will normally include a full decision-analytic model. It is also clear that cost-effectiveness considerations are an important part of the decision-making process, although NICE's Technology Appraisal Committee does consider evidence from clinical experts and patient organizations as well as the independent assessment report.

Unlike the HTA and reimbursement agencies in Australia and Canada, NICE does not currently consider every new drug for use outside hospitals. Its agenda is set by the Department of Health and tends to focus on new technologies (the majority of which are drugs) that are likely to have a major clinical or economic impact on the NHS.

In addition to NICE, the Scottish Medicines Consortium (SMC) issues guidance on the use of all new drugs for the Scottish NHS (Cairns 2006). Its mode of operation is very similar to that of the PBAC and CDR. Also, the All Wales Medicine Strategy Group issues guidance on the use of drugs to the Welsh NHS, particularly in cases where there is no NICE guidance.

Because there is considerable information in the public domain about NICE and its activities, it is probably the most widely studied HTA or reimbursement agency. In particular, the recent report of a Parliamentary Health Select Committee (2008) discusses the strengths and weaknesses of NICE and makes several recommendations for improvement. Principally, these relate to increasing the coverage of NICE guidance (to include a higher proportion of new drugs and other health technologies) and to reducing the time taken to issue guidance.

In addition, a recent report commissioned by the National Pharmaceutical Council examines the workings of NICE in detail and discusses its relevance to the United States (Sorenson et al. 2008). For further information, see Table 13.1.

13.3 COMPARISONS IN THE USE OF PHARMACOECONOMICS ACROSS THE FOUR COUNTRIES: THE CASE OF THE HUMAN PAPILLOMAVIRUS VACCINE

The case study being used in this chapter is the HPV vaccine. It is, however, important to note that vaccines differ from pharmaceuticals in several ways. While vaccines have many similarities to pharmaceuticals in general, they also raise additional

TABLE 13.1

Comparative Use of Pharmacoeconomics in Australia, Canada, and the United Kingdom, 2008

	Australia	Canada	United Kingdom
Key Decision Bodies	*Pharmaceutical Benefits Advisory Committee (PBAC)*: Reviews evidence and makes reimbursement recommendations. Ministry of Health: Makes final listing decision.	*Canadian Agency for Drugs and Technologies in Health (CADTH)*: Oversees the CDR and all HTA–related activities in Canada. *Canadian Immunization Committee (CIC) and National Advisory Committee on Immunization (NACI)*: Provides advice and recommendations on implementation of the National Immunization Strategy and related programmes.	*National Institute for Health and Clinical Excellence (NICE)*: Produces guidance on health technologies and interventions for the NHS. *National Coordinating Centre for Health Technology Assessment (NCCHTA)*: Coordinates HTA activities in the UK and administers contracts for NICE. *Scottish Medicines Consortium*: Issues guidance on the use of new drugs for the Scottish NHS. *Joint Committee on Vaccination and Immunization (JCVI)*: Provides recommendations on all matters related to immunization of communicable diseases.
Pharmacoeconomic Evidence and Review Requirements	Submissions must adhere to PBAC guidelines and be reviewed by an independent review group.	Submissions for the CDR must adhere to CADTH guidelines for economic evaluation.	Submissions must adhere to NICE guidelines and be reviewed by an independent review group. (NICE) Extensive use of pharmacoeconomics and cost–effectiveness evidence. (NICE)

Applications of Pharmacoeconomic Evidence	Used to make decisions on inclusion in the benefit schedule and any pricing/ reimbursement conditions. Review and decision made on every new drug for use outside hospitals.	Used to make decisions on inclusion in the benefit schedule and any pricing/ reimbursement conditions. Also plays a role in establishing clinical guidelines, especially for cancer care. Review and decision made on every new drug for use outside hospitals.	Used to make recommendations or render guidance on use of a technology or intervention in the NHS; does not control pricing/reimbursement (although, does have an indirect influence). (NICE) Review and recommendations made on select drugs (e.g., high cost). (NICE)
Key Challenges to Effective Use of Pharmacoeconomics	Where restricted use of a product is recommended, it needs to be followed by practitioners.	Adoption of CADTH recommendations by all individual provinces; ensuring quality of manufacturer submissions; and, reviewing drugs for rare diseases.	Consistent uptake of NICE guidance amongst different regions; speeding up time to issue guidance; expanding topics covered by NICE review.

analytic challenges, such as the need to model disease transmission. In most jurisdictions, the reimbursement of vaccines is handled by a separate decision-making
structure, and it is common for payers to place a contract for supply in countries with
a single payer (e.g., government). Nevertheless, pharmacoeconomic assessments,
along the lines of those discussed above, are frequently made and these often have
an impact on decision making

13.3.1 AUSTRALIA

The Australian government has invested heavily in the prevention of cervical cancer,
supporting one of the most successful national cervical screening programs in the
world. The program has played a central role in the approval and use of vaccines to
protect against HPV.

In mid-2006, Gardasil®, the first HPV vaccine approved for use in Australia, underwent consideration by the PBAC to attain public funding (Pharmaceutical Benefits
Advisory Committee 2006). The manufacturer's submission indicated current management involving screening for cervical cancer via the national screening program as the
main comparator, and presented six randomized trials comparing Gardasil and placebo.
Based on the efficacy analysis, Gardasil was deemed significantly more effective than
standard treatment (screening), but with similar or greater toxicity. Several economic
models were provided to estimate relevant costs and outcomes over the long term.
Incremental cost-effectiveness ratios ranged from $16,000 to $70,000, depending upon
the cohort. The total cost of the vaccine program in the first 4 years of operation was estimated to be more than $100 million. Based on the available evidence, the PBAC rejected
the application for Gardasil, given unacceptable and uncertain cost-effectiveness at the
price requested. Other considerations central to PBAC's decision included the fact that the
magnitude of the per patient clinical benefit was considered small across the vaccinated
population; the lack of estimation of potential costs associated with implementation; and,
the significant total cost of an HPV vaccination program. Subsequent to PBAC's decision, the Minister of Health requested that it consider a minor resubmission addressing
the main issues of concern identified by the initial review. The resubmission provided a
reduced vaccine price, further evidence to support the original cost-utility analysis, and
the potential for a risk-sharing agreement and additional surveillance between the sponsor and the Australian government. The PBAC considered these modifications sufficient
to subsidize Gardasil for use in 12–26-year-old females enrolled in school- and community-based programs under the auspices of the National Immunization Programme
(NIP). Consequently, the commonwealth government funds the purchase of the vaccine,
while the state and territory governments manage the immunization program, administering the vaccine in schools and local communities.

About a year later, another HPV vaccine, Cervarix®, was reviewed by the PBAC,
with Gardasil as the comparator.* The submission presented Cervarix as equivalent

---

* Submission presented an indirect comparison based on three randomized trials of Cervarix versus
placebo and three randomized trials of Gardasil versus placebo. A formal direct comparison was not
provided, only the results from the two sets of trials.

to Gardasil in terms of both comparative efficacy and safety and, based on a cost-minimization analysis, proposed that Cervarix be included on the NIP for the same treatment population and at the same price as Gardasil. However, due to uncertainty regarding the assumptions and data inputs used, the PBAC did not accept the sponsor's claim of cost-minimization and was therefore unable to determine a cost-effective price for Cervarix. Moreover, while Cervarix does not offer protection against genital warts (a broader benefit of Gardasil), the submission did not provide a full economic evaluation of the impact of the health forgone when Cervarix is used in place of Gardasil. Based on these considerations, PBAC rejected the submission on the grounds of uncertain cost-effectiveness.

13.3.2 Canada

In 2008, the Canadian Immunization Committee (CIC) published its recommendations on HPV vaccines, which are used by federal, provincial, and territorial jurisdictions to develop and implant their immunization programs (Canadian Immunization Committee 2008). A multidisciplinary, joint National Advisory Committee on Immunization (NACI)-CIC HPV Vaccine Expert Working Group, comprising a wide range of experts and key stakeholders, was established about a year prior to develop comprehensive recommendations for HPV vaccine programs. In developing its recommendations, the group examined the existing clinical data on the efficacy of Gardasil and Cervarix, as well as international and Canadian cost-effectiveness studies to determine the relative long-term epidemiologic and economic consequences of HPV vaccines. Cost-effectiveness estimates for HPV vaccination ranged from $15,000 to $37,000 in both international and Canadian studies, depending on the model used, the duration of vaccine protection, the age at vaccination, and other assumptions (e.g., use in both males and females vs. females only). The working group also considered evidence on the acceptability of HPV immunization, feasibility of eventual HPV immunization, ability to evaluate the impact of such programs, and equity and ethical concerns. Based on the aforementioned evidence, the working group recommended the use of Gardasil (Cervarix is not licensed for use in Canada), specifically for females aged 9 to 26 years.* Moreover, in order to achieve higher coverage at lower cost, vaccinations should be administered prior to the onset of sexual activity and in primary school. As immunizing all Canadian females aged 9 to 26 years upon initial implementation of the program was unfeasible, it was recommended that school-based HPV vaccination of one female cohort be implemented in all Canadian provinces and territories, so that 80% to 90% of school-aged girls in select grades were immunized within 2 to 5 years. Given that the level of benefit (in both health and economic terms) associated with HPV vaccines was greatly influenced by the duration of vaccine protection, the recommendations also called for evaluation procedures to be put in place to measure the persistence of effectiveness and develop strategies for reaching vaccinated females for additional doses, if required.

---

* Recommended only for females aged 14 to 26 years (even if already sexually active) if they have had previous Pap smear abnormalities or a previous HPV infection.

Following the CIC-NACI recommendations, the government provided $300 million to the provinces and territories through a third-party fund to launch HPV vaccine programs, specifically through supporting the purchase of HPV vaccines. Similar to Australia, the provinces and territories are responsible for the delivery of the immunization program(s) and are granted flexibility in decisions about their implementation.

13.3.3 UNITED KINGDOM

In the U.K., the Joint Committee on Vaccination and Immunization (JCVI) serves as the statutory expert on vaccine use. It provides advice to the secretaries of state for health for England, Scotland, Wales, and Northern Ireland on matters related to the immunization of communicable diseases. In 2006, the JCVI was commissioned by the Department of Health to systematically review the available evidence on the use of HPV vaccines and their potential benefit (Joint Committee on Vaccination and Immunization 2008). The committee examined both published and unpublished evidence sources, including efficacy and burden of disease studies, cost-effectiveness analyses, feasibility studies on implementing an HPV program, and research on HPV vaccination. Much of the efficacy evidence considered by the JCVI was submitted by the manufacturers of Gardasil and Cervarix, and included clinical trial data and post-marketing surveillance reports. In their review, the JCVI concluded that both vaccines are highly effective (especially in 10- to 14-year-olds), with good safety profiles, and offer an expected immunity of about 10 years. Again, only Gardasil demonstrated effective protection against genital warts. Upon initial review of existing burden of disease and economic modeling studies, the JCVI concluded that the available evidence was not sufficient to make a recommendation, especially as the models were not U.K. specific. Consequently, the JCVI considered two particular studies commissioned to two local institutions. The cost-effectiveness analyses used followed NICE guidelines and underwent a robust review process.

Following the review, the committee recommended to the secretary of state that routine HPV vaccination of females aged 12 to 13 years would be the most cost-effective, assuming the average duration of vaccine protection is at least 10 years. In addition, it would be feasible to include a time-limited "catch up" vaccination for girls aged 13 to 17 years. Vaccination of females above this age was not cost-effective given the assumed cost of vaccine and administration, and the increase in prevalence of previous infection in this age group. The JCVI recommended that the vaccine be delivered through schools, except for certain groups that may be difficult to reach (e.g., home-schooled females), in which case GPs should assume a role in delivery of the vaccine. It was considered whether Gardasil or Cervarix should be recommended for use over the other, with the committee concluding that the choice of vaccine to be purchased should be determined primarily by cost-effectiveness and, in relation, the negotiated cost of the vaccines. If offered at the same price, Gardasil was recommended due to its protection against genital warts. As with Canada, the JCVI recommended that a comprehensive monitoring and evaluation program be fully funded and implemented as an integral part of the vaccine program. The vaccination program is currently being implemented throughout the U.K. based principally on the JCVI recommendations. However, Cervarix is the sole vaccine being used in the program, following a U.K.-wide competitive procurement bid for supply of the HPV vaccine to the NHS.

13.3.4   UNITED STATES

In 2006, the Food and Drug Administration (FDA) approved the use of Gardasil in females 9 to 26 years of age, based on a review of the vaccine's safety and effectiveness.[*] The Advisory Committee on Immunization Practices of the Centers for Disease Control and Prevention (CDC) subsequently recommended that girls ages 11 and 12 receive the vaccine (in three separate doses),[†] with a temporary "catch-up" vaccination provided to women between 13 and 26 years of age who have not yet been vaccinated or completed the full vaccine series. The recommendation was based predominantly on efficacy and safety evidence, although available cost-effectiveness estimates were considered, albeit not formally.[‡] Thereafter, the CDC advised that Gardasil be added to the routine vaccination schedule for children and adolescents. Many states also introduced legislation to require girls to be vaccinated before entering the relevant grade in school.[§] While an "opt-out" policy generally accompanied most of these bills, such proposals generated considerable public debate and most were not passed. In another highly contested move, the U.S. Citizenship and Immigration Service (USCIS) recently agreed to mandate Gardasil for every age-appropriate female seeking to become a legal resident of the United States.

The CDC's guidelines arguably influenced insurance coverage of Gardasil, with many private health plans providing coverage for the vaccine. However, the extent and rates of coverage vary at both the plan and individual level. Indeed, one of the main concerns in a more fragmented system such as that of the United States is that vaccine coverage may not be at the desired or appropriate level. To narrow existing gaps in coverage, the Vaccines for Children (VFC) program added Gardasil onto its roster of vaccines provided at no or low cost to uninsured children aged 18 and younger. All of the state immunization projects have also adopted Gardasil, which provides the vaccine at $30 versus $360 (full cost) for the complete series of three injections. In addition, Merck has a patient assistance program to provide the vaccine to those 19 years and older who are uninsured and unable to afford the vaccine.

Despite such efforts and significant support for its use by a variety of stakeholders, a recent study conducted by the CDC found that while nearly 2.5 million of the country's 10 million girls had received at least one dose of the vaccine, only a

---

[*] Cervarix is still under FDA review and is unlikely to be on the market until 2009, at the earliest.

[†] This recommendation was based on several considerations, including age of sexual debut in the United States, cost-effectiveness, and the established young adolescent health care visit at ages 11–12 when other vaccines are also recommended (Javitt et al., 2008).

[‡] As intimated in the introduction, cost-effectiveness analysis has not assumed a formal role in coverage decision or practice guidelines in the United States, unlike the other countries highlighted in this chapter. For example, the government run vaccine fund for uninsured children (Vaccines for Children program) does not use cost-effectiveness to develop its recommendations and policies.

[§] The United States has a robust state-based infrastructure for mandatory vaccination, which became a condition of school entry in the 19th century.

quarter of that group had received all three recommended doses (CDC, 2008).* The low rate of completed vaccination with Gardasil has raised several concerns about its use, although investigators have noted that the vaccination series takes 6 months and thus not many of the participants studied would have had time to complete the full schedule (Drug Information Association, 2008). Moreover, the survey covered only girls between the ages of 13 and 17 years. Other contributing factors to the low vaccination rate may include limited public understanding that HPV causes cancer, difficulty in encouraging young women to visit the doctor, and the high cost of the vaccine, if not covered in some manner. Moreover, there has been some skepticism among parents and experts about use of the vaccine, particularly in the youngest girls (e.g., 9- and 10-year-olds), for a variety of social, economic, ethical, and health reasons. Such sentiments have generally been accompanied by requests for more parental control over HPV vaccination and additional studies to evaluate the long-term effectiveness, especially in terms of the duration of vaccine immunity, and safety of Gardasil.

It has also been recognized that additional evidence on the cost-effectiveness of HPV vaccines is needed to support appropriate guidelines for their use in the United States. A recent study by Kim et al. (2008) at Harvard University found that Gardasil is cost-effective in pre-adolescent girls aged 11 and 12 years at $43,600 per QALY, an estimate that falls below the $50,000–$100,000 per QALY threshold often used in the United States to ascertain maximum cost-effectiveness. However, this result assumes lifelong immunity, which has not yet been demonstrated in clinical studies. Cost-effectiveness declines significantly among older females (19 to 26 years old), with vaccination for girls and women up to age 26 estimated at $152,700. The results of this study, coupled with the recent CDC report, have been used to highlight the need for further evidence on the long-term costs and benefits of Gardasil, especially before mandates for vaccination are put into place.

13.4   WHAT CAN THE UNITED STATES LEARN FROM EXPERIENCE OVERSEAS?

It is well known in health policy circles that the devil is in the details and that policy solutions are very context-specific. Therefore, it is highly unlikely that approaches from particular countries could simply be uplifted and transported to other jurisdictions, such as the United States. In particular, models in Australia, Canada and the U.K., and many similar approaches in other European countries, reflect a policy response designed to meet the needs of a predominantly public, single-payer healthcare system. This contrasts sharply with the United States, which has a multifaceted healthcare system, involving public, private not-for-profit, and private for-profit payers.

More fundamentally, there are important social and cultural differences among Australia, Canada, and the U.K. and the United States, which may impact on efforts

---

* Estimates were derived from the CDC's annual National Immunization Survey for Teens, where nearly 3,000 teens were interviewed by telephone and their answers confirmed by vaccination records from physicians.

to introduce approaches based on economic evaluation. These include the willingness to accept explicit restrictions on the access to services, which is arguably absent in the United States, and the concern about extensive government involvement in healthcare, which is arguably greater in the United States (Kohut and Stokes 2006). Another major difference between the United States and elsewhere, which partly reflects these cultural differences, is the much greater level of patient copays in the U.S. healthcare system, especially for pharmaceuticals (Cohen et al. 2007; Cohen et al. 2006).

However, despite the differences between the United States and other countries, much can be learned from the successes and failures of systems elsewhere, and these lessons will be important to acknowledge as the debate on the role of HTA progresses in the United States. Here the comments are organized under the following headings: governance, funding, and organization; assessment methods; decision-making processes; and communication and implementation of guidance.

13.4.1 GOVERNANCE, FUNDING, AND ORGANIZATION

13.4.1.1 Structure and Composition

Experience from elsewhere suggests that an appearance of independence is important for HTA agencies or entities, as the findings of HTA reports are often controversial. A survey of general practitioners in the U.K. (Conn 2006) showed that NICE was perceived as being independent from industry, but not independent from government. Also, when NICE guidance is considered by the media, the institute is normally referred to as "the government's health watchdog" or, occasionally, as "the NHS's rationing body."

Therefore, despite their quasi-independence, bodies such as CADTH, the PBAC, and NICE are perceived as pursuing a payer's agenda. However, on occasion, they do make recommendations that are, at best, inconvenient for government. For example, NICE twice rejected beta-interferon for multiple sclerosis. Fearing a political backlash, the government brokered a risk-sharing scheme with the manufacturers in order to ensure that the drugs were available for patients (Department of Health 2002).

Reimbursement and HTA agencies also take other measures to increase public perceptions of independence. These include the use of expert committees, extensive patient representation on its committees, and stakeholder involvement.

In the United States, the primary decision affecting the governance, funding, and organization of any HTA entity would be where it is located. That is, should it be a new federal agency, part of an existing agency, or outside of government (Wilensky 2006; Orszag 2007)? Subsequently, it would need to be decided whether the entity was to be charged with informing the decisions of federal government alone, or the decisions of a wider range of payers.

In the former case, one could imagine a relationship similar to the ones that HTA and reimbursement agencies have with government in their respective countries. On the other hand, if any HTA entity were to be providing guidance to a broader range of healthcare decision-makers, a wide range of funding and organizational options would be possible. These could include a mixture of public and private funding, or a "virtual institute" involving a collaboration of several existing public and private organizations with expertise in HTA (Orszag 2007). Regardless of the governance arrangement(s), any public HTA entity will likely end up informing decisions of a whole range of payers, even if the entity is charged only with informing the decisions of the federal government. Indeed, currently the HTAs generated for the MCAC decisions are posted on the CMS website and are available for consultation by private health plans.

The precise nature of any HTA entity in the United States is still being decided. However, two observations can be made. First, it is difficult for any organization to develop an appearance of independence if its funding comes from a single source. From this point of view, multiple funding sources are preferred. Second, even where the HTA entity is charged with informing public decisions alone, it can also influence decisions in other sectors. For example, in Canada, the CDR was established by the federal government under the stewardship of CADTH. The federal government does not control the funding and availability of drugs. However, the outcomes of the CDR are influential in the decisions of the various provincial formularies, although the various provinces clearly take local factors into account (McMahon et al. 2006). Therefore, it would be unwise to assume that the influence of any HTA entity would be confined to a single sector of the healthcare system.

13.4.1.2 Remit

Regardless of the structure and composition of any new HTA entity in the United States, a critical feature would be its remit. NICE's remit is to consider all health technologies, and it seeks to apply the same methods of assessment to each. On the other hand, the CDR and PBAC processes focus on drugs, although CADTH's other activities cover other technologies. A broader approach is thought to be more policy-relevant than concentrating on one sector (e.g., drugs), although in practice a substantial proportion (around two thirds) of NICE technology appraisals have been of pharmaceuticals. Although the appraisal of devices, procedures, diagnostics, and public health interventions tends to be more challenging than the appraisal of drugs, it would make sense to have the same broad remit for any HTA entity in the United States.

The other element of an HTA entity's remit is the scope of the assessments it is asked to carry out. In particular, should it focus only on clinical outcomes (e.g., effectiveness), or should it also consider cost-effectiveness? In Australia, Canada, and the U.K., the remit of reimbursement and HTA agencies clearly obliges them to consider both clinical and cost-effectiveness. In the case of NICE, economic considerations have played a greater role in the guidance emanating from technology appraisals than that resulting from clinical guidelines or public health appraisals. This is mainly because of the increased difficulty in addressing the economic issues in the latter two programs, due to the breadth of the topics and the lack of available data.

The recent debate in the United States has been conducted using the term "comparative effectiveness." For many commentators, the study of comparative effectiveness would involve consideration of clinical outcomes only, usually through the conduct of clinical trials, comparing relevant technologies in a real-life (i.e., routine practice) setting (Wilensky 2006). On the other hand, some commentators (MedPac 2007; Orszag 2007) acknowledge that an assessment of comparative effectiveness could also consider costs. The definition given by MedPac is one of the clearest and most comprehensive. It cites the Academy Health (2005) definition that

> Comparative-effectiveness analysis evaluates the relative effectiveness, safety and cost of medical services, drugs, devices, therapies and procedures used to treat the same condition.

It also states that such studies may include:

- Clinical outcomes, including traditional clinical endpoints, such as mortality and major morbidity
- Functional endpoints, such as quality of life, symptom severity, and patient satisfaction
- Economic outcomes, including the cost of health care services and cost-effectiveness

In contrast to the MedPac definition, the majority of observers and policy initiatives employing "comparative effectiveness" deem that considerations of costs and cost-effectiveness should be undertaken by the payer, not the evaluator. Indeed, the term "comparative effectiveness" may have emerged and gained traction precisely because it avoids the mention of costs.

As the debate about comparative effectiveness progresses in the United States, the breadth, or restriction, in the scope of the required analyses will be a critical issue. At one end of the spectrum, the HTA effort could focus solely on the funding and conduct of clinical trials to compare alternative technologies. Unlike most of the trials currently funded by industry (e.g., Phase III for drugs), these trials are likely to compare two or more widely used therapies, enroll large numbers of patients, and have long-term follow-up. They are also likely to be quite costly, so their number will be limited, even with the budgets currently being proposed for the comparative effectiveness initiative, which at present range from $4–6 billion a year (Wilensky 2006).

A narrow definition of comparative effectiveness, excluding cost-effectiveness, has some appeal within the U.S. context. In particular, since healthcare organization, clinical practice patterns, costs, and, importantly, perspectives differ among the various payers, a centralized calculation of the cost-effectiveness of health technologies may have little meaning. Even in the context of one payer (e.g., CMS), it might be argued that the consideration of cost-effectiveness is not admissible within its remit. On the other hand, some feel quite strongly that costs should be considered, although such sentiments are generally promulgated by academics rather than decision makers. In a recent interview (Tunis 2007), David Eddy said, "I believe that our failure to explicitly consider costs in medical decision making is the single greatest flaw in our health care system … if we are not allowed to consider cost, there is no way to determine the value of any activity. We end up recommending everything that has any benefit, no matter how small." Nevertheless, it has been suggested that cost-effectiveness is an implicit consideration in some policies and private plans (Neumann and Sullivan 2006).

The other, more practical, argument is that cost-effectiveness considerations may eventually feature in decision-making, even if they are not explicitly considered. However, without a formal consideration of all the relevant economic factors, cost criteria might be considered inappropriately.

The best example of this comes from Germany, where the newly established Institute for Quality and Economic Efficacy in the Health Sector (IQWiG) was asked to provide advice to the Joint Federal Committee (Gemeinsamer Bundesausschuss, or G-BA) on the relative merits of insulin analogs as compared with regular insulin. At the time, the remit of the institute did not include a formal consideration of cost-effectiveness, so the comparison was limited to the clinical evidence, obtained from randomized controlled trials. The conclusion of the study was that all types of insulin were equally effective in controlling blood glucose levels.

Because the conclusion was one of comparative efficacy, the G-BA saw little reason to pay a premium price for insulin analogs. The problem was that the study, appropriately conducted within the institute's narrow remit, ignored most of the potential advantages of insulin analogs, which mainly relate to their greater potential to avoid hyperglycemic events and the associated costs and health outcomes. Therefore, if a formal consideration of cost-effectiveness is to be excluded, it is important that any differences between health technologies, in terms of their impact on quality of life and healthcare resource use, are estimated as part of the analysis. Otherwise, there is a risk that the eventual cost-effectiveness analysis, which must surely be conducted at some point in the decision-making process, will be a simple comparison of acquisition costs of the alternative technologies with the narrowly defined clinical effects.

13.4.2 ASSESSMENT METHODS

13.4.2.1 Priority-Setting and Scoping

Priorities for assessment by NICE are set by the government in the U.K., according to published criteria. If any HTA entity in the United States was also servicing the decision-making needs of the federal government, a similar process could apply. For example, the topics could relate to those technologies for which coverage decisions are required. If an HTA entity in the United States were seeking to be relevant to a wider range of healthcare decision-makers, the nature of the process for setting priorities is less clear, although many private health plans also cover Medicare enrollees. In the case of the CDR and the PBAC, the agenda is driven by the applications for reimbursement made by manufacturers. This is the model for most agencies dealing with the listing of drugs.

One clear message from international experience is the importance of the scoping stage, in particular, defining the alternatives to be compared. As in the case of priority setting, the scoping process is likely to be simpler if only the decision-making needs of the federal government are being considered. It may not be possible to specify a single analysis capable of meeting the needs of all the different payers in the United States, who may currently be sanctioning different treatment practices. However, it should be noted that the federal government is not a monolithic payer, and is not focused only on the elderly (via the Medicare program). As such, the lines drawn between the responsibilities of the various payers are not always so clear or distinct.

13.4.2.2 Methodological Guidelines

Most reimbursement and HTA entities have specified methodological guidelines for their assessments (Tarn and Smith 2004). These guidelines serve several purposes, including standardizing assessments and increasing transparency.

Although several aspects of the prescribed methods have been the subject of debate, the majority view is that it is better to have guidelines than not. An important feature of the NICE guidelines is that they embody the "reference case" concept, first proposed by the Panel on Cost-effectiveness in Health and Medicine (aka, the Washington Panel) established by the U.S. Public Health Service (Gold et al. 1996). The principle behind the reference case approach is that alternative analytic approaches are not excluded from consideration, as long as an analysis consistent with the reference case is also reported. Manufacturers submitting to NICE favor this approach; if they feel that they can improve upon the reference case, then they can submit an additional analysis. On the other hand, the reference case provides a clear statement of the minimum requirements.

As mentioned, several aspects of methodological guidelines have been the subject of debate. The most controversial aspects have been the perspective for costing (which often excludes productivity costs, costs to other government budgets, and costs falling on patients), the expression of health outcomes in terms of QALYs, the use of models to synthesize indirect comparisons in the absence of head-to-head studies, the ex-post analysis of patient subgroups, and the use of probabilistic sensitivity analysis.

If an HTA entity were established in the United States, it is likely that similar methodological debates would take place. Therefore, it would be necessary to establish a process to develop methodological guidelines that have the approval of the key parties (e.g., major payers and technology manufacturers). This effort would probably build on existing proposals, including the Washington Panel's reference case and the Academy of Managed Care Pharmacy (AMCP) Format (AMCP 2005).

13.4.2.3 Assessment Process

The assessments of HTA and reimbursement agencies overseas are mostly based on secondary research (i.e., systematic reviews and economic models), as opposed to primary research, such as large prospective studies. The main reason for this is the emphasis on the timeliness of the assessment. That is, since a decision has to be made (on the appropriate use of a health technology), the need is to develop the best possible guidance given currently available data.

If, in the United States, the emphasis in "comparative effectiveness" assessment were to be on large, long-term, controlled trials, this would have to be developed under a scheme similar to coverage with evidence development, because the technologies would have to be approved for funding to allow such trials to take place. Under coverage with evidence development, funding for the technology to be studied is contingent upon participation in the clinical trials. Therefore, more discussion of the design of such schemes, including study requirements, funding and risk-sharing arrangements (if any) is urgently required (Garrison et al. 2007; Drummond 2007). Beyond trials, other thought leaders envision the primary use of evidence syntheses of existing trials, complemented by retrospective data, where possible. To that end, the Medicare Modernization Act of 2003 contains language and funding for comparative effectiveness research that is now conducted by AHRQ, but the funding permits only syntheses of existing studies.

Another important feature of assessment processes is that technology manufacturers are invited to submit a dossier of data and analyses, consistent with the methodological guidelines existing in the jurisdiction concerned. Most manufacturers welcome this opportunity, as it provides them with the possibility to present the advantages of the product on their own terms. However, not all HTA entities provide for manufacturer submissions. In the U.S. context, drug companies are invited to submit dossiers to the Drug Effectiveness Review Project (DERP), which states that submitting a correctly completed dossier will ensure that the evidence submitted by a company will be fully reviewed (DERP 2007).

Many HTA entities overseas commission assessments from independent outside bodies (mainly academic groups), although they usually have a substantial internal staff to oversee and steer the HTA process. Given the controversy surrounding HTA findings, the process of independent external review is considered to be an important feature of the process. In the United States, any HTA entity would be wise to rely fairly heavily on external review, given the wide range of perspectives present in the healthcare system. There is also a large body of health services research expertise to draw upon in existing public and private organizations. Therefore, however the HTA effort in the United States is organized, it should be done in a way that provides sufficient funding for thorough scientific assessments to be conducted.

13.4.3 DECISION-MAKING PROCESSES

13.4.3.1 Assessment Versus Appraisal

In the U.K., NICE makes a clear distinction between assessments, where the technical analysis is undertaken, and appraisals, where the evidence is evaluated and the decisions made. The institute relies heavily on expert committees in its decision-making processes (e.g., appraisal committee, guideline review panels) and this adds somewhat to the appearance of independence. The experts are a mixture of academics (across several disciplines including medicine, statistics, and economics), NHS decision-makers and patient representatives. There is no reason that a similar approach should not work for an HTA entity in the United States, although it may be more of a challenge to secure adequate representation from the various decision-making groups, some of which are in competition with one another.

A more fundamental issue in the U.S. context is whether an HTA entity would have a decision-making role at all, given the diverse nature of the U.S. healthcare system. It is possible, indeed more likely, that the responsibilities of any entity in the United States would cease at the assessment stage. Assessments could then be made publicly available for the various payers to use (or not use) as they see fit.

13.4.3.2   Involvement of Stakeholders

In the U.K., NICE has arguably led the way in the involvement of key stakeholders in its decision-making processes, although most HTA entities have some form of stakeholder engagement. The main stakeholders are the technology manufacturers, professional societies, patient organizations, the health service, and government. In the case of NICE, all stakeholders have the opportunity to comment at key stages in the appraisal process. Although this involvement sometimes has the result of slowing down the appraisal process, it is generally regarded as a positive feature. Indeed, on some occasions, NICE guidance has been changed as a result of stakeholder comments. Therefore, this might be a feature to promote in any HTA effort in the United States, even if the HTA entity performed only assessments, as opposed to issuing guidance.

If they believe their comments have been ignored, in some jurisdictions, such as the U.K., stakeholders have the opportunity to appeal against decisions, mainly on the grounds that procedures were not properly followed. In other jurisdictions, such as Australia, the only option is to challenge decisions through the legal system.

13.4.3.3   Formulation of Guidance

Reimbursement and HTA agencies overseas often distinguish between patient subgroups in terms of cost-effectiveness and may recommend the new technology for some groups, but not for others. This may not be as acceptable in the United States, because it would likely be conceived as discriminatory. However, it is worth remembering that, in the presence of patient copays, a technology can be made available to all in the United States, providing the patient pays a substantial portion of the cost. Therefore, it may be possible, and acceptable, to discriminate by applying differential copay levels to different sub-groups. Such arrangements already exist in some three-tier pharmacy benefit programs.

13.4.3.4   Need for Transparency

The need for transparency arises from the fact that most HTA entities overseas are public bodies and, therefore, have to be accountable. Similar needs may arise if an HTA entity in the United States were a federal agency, for example.

It is worth noting that the need for transparency arises both in assessments and decision-making. Transparency in assessment methods and processes may also be important in the United States, even if the various resulting decisions may not be so transparent. For example, decision-making in for-profit health plans is unlikely to be transparent as a result of commercial sensitivities.

13.4.3.5   Cost-Effectiveness Threshold

To make an assessment of value for money, HTA entities need to take a view on whether the benefits of a new drug justify the costs. Over time NICE has come to base its decisions on a cost-effectiveness threshold, representing the maximum amount it is willing to pay for a QALY (i.e., unit of health gain). This has been made explicit by the Chair and Deputy Chair of NICE and is said to be in the region of £20,000 to £30,000 per QALY (Rawlins and Culyer 2004). The notion of thresholds has also been discussed in Australia, Canada, and a few other jurisdictions, but is rarely made explicit.

No such threshold exists for any public body in the United States, but in the health economics literature, a threshold of $100,000 per QALY is often referenced. Of course, in the United States, it is likely that the threshold, if one exists, will differ among the different sectors of the healthcare system, according to the level of budget available.

If there were ever an HTA entity in the United States issuing guidance (e.g., to CMS), it would probably be possible to infer a threshold from the decisions made, even if one were not explicitly stated (Devlin and Parkin 2004). However, as mentioned above, it is probably more likely that an HTA entity will restrict its role to undertaking assessments, rather than making appraisals.

13.4.4 COMMUNICATION AND IMPLEMENTATION OF GUIDANCE

Most HTA entities devote considerable effort to the communication and implementation of their guidance. Also, the implementation of NICE's technology appraisals is mandatory in the NHS. Even so, implementation of NICE guidance is patchy. The biggest problems arise when the guidance indicates use of the technology for some patient groups and not for others. In Australia, some drugs can be used only "on authority," which means that the physician needs to assure the authorities that the patient meets the required criteria for use of the drug. Similarly in the United States, for example with Medicaid (care of the indigent) in California (Medi-Cal), a treatment authorization request (TAR) may be necessary for certain procedures and services before reimbursement can be approved (http://www.dhcs.ca.gov/provgovpart/Pages/TAROverview.aspx). In general, though, one might expect the implementation of HTA findings to be easier in the United States, as this could be linked to coverage decisions, although no doubt difficulties would arise in practice.

Within the United States, it is likely that any HTA entity will have an extensive communication strategy, most likely for the results of its assessments, rather than guidance. How different decision-makers would react to this remains to be seen. It is already known that many payers in the United States consult the websites of NICE and other HTA entities, but the influence this has on decision-making is unclear. One option for some plans would be to use technology assessments as one way of engaging with enrollees about the trade-offs between more coverage, the extent of copays, and the level of premiums.

13.5 CONCLUSIONS

This brief discussion of the experience with the use of pharmacoeconomics in three countries illustrates that there is much to be learned from other jurisdictions. Although the precise models from elsewhere cannot simply be transported to another country, it is clear that some approaches work better than others and that elements of good practice can be specified. The debate about the extended use of pharmacoeconomics is currently taking place in many jurisdictions, including the U.S. Of course, as this debate progresses, it will become clearer as to which aspects of overseas experience are most relevant to the direction that is eventually taken.

However, despite the eventual outcome of the current debate about the use of pharmacoeconomics in the U.S. and other countries, the experience of other jurisdictions that have already implemented these policies contains several messages that have general relevance. Those in charge of the implementation of pharmacoeconomics in new settings should try to make good use of this accumulated experience.

REFERENCES

Academy Health. 2005. Placement, Coordination, and Funding of Health Services Research with the Federal Government. Washington, DC: Academy Health.

Academy of Managed Care Pharmacy. 2005. The AMCP Format for Evidence-Based Formulary Submissions. Version 2.1. Alexandria, VA: AMCP.

Anis, A., T. Rahman, and M.T. Schechter. 1998. Using pharmacoeconomic analysis to make drug insurance coverage decisions. Pharmacoeconomics 13(1): 119–26.

Cairns, J. 2006. Providing guidance to the NHS: The Scottish Medicines Consortium and the National Institute for Clinical Excellence compared. Health Policy 76(2): 134–43.

Canadian Agency for the Assessment of Drugs and Technologies in Health. 2006. Guidelines for the Economic Evaluation of Health Technologies: Canada (3rd Edition). http://www.ispor.org/PEguidelines/source/HTAGuidelinesfortheEconomicEvaluationofHealthTechnologies–Canada.pdf (accessed September 2, 2008).

Canadian Immunization Committee. 2007. Recommendations on a Human Papillomavirus Immunization Program. http://www.phac–aspc.gc.ca/publicat/2008/papillomavirus–papillome/pdf/CIC–HPV_Recommendations_Final.pdf (accessed October 18, 2008).

Centers for Disease Control and Prevention. 2008. Vaccination coverage for adolescents aged 13 to 17 years: United States 2007. MMWR 57(40): 1100–1103.

Cohen, J., L. Faden, S. Predaris, and B. Young. 2007. Patient access to pharmaceuticals: An international comparison. Euro J Health Econ 5(3): 177–87.

Cohen, J., C. Cairns, C. Paquette, and L. Faden. 2006. Comparing patient access to pharmaceuticals in the UK and US. Appl Health Econ Health Pol 5(3): 177–87.

Commonwealth of Australia. 2007. Guidelines for preparing submissions to the Pharmaceutical Benefits Advisory Committee. http://www.health.gov.au/internet/main/publishing.nsf/Content/pbacguidelines–index (accessed September 5, 2008).

Conn, F. 2006. A Survey for General Practitioners' Attitudes to Clinical Guidelines from the National Institute for Health and Clinical Excellence. PhD diss., London School of Economics.

Department of Health. 2002. "Payment by results" breakthrough ends years of uncertainty for MS patients: Agreement follows recommendations from NICE. Press release 2002/0056. London: Department of Health.

Devlin, N. and D. Parkin. 2004. Does NICE have a cost-effectiveness threshold and what others factors influence its decisions? A binary choice analysis. Health Economics 13: 437–52.

Drug Effectiveness Review Project. 2007. http://www.ohsu.edu/ohsuedu/research/policycenter/DERP/index.cfm (accessed August 23, 2008).

Drug Information Association. 2008. DIA Daily, October 10, 2008.

Drummond, M.F. 2007. Post-launch studies for drugs: The need for a reality check. Value in Health (in press).

Garrison, L. et al. 2007. Report of the ISPOR Good Practices Task Force on Real World Data. Value in Health (in press).

George, B., A. Harris, and A. Mitchell. 2001. Cost-effectiveness analysis and the consistency of decision-making: Evidence from pharmaceutical reimbursement in Australia (1991 to 1996). Pharmacoeconomics 19:1103–9.

Gold, M.R., J.E. Siegel, L.B. Russell, and M.C. Weinstein, Eds. Cost-effectiveness in Health and Medicine. New York: Oxford University Press. 1996.

House of Commons Health Select Committee. 2008. The National Institute for Health and Clinical Excellence: First Report of Session 2007–2008, Volume 1. London: The Stationary Office Limited.

Javitt, G., D. Berkowitz, and L.O. Gostin. 2008. Assessing mandatory HPV vaccination: Who should call the shots? J Law, Meds, Ethics 36(2): 384–95.

Joint Committee on Vaccination and Immunization. 2008. JCVI statement on human papillomavirus vaccines to protect against cervical cancer. http://www.advisorybodies.doh.gov.uk/jcvi/HPV_JCVI_report_18_07_2008.pdf (accessed October 19, 2008).

Kohut, A. and B. Stokes. America against the world. How we are different and why we are disliked. New York: Times Books. 2006.

Laupacis, A. 2006. Economic evaluations in the Canadian Common Drug Review. Pharmacoeconomics 24(11): 1157–62.

McMahon, M., S. Morgan, and C. Milton. 2006. The Common Drug Review: A NICE start for Canada? Health Policy 77: 339–51.

Medpac. 2007. Report to the Congress: Promoting greater efficiency in Medicare. http://www.medpac.gov/documents/jun07_EntireReport.pdf (accessed August 5, 2008).

National Institute for Clinical Excellence. Guide to the Methods of Technology Appraisal. London: NICE. 2008.

Neumann, P.J. and S.D. Sullivan. 2006. Economic evaluation in the US: What is the missing link? Pharmacoeconomics 24(11):1163–68.

Ontario Ministry of Health. 1994. Ontario guidelines for economic analysis of pharmaceutical products. Toronto: Ministry of Health Ontario.

Orszag, P.R. 2007. Research on the comparative effectiveness of medical treatments: Options for an expanded federal role. CBO Testimony, Subcommittee on Health, Committee on Ways and Means, US House of Representatives. Washington: Congressional Budget Office.

Pharmaceutical Benefits Advisory Committee. (2006). Quadrivalent human papillomavirus (Types 6, 11, 16, 18) recombinant vaccine, injection, 0.5 mL, Gardasil®. http://www.health.gov.au/internet/main/publishing.nsf/Content/pbac–psd–gardasil–nov06 (accessed October 14, 2008).

Rawlins, M.D. and A.J. Culyer, (2004). National Institute for Clinical Excellence and its value judgments. BMJ 329: 224–27.

Sorenson, C., M. Drummond, P. Kanavos, and A. McQuire, 2008. National Institute for Health and Clinical Excellence (NICE). How does it work and what are the implications for the U.S.? Arlington: National Pharmaceutical Council.

Tarn, T. and M.D. Smith. (2004). Pharmacoeconomic guidelines around the world. ISPOR Connections 10(4): 5–12. http://www.ispor.org/news/index_new.asp (accessed October 10, 2006).

Tunis, S.R. 2007. Reflections on science, judgment, and value in evidence-based decision-making: A conversation with David Eddy. Health Aff 19: 500–15.

Wilensky, G.R. 2006. Developing a center for comparative effectiveness information. Health Aff, 25(6): 572–85.

14 Pharmacoeconomics in Disease Management
Practical Applications and Persistent Challenges

Ryung Suh and David Atkins

CONTENTS

14.1 INTRODUCTION

Disease management (DM) programs refer broadly to programs that seek to improve the care of patients with specific chronic diseases by complementing their usual primary and specialty care with some variety of additional services. Also called care management and care coordination, DM aims to address the common failures of traditional episodic, symptom-based care of chronic diseases such as asthma and heart failure by teaching patients to manage their own disease, increasing communication among multiple providers, and emphasizing proactive prevention of exacerbations and complications of chronic disease. Disease management programs typically target high-risk or high-cost patients, emphasize clinical practice guidelines, employ telephone support to monitor and motivate patients, and aim to be cost effective by reducing costly complications, hospitalizations, or emergency visits.[1]

The promise of DM rests on the observation that many patients with chronic disease do not get all the evidence-based interventions that are indicated[2] and often lack the understanding and skills they need to know how to manage their disease, including how to adhere to their medication, when to seek out care, and how to modify their lifestyle to slow disease progression. The DM industry has grown because various programs have claimed positive financial returns on investment, but the methods to assess the economic returns remain controversial. There have been many recent initiatives to develop a consensus standard for the economic evaluation of disease management programs. Pharmacoeconomic approaches have been applied to DM programs and to component interventions—largely through observational studies offered by health plans, DM vendors, and academic researchers—but the reliability and validity of many of the studies have been questioned.

14.1.1 Evaluations of DM Programs

A number of comprehensive reviews of the literature on the cost implications of DM programs have pointed out frequent flaws in published literature claiming cost savings. The Congressional Budget Office examined peer-reviewed studies of DM programs for congestive heart failure, coronary artery disease, and diabetes mellitus and determined in 2003 that there was insufficient evidence to conclude that DM programs reduced overall health spending.[3] A systematic review of the literature by Ofman and colleagues in 2004 found that relatively few studies of DM programs evaluated the effects on healthcare utilization and costs and that, among the few studies that demonstrated reductions in utilization or costs, findings were inconsistent, modest, or failed to include program development and implementation costs. A review by Goetzel found that DM programs may reduce direct costs in heart failure and could be cost-saving in depression if productivity gains were included.[5] A RAND Corporation literature review in 2007 examined 317 unique studies and found no evidence of improved cost savings from DM programs.[6]

The introduction of the Medicare Health Support (formerly the Voluntary Chronic Care Improvement) Pilot Program raised hopes that a more rigorous economic evaluation methodology using a randomized design with intervention and comparison groups would lead to a definitive conclusion on the financial benefits of DM. Many programs, however, had difficulty enrolling beneficiaries, and preliminary data indicated that the programs were unlikely to generate sufficient savings to cover the program costs, leading Medicare to end the program earlier than planned and resulting in continued controversy about whether this constituted a good model of economic evaluation principles for DM programs.[7]

This chapter outlines how pharmacoeconomic (PE) principles, discussed in detail elsewhere in this book, have been applied with respect to DM programs. It will begin with an introduction to DM and the characteristics of DM programs that make it unique in the context of economic evaluation. Next, the chapter will examine different approaches and applications of PE principles in the context of DM programs. The final section will discuss challenges inherent in integrating these disciplines as the field moves from theory to practice.

14.2   DM PROGRAMS

DM programs have been in existence at least since the 1990s and have been proposed as a way to address the failings of the traditional approach to clinical medicine.[8] By providing a standardized, disease-focused approach to patient care, it was envisioned that chronic disease could be managed better through prevention so that acute episodes of illness (usually manifested as hospitalizations and emergency department visits) would be reduced or avoided altogether. Furthermore, DM programs would facilitate knowledge and application of standard of care medicine and improved coordination of care.[6]

The term "disease management" has been used to describe a number of component interventions, but the Disease Management Association of America (DMAA) has established a definition that includes a core set of required components.[9] In addition to the use of evidence-based clinical practice guidelines as mentioned, effective programs must identify the population at risk. Typically, a clinic, health system, or health plan uses administrative or clinical databases to identify a target population with a specific diagnosis based on diagnoses, procedures, medication use, lab results, or patient survey data. Commercial DM vendors typically also use administrative data on costs and utilization to target high-risk and high-cost populations who may benefit the most from better management. DM programs also require patient involvement and patient self-management education (to include primary prevention, behavior modification programs, and compliance/surveillance) to equip participants to take a more active role in managing their condition. Beyond the patient-program dynamic, DM authorities generally recognize the need for a collaborative effort among physicians, nurses, technicians, and other members of the care team to effectively manage chronic conditions. There must be efforts made to actively evaluate the programs using process and outcomes measurement, evaluation, and management. Finally, there must be routine reporting and feedback loops, including providing feedback to the patient and to the treatment team.

DM programs can be grouped into two general categories: integrated programs (those built into health plans or health systems) and non-integrated programs (stand-alone commercial products).[10] While many variations exist, the latter programs are designed, marketed, and implemented by third-party vendors with no formal connection to a particular health plan, system, or clinic. This has a significant impact on evaluation strategies, as who is purchasing the DM services, whether patients are embedded within the practice, and whether outreach, recruitment, and coordination costs are included or not have important impacts on the economic costs being measured.

DM programs have been applied to a number of diseases, with diabetes, heart failure, asthma, hypertension, cancer, and depression demonstrating encouraging outcomes data. Other diseases and conditions—for arthritis, pain management, HIV/AIDS, chronic obstructive pulmonary disease, lipid disorders, and others—have been evaluated less frequently but show the potential for benefits as well. With chronic illnesses accounting for nearly 75% of total healthcare expenditures, the expansion of DM programs has accelerated in recent years.

14.3   APPLICATION OF PHARMACOECONOMIC PRINCIPLES IN DM PROGRAMS

Despite their intuitive appeal and apparent simplicity, DM programs are highly variable in design and complex in implementation, and have proven difficult to evaluate. PE, in the strictest sense, evaluates cost-effectiveness of drug therapy in terms of the long-term costs and benefits to the patient, to the payer, or to the system. PE principles can be applied to DM programs, inasmuch as the DM program could be viewed like a pharmaceutical treatment and the costs and economic impacts of the treatment can be calculated. Unlike a medication, however, a DM program has multiple targets, including the behavior of patients and multiple providers, each of which have multiple different impacts on healthcare utilization, costs, and health outcomes. This makes a typical PE approach to DM programs difficult. The following section takes a look at different applications of PE principles to DM evaluation.

14.3.1   The Central Role of Pharmaceuticals

Many DM programs target the appropriate use of evidence-based drug therapy as a way to improve outcomes and reduce costs related to disease exacerbations or progression. For example, heart failure and asthma DM programs all include guidelines that specify the routine use of drugs such as angiotensin-converting enzyme (ACE) inhibitors for congestive heart failure (CHF) or inhaled corticosteroids for asthma, since these have been shown to reduce emergency room visits and hospitalizations. For depression and diabetes, guidelines promote treatments that have been proven to improve symptoms and prevent worsening of the disease and attendant hospitalizations. Effective DM programs assess whether patients are on appropriate therapy and dose, whether they are taking medications as directed, and whether they are responding as hoped.

14.3.2   Cost Analyses of Pharmaceutical Interventions

The crudest justification for DM programs and for pharmaceutical interventions are simple cost of illness (COI) studies (see Chapter 3 for more information on COI). Although COI studies can be useful in identifying candidate conditions with potential for reducing costs, they do not define alternative choices. Using average costs in patients with a given diagnosis (as opposed to marginal costs associated with having the diagnosis on top of other conditions) to assign direct costs of an illness often leads to overestimation of burden attributable to the disease in question and overestimation of the savings from better management of that single condition. Such studies have relatively limited roles in evaluating DM programs themselves, but articulating the burden of illness in financial terms has often been effective in justifying the need for some intervention, especially among health care purchasers.

Cost-minimization analysis (CMA) compares the costs of alternative interventions that are assumed to achieve the same target outcome (see Chapter 6 for more information on CMA). This analysis is most easily applied to pharmaceuticals where there may be evidence that several alternatives are equivalent in relieving symptoms or improving some physiologic endpoint—for example, a specific improvement in blood pressure. A DM program designer or manager may generate a list of all phar-maceuticals approved for use in a particular application within a DM program and identify the least expensive, accounting for direct, indirect, and intangible costs, while accounting for time horizon and discounting to present value (see Chapter 10 on discounting). An example would be to analyze currently approved HMG CoA reductase inhibitors (commonly referred to as statin drugs). While there are distinc-tions among these drugs in terms of cost, dosing, and evidence on long-term out-comes, if one assumes that there is no clear superiority among available statins (or among a selection of statins) on important outcomes, a simple CMA comparing the various drugs could identify cost-saving strategies for disease managers.

Cost-effectiveness analysis (CEA) calculates both the costs for a series of equiva-lent treatment or preventive options and the effectiveness expressed as change in a single common dimension of health outcomes, e.g., cases avoided, admissions avoided, life-years gained, deaths avoided, cases identified, etc. (see Chapter 7 for more information on CEA). Researchers in the U.K. have compared a group of statin medications with regard to the cost to achieve a certain reduction in LDL cholesterol and total cholesterol.[11,12] In these studies, researchers were able to name a specific drug as being the most cost-effective in the cohort examined. Such information can be useful in choosing among different interventions that may vary in effectiveness (for example, in formulary decisions). CEA can also be used to decide if a new inter-vention, such as a DM intervention, provides reasonable "value" relative to other health programs, even if it is not strictly cost-saving.

Cost-benefit analysis (CBA) is distinct from the previous analytic methods described as it strictly adheres to costs and benefits in monetary terms.[13] These tend to be comprehensive comparisons of all social costs and consequences, taking a societal perspective to maximize social welfare; these are not routinely used in the evaluation of DM programs as they require assigning monetary values to all health outcomes.

Cost-utility analysis (CUA) compares alternative interventions using the health outcome of individual "utility" based on preferences for different states of well-being (see Chapter 9 for more information on CUA). As mentioned previously, the quality-adjusted life year (QALY) is a common unit of measurement in North American studies. Unlike CEA, CUA can account for a variety of disparate outcomes, such as effects on symptoms, mortality, and unanticipated harms of treatment. Several chal-lenges complicate the use of CUAs: utilities must be assigned to a comprehensive set of outcomes; a small change in the disutility assigned to a common outcome (for example, the inconvenience of monitoring one's blood sugar regularly) can have big effects on overall assessments; and finally, the results can be hard for lay people to interpret. There is also no consensus about what cost per QALY represents a "rea-sonable" value. That is, there are generally no hard cut-offs for an acceptable cost to save one QALY. A common cut-off in the United States is $50,000, but lower thresholds are used in the U.K. and other European countries.[14] A conference on evaluation of DM sponsored by the Agency for Healthcare Research and Quality (AHRQ) in 2002 recommended the use of natural history models that combine the expected benefits of improvement from multiple outcomes measures into a single composite measure (the QALY), with the need for data validation and appropriate case-mix adjustments.[15]

14.3.3 Actuarial Analysis of DM Programs

Actuarial approaches to DM evaluation are more common than health economic approaches. Actuarial methods allow for analyses of DM programs that have been applied to an entire target population and where there is no concurrent comparison group. Actuarial analysis, instead, analyzes historical trends and relies on a set of methodological tools and techniques applied to financial risk and uncertainty. Actuarial analysis has a number of features: a financial focus, an interest in long-term outcomes, prediction based on historical experience, sensitivity testing on assumptions, the use of sophisticated statistics, and a marriage of pragmatism and theory.[16] Predictive modeling and assessments of DM interventions in terms of impacts on actuarial trend lines have become the dominant evaluation model. In its simplest form, actuarial analysis measures cost trends before and after a DM intervention and calculates the savings from the project cost trend line. The evaluation strategy is straightforward and unbiased as long as the analysis is applied to all eligible patients, but assumes that models can adjust for other secular factors that may affect cost trends. Trends (and estimated savings) can also be influenced by the duration of baseline data.

14.3.4 Recent Developments in the Economic Evaluation of DM Programs

Although actuarial analysis predominates with commercial programs, a number of other reports have sought economic evaluations with more reliable concurrent controls. The Medicare Prescription Drug, Improvement, and Modernization Act of 2003 (MMA) instituted a Chronic Care Improvement Plan for traditional fee-for-service Medicare beneficiaries. This is a volunteer program to evaluate the use of DM programs in the Medicare population. The name for this initiative was later changed to the Medicare Health Support (MHS) program. Briefly, this program called for DM vendors—selected vendors are henceforth referred to as Medicare Health Support Organizations (MHSOs)—to target enrollees with the selected conditions of heart failure and/or diabetes and to provide services incorporating those already in use in commercial DM and case management programs. Thirty thousand participants were identified and randomized into either the intervention group (enrolled in an MHSO program) or the control group.

The first of four reports to Congress was released in 2007 and presented preliminary findings from the first 6 months of the trial.[17] There were no significant differences between the intervention and the control groups in processes of care, acute care utilization (outcomes), or changes in Hierarchical Condition Code (HCC). Additionally, the authors of the first report did note as key findings that the cost per beneficiary in the intervention and comparison groups drifted apart between randomization and the start dates of the pilot; the intervention group (those that volunteered to participate) tended to be healthier and less expensive than the intervention group as a whole, and that the programs have generally not been cost effective for Medicare. While this initial report did not offer promising information for supporters of DM programs, additional data is needed to draw firm conclusions. The recently released 18-month interim report on MHS again failed to identify financial cost savings and continues to create controversy. The MHS experience illustrates a fundamental challenge of non-integrated DM programs in effectively engaging the sickest patients.

The RAND Corporation conducted a literature review on the available evidence for the impacts of DM programs.[5] The authors reviewed three evaluations of large population-based programs, ten meta-analyses, and sixteen systematic reviews. In total, 317 unique studies were included in the review. The report concluded that there is no evidence for improved cost savings by using DM programs despite improvements in processes of care and, in a very limited number of circumstances, reduced utilization. The overarching theme of the review was that scientific evidence had not kept pace with the growth of the DM industry. The report also contained a useful perspective on how to classify DM programs, as the authors recommended analyzing a DM program by both the severity of illness and by the intensity of the intervention. This perspective may prove useful for future work using economic evaluation applied to DM programs, as programs can be grouped and compared more easily if they are classified according to what they have in common.

AHRQ's report on Patient Self Management Support Programs also addressed evaluation issues in DM.[19] As discussed previously, DM programs depend on patient education as a key component of their approach to managing disease. Many of the observations here are applicable not only to patient self-management efforts, but also to DM programs as a whole, in that both focus on changes in behavior. These observations also provide opportunities for inclusion of PE techniques into the development, implementation, and evaluation of DM programs. The most specific example of how PE analysis may play a role in promoting positive behavior change pertains to medication compliance. This in turn belongs to a broader set of evaluation measures that help program managers determine the success of their program as well as areas for improvement. The authors emphasized the importance of aligning program objectives with measured objectives so that the results are meaningful. This is an area where PE analysis may be particularly useful. For example, when planning what to measure, managers may desire to perform a CEA specifically related to medication use within the DM program. Program managers working closely with PE experts in the development process will ensure that their program is generating appropriate data easily analyzed in future work, hence opening the door for meaningful program evaluation and improvement.

DMAA has also made significant contributions to developing practical approaches to the economic evaluation of DM programs. Their Outcomes Guideline Report (Volumes I and II) outlined recommended practices for measuring outcomes in DM and other population-based programs to include key clinical measures, applications to wellness programs, and approaches to small populations. Volume III expanded on the clinical and financial measures from the preceding volumes, validated an identification methodology, recommended a measure of medication possession ratio, and outlined principles for evaluating programs for more than one chronic medical condition.[20]

14.3.5   EFFECTIVE USE OF PHARMACOECONOMIC DATA

DM programs depend on the selection of best medications, their use in a correct regimen, and patient and provider compliance. Patient compliance alone may directly tie to the patient's ability to pay for the medication, an important area for pharmacoeconomics if patient cost sharing is a factor. All of the following examples demonstrate the role pharmacoeconomics can play in guiding DM programs, potentially at more than one stage of the program life cycle.

For example, clopidogrel is an antiplatelet agent used to treat a variety of vascular diseases, including the FDA-approved indications of acute coronary syndrome, stroke, and peripheral artery disease, all within specified time frames with respect to hospitalization or diagnosis. A recent study by Choudhry found that as many as 40% of a 5,000-person Medicare population were recently prescribed the drug despite its having no clear advantage over alternate or no therapy.[21] Many of the patients in this cohort would have been equally well treated by using aspirin. In this particular example, there is abundant literature on use of clopidogrel to include good scientific understanding of which specific patients benefit from its use versus aspirin alone. This information is important from an economic perspective as there is a great difference in price between clopidogrel and aspirin, with clopidogrel costing as much as several hundred times that of aspirin per tablet.[22] Choudhry estimated that potentially inappropriate use of clopidogrel cost the state of Pennsylvania as much as $2.87 million in 1 year (using FDA indications for clopidogrel use). It is then reasonable to suppose that were PE data such as these applied to DM programs, real and substantial cost savings could be achieved in a short time. Operationally, it would not be difficult to assign DM program participants into categories based on the clinical indicators for particular treatments, as risk stratification is already a part of some DM programs.

Seen from a different angle, the ability of a DM program to support medication compliance may be significantly enhanced by provision of payment for medications where there is strong evidence for their use in treating specific conditions. In another recent work, Choudhry examined how providing full coverage for drugs enhanced compliance with treatment regimens for post-myocardial infarction patients.[23] He found that among Medicare beneficiaries, eliminating patient responsibility for paying for essential drugs such as aspirin, beta-blockers, ACE inhibitors or angiotensin receptor blockers, and statins that there was an improvement in cost-utility of $7,182 per QALY saved despite the program's not being strictly cost saving. Choudhry made the macroeconomic argument that, from a societal perspective, this is beneficial. An application to DM programs might be offering enrollees full or partial drug coverage for those medications included within the DM program requirements.

In addition to these two examples of PE analysis playing an important role in DM programs, there has been work in gathering similar data from the treatment of illnesses less commonly thought of in the context of a DM program. In 2005, Dubinsky examined the cost effectiveness of various strategies for treating Crohn's disease, including a comparison of traditional methods with those more tailored to individual patients based on individual variance in metabolism of the main therapeutic drug.

She concluded that costs were significantly greater for non-tailored care and that time to reach a response to treatment was longer.[24] Treatment of Alzheimer's disease with a new drug was the topic of a recent pharmacoeconomics review by Lamb.[25] She showed that a specific acetylcholinesterase inhibitor, rivastigmine, was associated with cost savings (not including the cost of the drug itself), which became more significant over time and when initiated early in the progression of the disease. Both of these examples demonstrate situations where cost-effectiveness of a pharmaceutical intervention will be greatest if the drug is prescribed in a controlled environment, such as within a DM program, where patients and their use of particular medications are closely monitored and where changes in therapeutic regimens are potentially simpler to institute, monitor, and modify.

14.4   FROM THEORY TO PRACTICE

The application of PE theory into DM evaluation practice is beset by a number of challenges. Interventions and the components of DM programs that one strives to evaluate take place within complex health systems and our PE techniques tend to be rather crude, with fundamental biases when applied to DM programs.

14.4.1   EVALUATION STRATEGIES

The purpose of any evaluation is to demonstrate value in terms of cost savings, clinical improvements, or increased quality of care. Effective evaluations allow one to improve how the program is designed or delivered and help to sustain support for the program within the limitations of time, data, and resources. Good evaluation strategies aim to accurately reflect the impact of programs, avoid measures that conceal or mislead, and use resources for efficient measurement. Hence, the selection of measures and evaluation strategies must balance process and outcomes measures, consider the feasibility of data collection, and the importance of the measure in promoting actual improvements in the program.

Measuring the financial or economic impact of DM programs requires one to recognize the inherent challenges (e.g., allowing a sufficient time horizon for improvements, the turnover of subjects within the program, defining the population and the denominator). One must have realistic expectations about how much evaluation can be achieved in a given DM program and the value of longer, more contentious, and more expensive evaluations. Estimates of costs must be sure to include the costs of the DM program itself and the costs of increased medical care and pharmaceutical interventions. Accurate estimations of cost savings require a reliable comparison group, and certain comparisons are likely to be biased. For example, pre-post comparisons in high-cost patients are subject to regression to the mean. Likewise, unadjusted comparisons between patients who remain in a given DM program and those who do not are subject to selection bias.

Practical evaluation strategies call for the development of a standardized methodology, but this is beset by a number of conflicting dichotomies. Simplicity in practice comes at the price of accuracy, and practicality is at odds with evaluation granularity. The search for comparability makes it difficult to achieve customizability.

14.4.2 Persistent Challenges

Data availability varies considerably from DM program to DM program, and evaluations are often limited to administrative claims data. Beyond actuarial models that focus on financial risk, it is difficult to access data that relate to the broad definitions of economic value. For example, patient quality of life, worker productivity, and patient satisfaction are important, but these data are often unavailable. Case-mix adjustments are required, and one needs to identify all vendor fees and administrative costs associated with a given DM intervention, but data to support these evaluations are not always available.

The perspectives of different payers (e.g., Medicare, Medicaid, employers, health plans, etc.) may differ substantially and may have conflicting objectives—who captures the savings and when have important implications. Patients and clinicians often view impacts over an entire lifetime, while purchasers and health plans may prefer shorter time horizons that relate to turnover rates. Also, given that significant cost shifting (delays in cost burden) may occur across time, different purchasers are concerned with different analytical approaches that capture this perspective.

Measurement challenges are common and well-established in DM evaluation. Regression to the mean resulting from the targeted evaluation of high-risk or enrolled subpopulations only and selection bias resulting from selective enrollment or turnover remain critical challenges. Pre- and post-study designs without a control group are most practical, although evaluations with whole populations or probability sampling with case-mix adjustment and a comparison group would be more valid. Secular trends, technology changes, medical inflation, differential program ages, local pricing or accounting differences, enrollee turnover, treatment interference, and other factors may be significant confounders.

The generalizability of results from economic evaluations remains limited. It is difficult to attribute conclusions and results from specific interventions given that diseases, populations, and settings vary considerably. Multiple co-morbidities add complexity, although most chronic diseases have significant co-morbidities that must be managed concurrently. In addition, different diseases may have varying timelines for long-term economic returns.

14.5 CONCLUSIONS

The economic evaluation of DM programs depends largely on the structure of the DM programs and the objective of the evaluation. DM programs target multiple levels—patient behaviors, provider behaviors, and health system change—and each level must be appropriately incentivized. Patient self-management practices work only on those willing to be engaged. Moreover, incentives to change provider behavior depend on the model or embedded system of care within which providers operate. Systems integration and measurement depend on whether DM programs are standalone or integrated, and all DM interventions take place in complex health systems.

The practical application of PE principles often relies on over-idealistic assumptions about DM. It is important to recognize that economic evaluations are not simple and that they are not cheap. The analytic strategies that one chooses must recognize the fundamental limitations of traditional PE approaches and the need to select appropriate approaches and models in evaluating DM. Actuarial analysis and predictive modeling are likely to remain the dominant analytical strategy, both for their reliance on relatively easily accessible data and their relative simplicity, but one must also recognize that the challenge of evaluating practice change at multiple levels within complex health care systems requires the use of different analytical tools and approaches as needed.

REFERENCES

1. Norris SL, Glasgow RE, Engelgau MM, O'Conner PJ, McCulloch D. Chronic disease management: A definition and systematic approach to component interventions. *Disease Management Health Outcomes*;11(8):477–488.
2. McGlynn EA, Asch SM, Adams J, Keesey J, Hicks J, DeCristofaro A, Kerr EA. 2003. The quality of health care delivered to adults in the United States. *New England Journal of Medicine* 348(26):2635–2645.
3. Congressional Budget Office. Report to Congress. An Analysis of the Literature on Disease Management Programs. *Health Care Financing Review* October 14, 2004.
4. Ofman JJ, Badamgarav E, Henning JM, et al. 2004. Does disease management improve clinical and economic outcomes in patients with chronic diseases? A systematic review. American Journal of Medicine 117(3):182–92.
5. Goetzel RZ, Ozminkowski RJ, Villagra VG, Duffy J. 2005. Return on investment in disease management: A review. *Health Care Financing Review* 26(4):1–19.
6. Mattke S, Seid M, Ma S. 2007. Evidence for the effect of disease management: Is $1 billion a year a good investment? American Journal of Managed Care; 13: 670–676.
7. Peikes D, Chen A, Schore J, Brown R. 2009. Effects of care coordination on hospitalization, quality of care, and health care expenditures among Medicare beneficiaries. *Journal of the American Medical Association* 301(6):603–618; and McCall N, Cromwell J, Shulamit B. Evaluation of Phase I of Medicare Health Support (Formerly Voluntary Chronic Care Improvement) Pilot Program Under Traditional Fee–For–Service Medicare. June 2007.
8. Congressional Budget Office. Report to Congress. An Analysis of the Literature on Disease Management Programs. October 14, 2004.
9. Disease Management Association of America. http://www.dmaa.org/dm_definition.asp. Accessed December 29, 2008.
10. Geyman J. 2007. Disease management: Panacea, another false hope, or something in between? *Annals of Family Medicine* 5:257–260.
11. Wilson K, Marriot J, Fuller S, Lacey L, Gillen D. 2003. A model to assess the cost effectiveness of statins in achieving the UK National Service framework target cholesterol levels. *Pharmacoeconomics*, Suppl 1:1–11.
12. Palmer S, Brady A, Ratcliffe A. 2003. The cost-effectiveness of a new statin (Rosuvastatin) in the UK NHS. *International Journal of Clinical Practice* 57: 792–800.
13. Lee R. *Economics for healthcare managers*. Chicago: Health Administration Press, 2000.
14. Rascati K. 2006. The $64,000 question—What is a quality-adjusted life-year worth? *Clinical Therapeutics* 28: 1042–1043.
15. Selby JV, Scanlon D, Lafata JE, Villagra V, Beich J, Salber PR. 2003. Determining the value of disease management programs. *Joint Commission Journal on Quality and Safety* 29(9):491–499.

16. Adler J. Actuarial Forecasting for Health, September 12, 2007. Southeast Public Health Observatory.   http://www.sepho.org.uk/download.aspx?urlid=10963&urlt=1. Accessed December 29, 2008.

17. Centers for Medicare and Medicaid Services. Report to Congress. Evaluation of Phase I of Medicare Health Support (Formerly Voluntary Chronic Care Improvement) Pilot Program Under Traditional Fee-for-Service Medicare. June 2007.

18. Mattke S, Seid M, Ma S. 2007. Evidence for the effect of disease management: Is $1 billion a year a good investment? *American Journal of Managed Care* 13: 670–676.

19. RAND Health. Patient self–management support programs: An evaluation. Final contract report to the Agency for Healthcare Research and Quality. Rockville, MD: AHRQ, November 2007.

20. Disease Management Association of America. Outcomes guidelines reports, Vol. I–III.

21. Choudhry N, Levin R, Avron J. 2008.The economic consequences of non-evidence-based Clopidogrel use. *American Heart Journal* 155: 904–909.

22. Drugstore.com. http://www.drugstore.com. Accessed December 28, 2008.

23. Choudhry N, Patrick A, Antman E, Avon J, Shrank W. 2008. Cost-effectiveness of providing full drug coverage to increase medication adherence in post-myocardial infarction Medicare beneficiaries. *Circulation* 117:1261–1268.

24. Dubinsky M, Reyes E, Ofman J, Chiou C, Wade S, Sandborn W. 2005. A cost-effectiveness analysis of alternative disease management strategies in patients with Crohn's disease treated with Azathioprine or 6–Mercaptopurine. *American Journal of Gastroenterology* 100: 2239–2247.

25. Lamb H, Goa K. 2001. Rivastigmine. A pharmacoeconomic review of its use in Alzheimer's disease 19: 303–318.

15 Computer-Aided Decision Making from Drug Discovery to Pharmacoeconomics

Sean Ekins and Renée J.G. Arnold

CONTENTS

15.1 INTRODUCTION

It is logical to expand decision-analytic/mathematical modeling beyond individual patient or population decisions to encompass the whole drug discovery and development process. Successful biomedical drug discovery, to a great extent, requires us to answer what is the key biological target(s) that will change the disease outcome, and how much of the biological target(s) can my drug afford to perturb without causing intolerable harm to the patient population being treated? The focus has perhaps for too long been on the former, finding validated clinical targets, while the latter question relating to dose and toxicity has been avoided. At the molecular level, a coordinated system of proteins, including transporters, channels, receptors, and enzymes, act as gatekeepers to foreign molecules with toxicology implications. The understanding of small molecule–protein interactions would enable us to predict these interactions with targets of interest. Simultaneously, this would also improve our ability to predict the toxic consequences responsible for withdrawal of numerous marketed drugs and late-stage clinical failures that are having a devastating effect on bringing safe and effective treatments to patients.[1] Because of the complexities of different model systems, whether in vitro or in vivo, currently in use, better predictive approaches are needed overall. Accurate predictions for toxicity mechanisms are also complicated as the whole organism is involved, with possibly hundreds to thousands of endogenous (endobiotic) and foreign (xenobiotic, e.g., drug) molecules interacting in different cellular organelles of tissues. Species differences in protein expression and the small endobiotic or xenobiotic molecules that will bind to these (ligand specificity), should also be considered as complicating our understanding, as what happens in a mouse model may not relate to humans. It is also important to understand that both the parent molecule and the products of metabolic pathways may also be involved in favorable or unfavorable drug interactions, where they interfere with the metabolism of endogenous or other co-administered compounds. Such drug–drug interactions, or other adverse drug reactions, can have potentially fatal consequences for the patient or be very costly for health care providers.[2–6]

The above is just one small but critical part of the drug discovery and development process that generates a huge amount of data and has done so for decades. Information systems for data analysis and management within pharmaceutical companies have had to evolve to answer more complex questions as the data has flooded in, and these systems themselves have the potential to deliver increased value to the organization.[7,8] We should be learning from our past experiences and using computational tools extensively to make decisions in this inherently highly dimensional space. The increasing generation of biological data using highly parallel automated screening and analytical systems (such as high throughput methods) in drug discovery complements the use of computational technologies and provides a foundation for model generation. Computational models are becoming more widely available based upon quantitative structure activity relationships (QSAR), or docking methods[9] (see Section 15.2.2) with individual proteins known to be important therapeutic targets or that have some relationship to toxicity.

In reality, drug discovery is a multi-criteria process in which the lead molecule (or series) is optimized and where on-target, off-target, and pharmacokinetic properties can be assessed in parallel.[10] Within drug disposition and toxicology, in vitro approaches for generating data with drug metabolizing enzymes, transporters, ion channels, and receptors can be used for predictive computer model generation.[11] More generally, within the pharmaceutical industry computers are used for electronic data capture, data analysis, data management, statistical modeling, bioinformatics, systems biology, information management, chemoinformatics, electronic laboratory notebooks, management decision-making, computer-aided drug design, drug metabolism, toxicology, risk assessment, optimization of biopharmaceutical properties, pharmacokinetics/pharmacodynamics, optimizing trial design, medical decision-making, clinical data collection and management, analyzing adverse drug events and pharmaceutical formulation, as well as many other areas.[12] For example, the pharmacokinetic/pharmacodynamic (PK/PD) modeling and simulations component can be used in preclinical through development, with utility in suggesting a dose range for clinical trials, predicting drug–drug interactions and ultimately allowing the selection of the optimal clinical candidate.[13]

The following sections illustrate some of the software tools that have been applied successfully in computer-aided molecular design and can be used to rapidly identify leads, as well as optimize them. In addition, we will describe some applications of software in pharmacoeconomics and ultimately suggest how we could use such approaches to create a decision-making algorithm for pharmaceutical research and development.

15.2   LEARNING FROM COMPUTER-AIDED MOLECULAR DESIGN

An understanding of the molecular properties required for a lead-like or drug-like[14,15] small molecule interacting with a target is important for drug and combination device development[16] and generally does not require sophisticated software. For example, many Web-based tools will calculate molecular properties from an input 2D molecular structure, as well as other open access tools, e.g., ChemSpider (www.chemspider.com, Figure 15.1A).[17,18] In addition, the development of new Web-based biology and chemistry databases such as the Collaborative Drug Discovery database (CDD Inc. www.collaborativedrug.com) includes such molecular property calculators[19] (Figure 15.1B). This would allow the user to mine molecules by similar physicochemical properties. More sophisticated, commercially available computational methods that can be used for virtual screening when either the scientist possesses some hits or lead molecules with biological data or the structure (or a model) of the target protein of interest are described here.

15.2.1   Quantitative Structure-Activity Relationships (QSARs)

QSARs are mathematical models relating a molecular structure to a chemical property or biological effect using statistical techniques. When a significant correlation is achieved for a set of training molecules with available biological data, the model can then be used to predict the biological effect for other molecules, although there may be some limitations to model applicability.[20] QSAR is a key component of modern medicinal chemistry and pharmacology, with much of the early work in the field published by Hansch and co-workers in the 1960s onward;[21] since this time there have been thousands of models generated.[22,23] QSAR uses a wide array of molecular descriptors (1D, 2D, and 3D) as numerical representations of chemical structures[24,25] and methods to select those that are most relevant.[26] 3D-QSAR methods, including comparative molecular field analysis (CoMFA)[27] and comparative molecular similarity indices analysis (CoMSIA),[28] are perhaps the most widely used. Of course, the real value of these QSAR methods is in using them to make predictions for new molecules or as frequently used in the process of scoring and ranking molecules in large chemical libraries for their likelihood of possessing affinity for a target of interest (also known as virtual screening).[29] The pharmaceutical industry has learned to accept that virtual screening methods represent an efficient complement to high throughput screening.[30–32] Virtual screening requires either a ligand-based model of the protein of interest, a QSAR or pharmacophore, or the target itself (target-based virtual screening).[33,34]

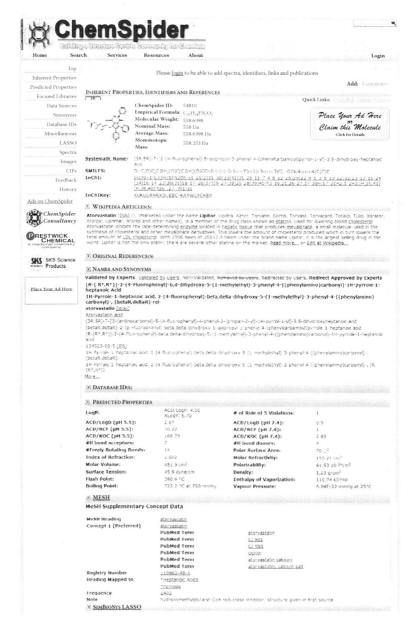

(a)

FIGURE 15.1 Screenshots of software used for molecular property prediction and searching. (a) ChemSpider, (b) CDD, and (c) Accelrys DiscoverStudio 2.0 (www. accelrys.com) showing a pharmacophore (top right panel) with a mapped hit after searching a database of over 1000 drug-like compounds.

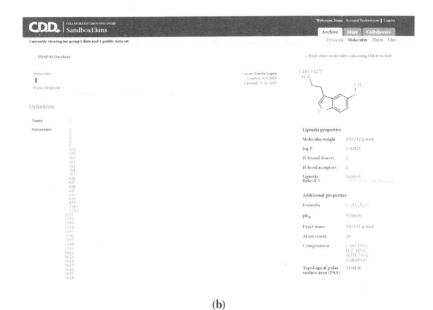

(b)

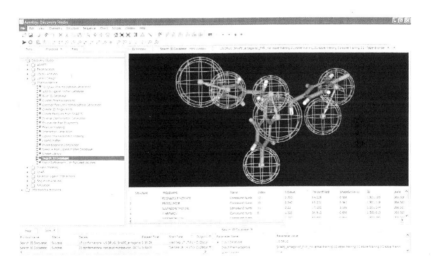

(c)

A diverse range of ligand-based virtual screening methods is available[35] (for more details, see reviews[20,36]). Perhaps the most widely employed methods requiring 3D structure representations of molecules are those exploiting the concept of pharmacophore similarity,[37] where a pharmacophore is the 3D arrangement of molecular features necessary for bioactivity.[38–42] Pharmacophore approaches have subsequently been applied to many therapeutic targets for the virtual screening of compound databases.[43–45] Successful pharmacophore applications include the identification of hits for a variety of targets[46,47] such as absorption, distribution, metabolism, excretion, and toxicity (ADME/Tox)-related proteins, using database searching protocols (Figure 15.1C).[11,48–50] Hence, pharmacophore-based approaches have considerable versatility and applicability.

15.2.2 Target-Based Methods

Target-based virtual screening methods require structural information on the target, either determined experimentally or computationally (using homology modeling techniques in which homologous proteins with known sequences and structures are compared).[51,52] These methods aim at providing an approximation of the expected conformation and orientation of the ligand into the protein cavity and an estimation of its binding affinity. This is a challenge and the performance of different software has been found to vary widely, depending on the target.[53] To alleviate this, the use of multiple scoring functions has also been recommended to improve the number of true positives in virtual screening.[54] Target-based virtual screening has also been used successfully for identifying and generating novel bioactive compounds. For example, docking methods that automatically position the small molecules in the postulated protein binding site and score the ligand–protein interactions have resulted in the discovery of novel inhibitors for several kinase targets,[55] as well as being applied to targets for which experimentally determined structures are not available, e.g., G protein-coupled receptors.[56] In these cases, structural information is generated computationally by modeling the structure of the target of interest on the basis of a template structure of a related target,[57] with the result that novel antagonists have been identified for the neurokinin-1 and the α1A adrenergic receptors[58,59] as well as other targets.[60] These methods represent just some of those available that can be used to suggest molecules to test for a particular bioactivity in order to increase efficiency of drug discovery in the earliest stages.

15.3 LEARNING FROM PHARMACOECONOMICS: COMPUTER-AIDED DECISION MAKING

In order to succeed, the pharmaceutical industry and pharmaceutical researchers have to promote internal collaboration and the sharing of data that can be mined efficiently rather than generating silos of impenetrable information. Data mining is just a part of the drug discovery and development process, as ultimately the information retrieved has to be integrated into an overall decision making process. This requires what has been termed a "seamless product flow process" from lab bench to patient.[61] Some have suggested the industry should learn from other engineering-based industries, such as the auto industry, that have revolutionized productivity using simulations.[62,63] At a meeting, Janet Woodcock from the FDA remarked that "the pharmaceutical industry needs to be more like engineering" (PharmaDiscovery, Maryland, May 10th, 2006) but it is also important to remember that engineers occasionally fail, buildings and bridges collapse, and planes crash due to structural failure, so they are certainly not infallible.

Drug discovery and development has been suggested to be composed of distinct decision gates,[64,65] where key questions can be asked of a candidate molecule and answers may be provided using experimental studies. One could imagine that these decision gates could represent individual computational models that ultimately lead to the development of decision analytic methods, which will be useful to determine whether a molecule should progress through additional steps of the drug discovery and development process. The decisions suggested in such an approach could be based on one of a number of algorithms such as a decision tree approach that has been used widely in health economic analysis[66] and drug innovation assessment algorithm analysis[67] and that incorporates probability models and weights at each step. This may represent an opportunity for the industry to consider predictions from many computational simulations in different areas of research alongside experimental data.

15.3.1 TYPES OF DECISION-MAKING MODELS

Perhaps drug discovery and development should look closer to home to improve success by employing some of the tools used in pharmacoeconomics.[68] In fact, decision analysis and valuation of alternate outcomes has already been suggested as applicable to target selection.[69] Indeed, continuous risk and uncertain timing of events may depend on when events occur. Special types of decision-analytic models, such as Markov models,[70] account for issues of time-sensitivity. For example, Lewis and colleagues[71] employed a Markov model to discern the relative cost-effectiveness of Sandimmune® (an older formulation of cyclosporine) versus Neoral® (a newer formulation of cyclosporine) in the first 3 months following renal transplantation. Using results from one of the multiple sources that informed the model, Neoral was shown to be both more effective and less costly than Sandimmune for both effectiveness criteria—non-functioning graft and rejection-free clinical course; thus, Neoral was the dominant strategy, a result that the pharmaceutical manufacturer would embrace. The practical application of these data for the healthcare providers would be that with a $10 million budget, it would be possible to transplant 115 patients on Sandimmune or 124 patients on Neoral; 49/115 (43%) patients on Sandimmune vs. 84/124 (68%) patients on Neoral would have a rejection-free clinical course. This market evaluation bodes well for future sales of the more cost-effective agent.

Risk assessment data from pre-marketing and post-marketing studies can also be linked using statistical analyses to determine the nature of the side effects that are observed and whether they represent sentinels for more serious events that may only occur in very large trials.[72] The influence of mathematical modeling has also reached pharmaceutical pricing and go/no-go decision-making for licensing.[73] A decision-analytic model was used to estimate the average cost per patient with heparin-induced thrombocytopenia (HIT) with or without thrombosis[74] (Figure 15.2a). Probability data used to populate the model were obtained from trials and from published clinical literature. Resource utilization data and cost data were also obtained from available literature, the 2003 Physician's Fee Reference, the Healthcare Cost and Utilization Project 2000, the 2003 Drug Topics RedBook, and a modified Delphi panel. The total per-patient cost included: hospital days, diagnostic tests, drug costs, major hemorrhagic events, and patient outcomes (i.e., amputation, new thrombosis, stroke, or death), multiplied by the probability of each event. The incremental cost-effectiveness ratio (ICER) was calculated by dividing the incremental cost between patients with and without treatment by the incremental effectiveness, or the cost per new thrombosis event avoided.

Moreover, data mining is an integral component of decision-analytic modeling as it is employed in pharmacoeconomic analyses. Data sources routinely employed in these types of analyses include patient charts,[75,76] individual or meta-analyses of clinical trials in the literature,[77–81] medical and pharmacy claims data,[82,83] Medicare databases,[71,84] and other large, publicly available data sets such as the National Center for Health Statistics' National Health Care Survey and National Health Interview Survey and the Agency for Healthcare Research and Quality's Medical Expenditure Panel Survey and Healthcare Cost and Utilization Project, among others. Claims or administrative databases have, in particular, recently gained favor as they are frequently computerized and reflect actual charges and payments for specific plans and populations (see Chapter 5 on review of data sources for analysis). The advantages of these databases include the fact that they are relatively inexpensive, quickly available, reflective of different populations, encompass a realistic time frame, are organizationally specific, can be used for benchmarking purposes, include large sample sizes, and can capture real-world prescribing patterns.[85] The disadvantages of these databases are missing data, the inability to retrospectively interpret data, diagnosis and procedure codes that may reflect reimbursement strategies instead of clinically accurate diagnoses, limited information on important covariates, sparse outcomes data, the lack of representation, and the lack of structure for research purposes.

15.3.2 APPLYING THE MODELS THROUGHOUT DRUG DISCOVERY

We and others[86] suggest that computer software has a significant role to play in informing the pharmaceutical decision-making process. From our analysis of the situation it is apparent that, alone, none of the software tools described earlier provides the major integrated functions needed to assist in drug discovery and development, to minimize attrition, or aid in decision-making. In addition, these tools address only a narrow component of the drug discovery and development process, namely preclinical. As we have suggested, the availability of computational approaches and models to virtually all aspects of pharmaceutical research and development would indicate that the unification of the outputs would represent a means to prioritize molecule ideas.[62] For example, many facets to drug discovery and development are amenable

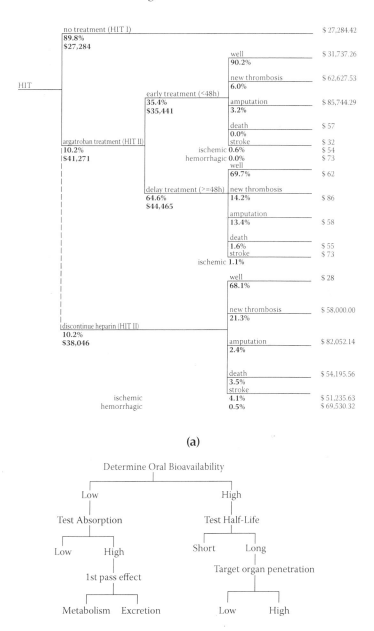

(a)

(b)

FIGURE 15.2 (a) A decision tree for patients with heparin-induced thrombocytopenia (HIT) without thrombosis, and (b) a typical decision tree for determining oral bioavailability (adapted from White R. A comprehensive strategy for ADME screening in drug discovery. In: Borchardt RT, Kerns EH, Lipinski CA, Thakker DR, Wang B, Eds. *Pharmaceutical profiling in drug discovery for lead selection*: AAPS Press, 2004).

to the use of computers and some of these can be further subdivided (Table 15.1) for the application of specific algorithms.

The information required and the questions to ask prior to candidate selection is a well studied area, consisting of primarily metabolism, safety, efficacy, and chemistry[64,65] that can be captured in simple flowcharts to identify molecules safe for human clinical testing.[65] The success of each of these areas can be used to track productivity.[87] The process of drug discovery and development can be thought of as consisting of many unique elements that may require the identification and quantitative evaluation of costs and benefits for each. Bayesian methods represent a robust approach to model estimation used already for clinical trials.[88] Monte Carlo methods for random sampling have also been used to simulate the probability of success, yet these methods have not until recently expanded into other areas of drug discovery and development decision-making. A simulation model using Bayesian probabilistic networks for statistical modeling of drug discovery has been described where nodes represent predicted, measured, or subjective properties to ultimately estimate future development value. It was also suggested that available capacity and flow could be modeled with this software, termed ARBITER (proprietary and patented by PA Consulting[86,89,90]).

TABLE 15.1
Examples of Preclinical Data (Measured and Predicted) that Can Be Captured and Used in the Pharmaceutical Decision-Making Process

Physicochemical Properties of Molecules	Efficacy Data	ADME Data	Toxicity/Safety Data
LogD	In vitro enzyme activity IC_{50}; Ki	In vitro metabolism in rat, mouse, dog, and human microsomes	In vitro selectivity – cytotoxicity
pK_a	Selectivity data against other targets or receptors	Identity of major metabolites	In vitro mutagenicity, computer based alerts, Ames, micronucleus, mouse lymphoma etc.
Solubility	Whole cell data	Potential for drug–drug interactions; inhibition of CYPs or other enzymes	In vitro cardiac toxicity hERG binding and telemetry
Stability	Animal data	Excretion balance data dog–monkey	Behavioral testing
Plasma protein binding		Absorption	Reproductive toxicology
		In vivo PK in rodent over therapeutic dose range—capture plasma half life, C_{max}, clearance V_d Oral bioavailability—role of transporters Human dose ranging	Animal toxicology single and multidose range finding

More recently, a Bayesian network approach sampled by Monte Carlo methods has been proposed to model the drug discovery and development process. Each stage in the process represents a discrete node with inputs (duration, cost, revenue, rate, transitional probability) and outputs (start, finish, cost, net present value, revenue, profit, completion probability) with probability distributions and costs. This model was implemented in Excel and Crystal Ball as a spreadsheet, with Monte Carlo simulation used to produce alternative scenarios. The presentation output from this method was in the form of bubble charts, where the diameter of bubbles was proportional to probability of successful completion. Ultimately, this method was proposed to model the risk/benefit analysis factors.[91] Bayesian analysis was also used to account for uncertainty in a diagnosis/prognosis and to allow the incorporation of differential specificity and sensitivity of diagnostic tests into the decision about which diagnostic method to employ.[92]

We propose the future design of an interactive tool that will allow pharmaceutical and biotechnology company researchers and executives to utilize preexisting/new conditional probabilities, costs, and other criteria to make the decision of whether to proceed in drug development at multiple points in the discovery and development cycle. The majority of steps in the drug discovery and development process will need to be captured as discrete nodes where decisions can be made. From a preliminary analysis, it is likely that this number could be in the hundreds, if not thousands, of possible unique data points. Modeling this process to enable prospective simulations would go significantly beyond the high-level simulation models previously proposed and described, which use a very small number (10–20) of inputs and do not subdivide each major stage in drug discovery and development (e.g., target identification, formulation, etc.).[89-91] Such a tool would need to include the key data that are gathered from target selection justification (e.g., validation of target) and estimated market size for a product through to the completion of clinical trials and cost-effectiveness analysis. Some of these steps have been outlined previously;[62,93] many are potentially predictable using computer algorithms, while others include discrete empirical information gathered in preclinical testing, such as the properties described in Table 15.1, which can be used in decision-making. It is worth noting that the ADME and safety data described in this table could take several months to generate at a considerable cost, depending on the number of questions that need to be answered. This is also a significant cost before a decision would normally be made to proceed to clinical testing. It is, therefore, immensely important to extract as much value as possible from these data as quickly as possible. Several monographs can be used to discern the different preclinical tests (which, in some cases, vary with therapeutic area) as well as requirements at different stages of drug development.[65,94-96]

Tables of pharmacokinetic and pharmacodynamic parameters also exist for many drugs,[95,97] which could aid in setting decision criteria. Depending on the molecules selected and whether they belong to a particular therapeutic area may require tailoring of the decision steps and data that need to be collected for effective modeling. It would be necessary to capture not only the types of data shown in Table 15.1, but also the acceptable values, time, and costs to obtain these data and associated properties related to the experimental or computational generation of this data. A relational database architecture would likely be required to store this information and this could serve as the foundation to develop a software system representing an interactive database of drug discovery and development processes. The data types at each step, as well as known requirements and links to other steps in drug discovery and development with many relationships between them, would need to be annotated. Any corresponding input data could then be linked to these steps by input from the user.

The use of decision-analytic, Bayesian, and other techniques would be important to develop the transparent, computational framework of such a tool alongside methods to visualize the tradeoffs necessary to follow a decision pathway that would make for the greatest value for effort. Problems encountered in preclinical studies usually result in systematic investigations and can be best illustrated by a simplistic decision tree for planning studies to identify potential problems related to poor oral bioavailability (Figure 15.2b).[98] This type of simplistic tree could be programmed into the software along with those that depend on particular molecular properties.[99] The combination of different algorithms that can learn from input data (such as machine learning methods) may also be advantageous (Figure 15.3); for example, tree-based methods have been previously combined with Bayesian networks for protein fold and structure prediction to provide an intuitive network structure that is more accurate than other discriminative methods.[100] The overall schematic design of the software is shown in Figure 15.3. The design of a user-friendly interface to the software that would allow non-computer-literate, as well as non-technical, individuals within healthcare companies to individualize the analysis for their own product development pathways cannot be underestimated. Such a user-friendly program would need to display the following types of modules:

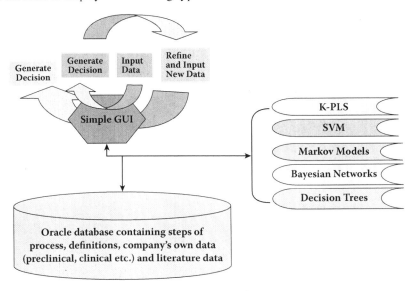

FIGURE 15.3   A schematic showing how the combination of multiple computer aided methods could be used to assist in the decision-making process.

- Premise and Assumptions—reiteration of data input by the end-user
- Methodology—transparency of decision-analytic and other methods composing the modeling framework
- Enumeration of baseline probabilities and costs used in the model
- Input and output screens (including any available "help" screens) in the program
- Any other interactive components of the program—e.g., sensitivity analyses, population modeling
- Final outcome results

The development of these modules would need to proceed with a pharmaceutical or biotechnology collaborator to provide a tool that would be accessible to research scientists, project managers, and senior management. The models could output decisions as color-coded symbols initially (red = do not progress further, green = progress, amber = need more data to decide), followed by prompting the user with directions to take next in the drug discovery and development pathway. Testing the predictive ability of the tool using retrospective predicted and empirical data from the pharmaceutical industry would be essential for multiple compounds to enable validation.

15.3   CONCLUSION

Computational tools should be used for computer-aided drug design and computer-aided decision making. These tools are usually used in isolation to make discrete decisions. There has been little research on when to select computational tools for use or even the optimal use and integration of numerous computational tools. It is important not to lose sight of the complexity of drug discovery and development that incorporates a complex decision-making process. Therefore, the integration of many computational approaches could allow unparalleled pharmaceutical decision-making. This appears to be an area that is underserved by software tools and could ultimately provide an adjunct to scientists at all stages of the research and development pipeline.

ACKNOWLEDGMENTS

S.E. gratefully acknowledges Accelrys for making Discovery Studio available, Dr. Barry Bunin for making the Collaborative Drug Discovery database available and Dr. Antony Williams for his considerable efforts to develop Chemspider and providing it freely.

REFERENCES

1. Rawlins MD. 2004. Cutting the cost of drug development? *Nature Rev* 3:360–4.
2. Doucet J, Chassagne P, Trivalle C, Landrin I, Pauty MD, Kadri N, et al. 1996. Drug–drug interactions related to hospital admissions in older adults: A prospective study of 1000 patients. *JAGS* 44:944–8.

3. Yee JL, Hasson NK, Schreiber DH. 2005. Drug-related emergency department visits in an elderly veteran population. *Ann Pharmacother* 39:1990–4.

4. Pezalla E. 2005. Preventing adverse drug reactions in the general population. *Manag Care Interface* 18:49–52.

5. Zhan C, Correa-de-Araujo R, Bierman AS, Sangl J, Miller MR, Wickizer SW, et al. 2005. Suboptimal prescribing in elderly outpatients: Potentially harmful drug–drug and drug–disease combinations. *J Am Geriatr Soc* 53:262–7.

6. Klarin I, Wimo A, Fastbom J. 2005. The association of inappropriate drug use with hospitalization and mortality: A population-based study of the very old. *Drugs Aging* 22:69–82.

7. Waller CL, Shah A, Nolte M. 2007. Strategies to support drug discovery through integration of systems and data. *Drug Discovery Today* 12:634–9.

8. Fay N. 2006. The role of the informatics framework in early lead discovery. *Drug Discovery Today* 11:1075–84.

9. Ekins S. *Computational toxicology: Risk assessment for pharmaceutical and environmental chemicals*. Hoboken, NJ: John Wiley and Sons, 2007.

10. Ullman F, Boutellier R. 2008. A case study of lean drug discovery: From project driven research to innovation studios and process factories. *Drug Discovery Today* 13:543–50.

11. Ekins S, Swaan PW. 2004. Computational models for enzymes, transporters, channels, and receptors relevant to ADME/TOX. *Rev Comp Chem* 20:333–415.

12. Ekins S. *Computer applications in pharmaceutical research and development*. Hoboken, NJ: John Wiley and Sons, 2006.

13. Rajman I. 2008. PK/PD modelling and simulations: Utility in drug development. *Drug Discovery Today* 13:341–6.

14. Oprea TI. 2002. Current trends in lead discovery: Are we looking for the appropriate properties? *J Comp-Aided Molec Des* 16:325–34.

15. Oprea TI, Davis AM, Teague SJ, Leeson PD. 2001. Is there a difference between leads and drugs? A historical perspective. *J Chem Info Comp Sci* 41:1308–15.

16. Hupcey MAZ, Ekins S. 2007. Improving the drug selection and development process for combination devices. *Drug Discovery Today* 12:844–52.

17. Williams AJ. 2008. Internet-based tools for communication and collaboration in chemistry. *Drug Discovery Today* 13:502–6.

18. Williams AJ. 2008. A perspective of publicly accessible/open-access chemistry databases. *Drug Discovery Today* 13:495–501.

19. Hohman M, Gregory K, Chibale K, Smith PJ, Ekins S, Bunin B. Novel web-based tools combining chemistry informatics, biology, and social networking for drug discovery. submitted 2008.

20. Ekins S, Mestres J, Testa B. 2007. In silico pharmacology for drug discovery: Applications to targets and beyond. *Br J Pharmacol* 152:21–37.

21. Hansch C, Fujita T. 1964. Rho-sigma-pi analysis. A method for the correlation of biological activity and chemical structure. *J Am Chem Soc* 86:1616–26.

22. Hansch C, Hoekman D, Leo A, Weininger D, Selassie CD. 2002. Chem-bioinformatics: Comparative QSAR at the interface between chemistry and biology. *Chem Rev* 102:783–812.

23. Kurup A. 2003. C-QSAR: A database of 18,000 QSARs and associated biological and physical data. *J Comp-Aided Molec Des* 17:187–96.

24. Karelson M. *Molecular descriptors in QSAR/QSPR*. New York: Wiley-VCH, 2000.

25. Todeschini R, Consonni V. *Handbook of molecular descriptors*. Weinheim: Wiley-VCH, 2000.

26. Walters WP, Goldman BB. 2005. Feature selection in quantitative structure-activity relationships. *Curr Opin Drug Disc Devel* 8:329–33.

27. Cramer RD, Patterson DE, Bunce JD. 1988. Comparative molecular field analysis (CoMFA). 1. Effect of shape on binding of steroids to carrier proteins. *J Am Chem Soc* 110:5959–67.

28. Klebe G. 1998. Comparative molecular similarity indices analysis: CoMSIA. *Persp Drug Disc Design* 12–14:87–104.

29. Oprea TI, Matter H. 2004. Integrating virtual screening in lead discovery. *Curr Opin Chem Biol* 8:349–58.

30. Stahura FL, Bajorath J. 2004. Virtual screening methods that complement HTS. *Combin Chem High Through Screen* 7:259–69.

31. Bajorath J. 2002. Integration of virtual and high-throughput screening. *Nature Rev Drug Disc* 1:882–94.

32. Bleicher KH, Bohm HJ, Muller K, Alanine AI. 2003. Hit and lead generation: Beyond high-throughput screening. *Nature Rev* 2:369–78.

33. Evers A, Hessler G, Matter H, Klabunde T. 2005. Virtual screening of biogenic amine-binding G-protein coupled receptors: Comparative evaluation of protein- and ligand-based virtual screening protocols. *J Med Chem* 48:5448–65.

34. Zhang Q, Muegge I. Scaffold hopping through virtual screening using 2D and 3D similarity descriptors: Ranking, voting, and consensus scoring. *J Med Chem* 2006.49:1536–48.

35. Lengauer T, Lemmen C, Rarey M, Zimmermann M. 2004. Novel technologies for virtual screening. *Drug Disc Today* 9:27–34.

36. Ekins S, Mestres J, Testa B. 2007. In silico pharmacology for drug discovery: Methods for virtual ligand screening and profiling. *Br J Pharmacol* 152:9–20.

37. Mason JS, Good AC, Martin EJ. 2001. 3D pharmacophores in drug discovery. *Curr Pharm Des* 7:567–97.

38. Wermuth CG, Ganellin CRL, P, Mitscher LA. 1998. Glossary of terms used in medicinal chemistry (IUPAC Recommendations 1997). *Annu Rep Med Chem* 33:385–95.

39. Martin YC. 1992. 3D database searching in drug design. *J Med Chem* 35:2145–54.

40. Martin YC, Bures MG, Danaher EA, DeLazzer J, Lico I, Pavlik PA. 1993. A fast new approach to pharmacophore mapping and its application to dopaminergic and benzodiazepine agonists. *J Comput Aided Mol Des* 7:83–102.

41. Guner OF, Ed. *Pharmacophore, perception, development, and use in drug design.* San Diego: University International Line, 2000.

42. Langer T, Hoffman RD. *Pharmacophores and pharmacophore searches.* Weinheim: Wiley-VCH, 2006.

43. Barnum D, Greene J, Smellie A, Sprague P. 1996. Identification of common functional configurations among molecules. *J Chem Inf Comput Sci* 36:563–71.

44. Sprague PW. 1995. Automated chemical hypothesis generation and database searching with catalyst. *Perspect Drug Disc Design* 3:1–20.

45. Sprague PW, Hoffman R. CATALYST pharmacophore models and their utility as queries for searching 3D databases. In: van de Waterbeemd H, Testa B, Folkers G, Eds. *Computer-assisted lead finding and optimization.* Basel: Verlag Helvetica Chimica Acta, 1997. p. 225–40.

46. Guner O, Clement O, Kurogi Y. 2004. Pharmacophore modeling and three dimensional database searching for drug design using catalyst: Recent advances. *Curr Med Chem* 11:2991–3005.

47. Ekins S, Kholodovych V, Ai N, Sinz M, Gal J, Gera L, et al. 2008. Computational discovery of novel low micromolar human pregnane x receptor antagonists. *Molec Pharmacol* (in press).

48. Chang C, Bahadduri PM, Polli JE, Swaan PW, Ekins S. 2006. Rapid identification of P-glycoprotein substrates and inhibitors. *Drug Metab Dispos: Biolog Fate Chem* 34:1976–84.

49. Chang C, Ekins S, Bahadduri P, Swaan PW. 2006. Pharmacophore-based discovery of ligands for drug transporters. *Adv Drug Del Rev* 58:1431–50.

50. Ekins S, Johnston JS, Bahadduri P, D'Souzza VM, Ray A, Chang C, et al. 2005. In vitro and pharmacophore based discovery of novel hPEPT1 inhibitors. *Pharmaceut Res* 22:512–7.

51. Shoichet BK. 2004.Virtual screening of chemical libraries. *Nature* 432:862–5.

52. Klebe G. 2006. Virtual ligand screening: strategies, perspectives, and limitations. *Drug Disc Today* 11:580–94.

53. Cummings MD, DesJarlais RL, Gibbs AC, Mohan V, Jaeger EP. 2005. Comparison of automated docking programs as virtual screening tools. *J Med Chem* 48:962–76.

54. Charifson PS, Corkery JJ, Murcko MA, Walters WP. 1999. Consensus scoring: A method for obtaining improved hit rates from docking databases of three-dimensional structures into proteins. *J Med Chem* 42:5100–9.

55. Muegge I, Enyedy IJ. 2004. Virtual screening for kinase targets. *Curr med chem* 11:693–707.

56. Bissantz C, Bernard P, Hibert M, Rognan D. 2003. Protein-based virtual screening of chemical databases. II. Are homology models of G–Protein coupled receptors suitable targets? *Proteins* 50:5–25.

57. Evers A, Gohlke H, Klebe G. 2003. Ligand-supported homology modelling of protein binding-sites using knowledge-based potentials. *J Molec Biol* 334:327–45.

58. Evers A, Klabunde T. 2005. Structure-based drug discovery using GPCR homology modeling: Successful virtual screening for antagonists of the alpha1A adrenergic receptor. *J Med Chem* 48:1088–97.

59. Evers A, Klebe G. 2004. Successful virtual screening for a submicromolar antagonist of the neurokinin-1 receptor based on a ligand-supported homology model. *J Med Chem* 47:5381–92.

60. Kubinyi H. Success stories of computer-aided design. In: Ekins S, Ed. *Computer applications in pharmaceutical research and development*. Hoboken, NJ: John Wiley and Sons, 2006. p. 377–424.

61. Hassan F. 2001. Being a modern pharmaceutical company: New paradigms for the pharmaceutical industry. *Clin Pharmacol Therap* 69:281–5.

62. Swaan PW, Ekins S. 2005. Reengineering the pharmaceutical industry by crash-testing molecules. *Drug Disc Today* 10:1191–200.

63. Kola I, Hazuda D. 2005. Innovation and greater probability of success in drug discovery and development—from target to biomarkers. *Curr Opin Biotechnol* 16:644–6.

64. Nwaka S, Ridley RG. 2003. Virtual drug discovery and development for neglected diseases through public–private partnerships. *Nature Rev* 2:919–28.

65. Pritchard JF, Jurima-Romet M, Reimer ML, Mortimer E, Rolfe B, Cayen MN. 2003. Making better drugs: Decision gates in non-clinical drug development. *Nature Rev* 2:542–53.

66. Goldberg Arnold RJ, Kim RB, Tang B. 2005. The cost-effectiveness of argatroban treatment in heparin-induced thrombocytopenia. *Cardiol Rev* 13:1–8.

67. Caprino L, Russo P. 2006. Developing a paradigm of drug innovation: An evaluation algorithm. *Drug Disc Today* 11:999–1006.

68. Goldberg Arnold RJ. 2007. Cost-effectiveness analysis: Should it be required for drug registration and beyond? *Drug Disc Today* 12:960–5.

69. Knowles J, Gromo G. 2003. Target selection in drug discovery. *Nat Rev Drug Disc* 2:63–9.

70. Beck J, Pauker S. 1983. The Markov process in medical prognosis. *Med Decis Making* 3:419–58.

71. Lewis R, Canafax D, Pettit K, DiCesare J, Kaniecki D, Arnold R, et al. 1996. Use of Markov model for evaluating the cost-effectiveness of immunosuppressive therapies in renal transplant recipients. *Transplant Proceed* 28:2214–17.

72. O'Neill RT. 1998. Biostatistical considerations in pharmacovigilance and pharmacoepidemiology: linking quantitative risk assessment in pre-market licensure application safety data, post-market alert reports, and formal epidemiological studies. *Stat Med* 17:1851–8. discussion 9–62.

73. Vernon JA, Hughen WK, Johnson SJ. 2005. Mathematical modeling and pharmaceutical pricing: Analyses used to inform in-licensing and developmental go/No-Go decisions. *Health Care Manag Sci* 8:167–79.

74. Arnold RJ, Kim R, Tang B. 2006. The cost-effectiveness of argatroban treatment in heparin-induced thrombocytopenia: The effect of early versus delayed treatment. *Cardiol Rev* 14:7–13.

75. Arnold RJ, Kaniecki DJ, Frishman WH. 1994. Cost-effectiveness of antihypertensive agents in patients with reduced left ventricular function. *Pharmacotherapy* 14:178–84.

76. Jubran A, Gross N, Ramsdell J, Simonian R, Schuttenhelm K, Sax M, et al. 1993. Comparative cost-effectiveness analysis of theophylline and ipratropium bromide in chronic obstructive pulmonary disease. A three-center study. *Chest* 103:678–84.

77. Podrid PJ, Kowey PR, Frishman WH, Arnold RJ, Kaniecki DJ, Beck JR, et al. 1991. Comparative cost-effectiveness analysis of quinidine, procainamide, and mexiletine. *Am J Cardiol* 68:1662–7.

78. Oster G, Epstein AM. 1987. Cost-effectiveness of antihyperlipemic therapy in the prevention of coronary heart disease. The case of cholestyramine. *JAMA* 258:2381–7.

79. Krumholz HM, Pasternak RC, Weinstein MC, Friesinger GC, Ridker PM, Tosteson AN, et al. 1992. Cost effectiveness of thrombolytic therapy with streptokinase in elderly patients with suspected acute myocardial infarction. *N Engl J Med* 327:7–13.

80. Barrett BJ, Parfrey PS, Foley RN, Detsky AS. 1994. An economic analysis of strategies for the use of contrast media for diagnostic cardiac catheterization. *Med Decis Making* 14:325–35.

81. Goldberg Arnold R, Kaniecki D, Tak Piech C, Puder K. An economic evaluation of HMG-CoA reductase inhibitors for cholesterol reduction in the primary prevention of coronary heart disease. 11th International Conference on Pharmacoepidemiology. Montreal, 1995.

82. Goldman L, Weinstein MC, Goldman PA, Williams LW. 1991. Cost-effectiveness of HMG–CoA reductase inhibition for primary and secondary prevention of coronary heart disease. *JAMA* 265:1145–51.

83. Iversen LF, Brzozoxski M, Hastrup S, Hubbard R, Kastrup JS, Larsen IK, et al. 1997. Characterization of the allosteric binding pocket of human liver fructose-1,6-bisphosphatease by protein crystallography and inhibitor activity studies. *Protein Sci* 6:971–82.

84. Thorn CF, Klein TE, Altman RB. 2005. PharmGKB: The pharmacogenetics and pharmacogenomics knowledge base. *Methods Mol Biol* 311:179–91.

85. Arnold R, Kotsanos J. 1999. Proceedings of the Advisory Panel Meeting and Conference on Pharmacoeconomic Issues: Panel 3: Methodological issues in conducting pharmacoeconomic evaluations—retrospective and claims database studies. *Value in Health* 2:82–7.

86. Chadwick A, Moore J, Hupcey MAZ, Purshouse R. Improving the pharmaceutical R & D Process: How simulation can support management decision making. In: Ekins S, Ed. *Computer applications in pharmaceutical research and development*. Hoboken, NJ: John Wiley & Sons, 2006. p. 247–73.

87. Cohen CM. 2003. A path to improved pharmaceutical productivity. *Nature Rev* 2:751–3.

88. Berry DA. 2006. Bayesian clinical trials. *Nature Rev Drug Disc* 5:27–36.

89. Chadwick A, Hajek M. 2004. Learning to improve the decision-making process in research. *Drug Disc Today* 9:251–7.

90. Chadwick AT. *Method and systems of enhancing the effectiveness and success of research and development.* Georgetown, KY: PA Knowledge Limited, 2005.

91. Tang Z, Taylor MJ, Lisboa P, Dyas M. 2005. Quantitative risk modelling for new pharmaceutical compounds. *Drug Disc Today* 10:1520–6.

92. Bree RL, Arnold RJ, Pettit KG, Kaniecki DJ, O'Haeri C, LaFrance ND, et al. Use of a decision-analytic model to support the use of a new oral US contrast agent in patients with abdominal pain. *Acad Radiol* 2001.8:234–42.

93. Ekins S, Shimada J, Chang C. 2006. Application of data mining approaches to drug delivery. Adv Drug Deliv Rev 58:1409–30.

94. Borchardt RT, Kerns.E.H., Lipinski CA, Thakker DR, Wang B, Eds. *Pharmaceutical profiling in drug discovery for lead selection.* Arlington,VA: AAPS, 2004.

95. Katzung BG. *Basic and clinical pharmacology.* San Francisco: Lange Medical Books/ McGraw-Hill, 2001.

96. Spilker B. *Multinational drug companies: Issues in discovery and development.* New York: Raven Press, 1989.

97. Thummel K, Shen DD. Design and optimization of dosage regimens: Pharmacokinetic data. In: Hardman JG, Limbird LE, Gilman AG, Eds. *Goodman & Gilman's the pharmaceutical basis of therapeutics.* New York: McGraw-Hill, 2001. p. 1924–2023.

98. White R. A comprehensive strategy for ADME screening in drug discovery. In: Borchardt RT, Kerns EH, Lipinski CA, Thakker DR, Wang B, Eds. *Pharmaceutical profiling in drug discovery for lead selection:* AAPS Press, 2004. p. 431–50.

99. Young SS, Gombar VK, Emptage MR, Cariello NF, Lambert C. 2002. Mixture deconvolution and analysis of Ames mutagenicity data. *Chemo Intell Lab Sys* 60:5–11.

100. Chinnasamy A, Sung WK, Mittal A. 2005. Protein structure and fold prediction using tree-augmented naive Bayesian classifier. *J Bioinform Comput Biol* 3:803–19.

16 Speculations on the Future Challenges and Value of Pharmacoeconomics

J. Jaime Caro, Denis Getsios,
and Rachael L. Fleurence

CONTENTS

16.1 SURVIVAL REQUIRES RELEVANCE

Pharmacoeconomics is a young field—the term itself did not exist when most of the authors of this book began their careers. And yet, it may die as quickly as it arose because we have largely failed to address the questions that actual decision makers ask. If pharmacoeconomics is to have as vibrant a future as has been its short past, it must meet the substantial challenges posed in providing the information that is really needed.

Pharmacoeconomics began as an applied field. It was an urgent practical response to a torrent of new products—especially pharmaceuticals—reaching the market at an unprecedented rate just before the turn of the century, and to the growing perception that healthcare budgets were being strained as a consequence of pharmaceuticals expenditures outpacing those in other healthcare sectors. Manufacturers were suddenly facing requests from payers to justify the price of their products, and they turned to an assortment of clinical experts, decision analysts, and economists for help in providing answers. Initially, most of these justifications were not guided by theory. They mainly involved documentation of the clinical effects—often in broader, more patient-oriented terms—and some attempt at quantifying the expected costs.[1,2] These were early examples of what came to be known as "cost-consequences" analysis and were in line with emerging recommendations for the evaluation of healthcare programs.[3]

Before long, however, a theoretical structure was imposed on the field.[4] This theory holds that the role of healthcare systems is to maximize collective health across the society within a fixed budget and that the worth of any new intervention can be appraised by estimating how much additional cost is required to produce an additional unit of health.[5] Furthermore, the practitioners proposed that health should be measured in quality-adjusted life years (QALYs)—a unit that conflates life expectancy with the expected quality of that life relative to some undefined "perfect" health.[6] Neither concept was built on strong theoretical foundations,[7,8] nor did they have an empirical basis.[9]

More importantly, the work guided by new notions did not respond to the decision-makers' actual questions.[10,11] Real decision-makers were not seeking to maximize aggregate health—they were trying to deal with illness and its consequences; they were bewildered by the unfathomable QALY, which was not something anyone pursued, measured, or valued before this. Worse, even after they grasped the ideas, they discovered that the resulting efficiency estimate didn't indicate whether the intervention was worth it.[12] They were no further ahead and now needed yet another element—a cost-effectiveness threshold[13]—that no one could tell them where to obtain or even what it was.[14] Thresholds that were and continue to be put forward have been arbitrary, inconstant[15] and are out of line with exploratory research on society's valuation of health outcomes.[16] The academics had responded to a question that kept their work within the safe confines of what they believed they could do, but did not address the majority of decision-makers' concerns.

16.2   A MORE MATURE FIELD

To survive and gain traction, pharmacoeconomics must mature and deal with the actual problems faced in making resource allocation decisions. This will require estimating the total additional costs an intervention will accrue in the population of patients who will be affected, not the per patient costs in some abstract context. The analyses will place much more emphasis on the near term, which is the time period of most relevance to actual decisions, and will have to consider how quickly and which patients take up the intervention. The analyses will call for using real cost offsets that can be expected by the healthcare system (not by other sectors), rather than hypothetical ones that might occur under ideal circumstances. It will be important to consider what interventions might the new ones actually replace and to what extent.

On the benefits side, similar questions will need to be answered. The benefits that can be expected with the intervention, in reality, for the full population of patients who will actually use it (not per patient), over the near term, with realistic estimates of the uptake will have to be estimated based on real data.

It will be important to compare effect profile and cost impact with those of the other interventions available for the condition at issue. In most instances, this will mean that not only new technologies are evaluated, but also the full array of available interventions. Then, the analysis will need to take up the question of what existing interventions would need to be given up to cover the new one, or what level of budget increases will be required if nothing is removed. Most important, new interventions will need to fit into the relevant practice guidelines and what effect the new intervention will have on the guideline.

There will be several consequences of the maturation of pharmacoeconomics, not only methodological developments, but also effects on other research areas such as efficacy clinical trials, and even on the structure of pharmaceutical companies.

16.3 CONSEQUENCES

16.3.1 MODEL SOPHISTICATION

Despite their moniker, current "decision-analytic" models tend not to address the actual decisions that need to be made. They do not contrast various realistic potential scenarios of use of a new intervention. Instead, they engage in the very artificial comparison of all patients using the new intervention versus all using some alternative (e.g., the most common one), and all starting at the same time. The models are typically conceptualized in terms of health states, that is, Markov models (see Chapter 4, Markov modeling), even though much of what happens in medicine is an event, so they don't correspond to what the clinicians are seeing in practice. But, the biggest problem is that they are set up in terms of the population as a whole ("cohort" models). This creates awkward problems because populations are not homogeneous and applying probabilities based on the average profile yields incorrect results. Moreover, the characteristics of the population change over time both because of the passage of time itself and due to the successive fragmentation of the population into subcohorts according to the characteristics themselves. It is the riskier subgroups that tend to transition to other states, leaving the original state with a different mix of risk factors, which is difficult to compute and integrate with the time changes. In the great majority of cases, analysts have opted to ignore this thorny problem. Thus, as the model analysis progresses, the cohorts depart further and further from reality. It is no wonder that models continue to be regarded with misgivings by decision-makers.

To handle real decision problems, models will need to be considerably more sophisticated than those being commonly produced today.[17] Conceptually, the models will have to incorporate all the relevant aspects of the decision problem—it will not be acceptable to select a cohort Markov technique and then force everything to fit the state-transition idea, leaving out key portions that are not amenable to the technique. The vast majority of models will simulate at the individual level, where risk factors and their evolution, competing risks, and natural variability can be taken into account properly. Suitably constructed, these models are more transparent, more readily checked for errors, and easier to convey to nontechnical audiences. Just as important, they allow a broader array of questions to be answered, such as what is the optimal mix of patients to treat, what might be the impact of suboptimal compliance, and what are the consequences of risk-sharing agreements between manufacturers and payers. The last remaining concern with these—that they require substantial power of calculation[18]—is already largely moot[19] but will surely disappear with continuing progress in computing. In any case, as the field opens up to other fields that have been constructing simulations for much longer, the models will be built to be more efficient and the implementation of variance reduction techniques[20] will further reduce computational needs.

As the activities and methods of health technology assessment agencies come under increasing scrutiny by stakeholders, including patients, their doctors, and families, it will become more and more unacceptable to declare that only certain modeling software is sanctioned, even if the choices made available force models to be so unrealistic that they do not properly inform the decisions.[21] The agencies will be forced to carry out their work using the best tools available, rather than whatever simplistic ones they have elected to train on. The agency's lack of expertise in its own areas of competence will not be tolerated by the public or even the healthcare community. On the side of manufacturers, pressure will increase not only to collect the appropriate data to populate these simulations, but to make these data available to scrutiny.

16.3.2 THE END OF THE QALY?

For more than two decades now, the predominant approach to pharmacoeconomics evaluation has been founded on the idea that the purpose of pharmaceuticals (indeed, of any health care) is to maximize total health across the population given scarce resources and that, to ensure this, a universal measure of health is required. By far the most common measure used in this pursuit is the aggregate of life expectancy and average predicted quality of that life—the QALY. Despite considerable methodological critique of this construct,[22,23] its proponents have been steadfast in its support on the grounds that "we have nothing better."[24,25]

This ultimate rationale for a potentially flawed measure cannot possibly stand much longer. Surely, that cannot be our field's collective response. The growing awareness outside dogmatic methodological circles of the implications of the QALY and the unreasonable decisions it can foster will result in outright revolt. It will not be acceptable to defend its use as a necessary evil, especially when it is not needed.

Recognition of the unethical nature of the QALY, which equates the value of life with the product of its expected duration and quality, should be enough to eradicate it. Use of the QALY as the scale of value implies discrimination against people with characteristics that diminish their quality of life or their life expectancy. Among these are those that our societies have legally banned from being used to discriminate: age, sex, disability, race, social status, and so on. It is immaterial that a QALY gained is valued equally regardless of who gains it if some people just cannot gain as many QALYs through no fault of their own.

If this immoral aspect is not enough to end the QALY's reign, then the fact that its use does not meet the requirements that led to the measure should remove the last excuse for it. Even if the QALY is perfectly computed and the questionable ethics are ignored, the cost per QALY ratio does not provide for efficient allocation of resources, fails to respect any budget limit, and does not even guarantee that aggregate health is maximized. The incremental cost-effectiveness ratio does not indicate what should be done—it isn't even clear whether a particular value is reasonable, or even how to go about determining whether it is reasonable. The common practice of referencing it to an arbitrary threshold does not improve the guidance provided and, in any case, provides no indication of which resources should be reallocated to cover the new intervention. If coverage is based on this capricious reference then the budget will simply increase.[26] Moreover, given that the incremental ratio is computed within a particular therapeutic area by comparison with an alternative intervention and not across areas, the result may support an intervention in an area that is providing very few QALYs (because few people are affected and the total cost is high) and thus may lead to fewer aggregate QALYs than the same investment in another area where more QALYs are produced (because many more people are affected but the total costs are no higher).

Given its discriminatory basis, its inability to consistently and reasonably guide decisions, and its theoretical weakness, the QALY will be relegated to the history of the early days of our field. In its place will be a return to consideration of the full profile of consequences (see Chapter 8, Budgetary Impact Analysis), with some explicit valuation of these profiles by citizens' committees. Decision-makers will consider efficiency as one factor, but this will be explicitly recognized as only the relative efficiency within a therapeutic area.

16.3.3   DEVELOPMENT OF THE EFFICIENCY FRONTIER APPROACH

The recently published first edition of the Institute for Quality and Efficiency in Health Care (IQWiG) Methods for Economic Evaluation in Germany[27] brings to the forefront the explicit depiction and use of the efficiency frontier approach. This technique involves assessing the interventions available in a given therapeutic area and plotting the value of their health effects against their net total costs. The resulting graph presents the current status of the market for that therapeutic area and indicates the relative efficiency of one intervention to another. The most efficient ones—those not dominated by others—form the efficiency frontier. This plot communicates to decision-makers what they are currently obtaining for investments in that area and reveals whether, and how, more can be obtained with that expenditure. In addition, the price requested by newer interventions for that condition can be assessed in terms of how consistent they are with the ongoing efficiency in that area.

While the efficiency frontier (Figure 16.1) does not pretend to address broader issues of resource allocation across the healthcare system, it does provide useful information in a clear, concise manner and, thus, can help guide decision-makers. Moreover, if a given jurisdiction wishes to explicitly assess how its citizens value a given profile of effects relative to those in other areas, this information can be readily incorporated to further appraise the worthiness of investments in that area. By the same token, should the decision makers be willing to express the amount they feel

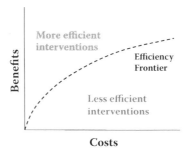

FIGURE 16.1   The Efficiency Frontier Plot.

is reasonable to spend for a given condition, this can be included in the efficiency frontier plot and more precise guidance will result.

As experience with the efficiency frontier grows, health authorities, as well as researchers, will realize its benefits and embrace the approach as more reasonable and tenable than the current one. Already, several jurisdictions beyond Germany are looking to implement their own versions of this technique. Much methodological development still needs to happen, however. This ranges from quantification and display of uncertainty to regression approaches for estimating the relation of declining efficiency to growing benefits (and costs). Valuation of the benefits on a cardinal scale will also require careful development.

16.3.4   More Extensive Validation and Verification

A major problem with many of the models that underlie today's economic evaluations is that they undergo very little validation. This is, to some extent, understandable given the very short timelines that are typical and the tendency for models to be for one-time use only. The result is that the models are error-prone and unreliable. Until now, this has not been very noticeable because no one has the time to check the models, and mistakes remain undiscovered. This is exacerbated by the practice of one-off models, developed and used over a brief interval, and then discarded, with new models being created to answer similar questions, often with little reference to previous work beyond a gross comparison of the cost-effectiveness estimates. This situation cannot continue, however. With increased scrutiny of decisions based on health technology assessments, errors will come to light and prove costly for all. What little confidence in models has been building among stakeholders will be rapidly lost and difficult to regain. It makes no sense to continue to construct one or more original models for every new product only to discard them as soon as the immediate analyses are complete.

The solution to this problem is to develop models with long-term use in mind. Instead of custom models built in a few months for one evaluation, we will see more investment in enduring models that can serve multiple purposes over years.[28,29] These ongoing models will become more sophisticated and comprehensive and eventually each therapeutic area will have a small set of well developed models available for evaluations, validated not only in terms of the integrity of mathematical formulae and calculations, but also in terms of their clinical appropriateness and predictive accuracy.

The more durable models may be commercial in nature, but it is likely that some jurisdictions will choose to develop and maintain their own in order to have more control over what happens to them and gain confidence in their predictions. Manufacturers would then be forced to submit their data to those models and abide by the resulting estimates. Consultancies and academic groups will also want to build these kinds of models and ensure they are high quality so that they can profit from their more solid reputation. Whether the business tactic will be to license the use of the models or use them to draw full consulting projects remains to be determined.

Given the much longer horizon and the intended uses for the tools, it will be imperative to validate them properly and there will be time to do so. This process will extend beyond the technical validation commonly implemented today. There will be more attention given to ensuring face validity—that the model reflects the disease and its management at a reasonable level. A full detailed influence diagram will be developed to guide the model design, with input from appropriate specialists. In addition, the technical validation will be much more extensive and will follow quality assurance standards, including those for documentation and reporting.

The biggest change, however, will be that researchers will engage in true predictive validation of their models. Datasets will be sought and many will be created expressly for the purpose of validation. Registries and other cohort studies will be designed so that they can be used to validate the related models, and clinical trial data will become more available for this purpose. This will be driven by reimbursement and regulatory authorities who will demand that this take place. Indeed, validation will become an ongoing process as models are continuously improved and adjusted to reflect new understandings of a particular disease and the appearance of novel interventions.

Not only will validation become comprehensive, it will also be standard practice to publish the results and the full details will be available online. A model without published validation will not be considered reliable enough for actual decisions.

16.3.5 MARKET-ORIENTED CLINICAL TRIALS

Despite two decades of pharmacoeconomics, clinical trials remain firmly focused on efficacy, with some attention to safety. This will remain the norm until regulatory authorities begin demanding that data be more relevant to the reimbursement and usage decisions that must be made before the product is marketed. With reimbursement authorities increasingly challenging the results of models based on flimsy data, extensive assumptions and even expert opinion, there will be increasing pressure to better leverage the enormous investments made in clinical trials and provide timely, market-ready information. This will involve some relaxing of the strict requirements for blinding, placebo-control, and so on, and improved analytic techniques to mitigate potential increases in bias.

Already, there is a strong movement toward effectiveness trials that contrast actual scenarios of practice.[30] These comparative effectiveness trials will massively strain resources, however, if they are not implemented efficiently. New designs that integrate Bayesian methodologies and pharmacoeconomic data will become more common. Adaptive designs used to speed up drug development[31] will be put to pharmacoeconomic use and simulations built to understand the trial design[32] will seamlessly transition to market-ready models.

Even before trials regularly implement pharmacoeconomic aspects, access to individual level data will be increasingly granted to analysts seeking to understand and quantify complex relationships between patient characteristics, time, compliance, and treatment effects. It is extremely wasteful to spend millions conducting these trials only to obtain a statistically significant estimate of efficacy and then relegate the data collected to storage. Much can be learned by taking full advantage of the wealth of available data. Doing so will also go hand in hand with adoption of simulation techniques capable of meaningfully accounting for these relationships.

16.3.6 IMPACT ON PHARMACEUTICAL COMPANY STRUCTURE

As the drug development process evolves to become more attuned to the needs of the reimbursement authorities and those of the market, the structure of pharmaceutical companies will also be transformed.[33] Pharmacoeconomics and related functions will move from the outskirts to the core of research and development and the structural separation between pre-approval work and market activities will be removed. Medical affairs are a strong candidate for this expanded, more central role.[34]

16.4 CONCLUSION

For pharmacoeconomics to survive, let alone prosper, it must rapidly mature into a discipline that addresses the needs of decision-makers, and does so with well-founded approaches. This will require development and adoption of new methods and abandoning those that have little basis for carrying on. In particular, the use of the cost per QALY ratio as the key to reimbursement decisions will fade away, to be replaced by more direct methods that consider fully the relevant aspects of the difficult decisions that must be made. Although efficiency will remain an input, it will be confined to the much smaller role of ensuring that prices are reasonably consistent within a therapeutic area. Models will need to be increasingly sophisticated to be able to inform this broader array of questions. They will need to be extensively and continuously validated so that decision-makers trust the results enough to defend the decisions that rely on them.

These developments will pose significant challenges that need to be met for pharmacoeconomics to retain its relevance. As with any field, advancement in methods is essential, but pharmacoeconomics is faced with the more unique challenge of training and education in methods whose development is ongoing.

REFERENCES

1. Caro JJ, Trinadade E, C.E.T.S. Evaluation of low vs. high osmolar contrast media. Technical Report. Quebec: Gouvernement du Quebec, 1989.

2. Caro JJ, Trindade E, McGregor M. 1992. The cost-effectiveness of replacing high-osmolality with low-osmolality contrast media. *Am J Roent.* 159:869–74.
3. Drummond, MF, O'Brien, BJ, Stoddart, GL. *Methods for the Economic Evaluation of Health Care Program,* 1st ed. Oxford University Press. 1987.
4. Weinstein MC, Stason WB. 1977. Foundations of cost-effectiveness analysis for health and medical practices. *N Engl J Med* 296:716–21.
5. Gold MR, Russell LB, Siegel JE (Ed.). *Cost-effectiveness in health and medicine.* New York: Oxford Univ. Press. 1996.
6. Brouwer WBF, Koopmanschap MA. 2000. On the economic foundations of CEA. Ladies and gentlemen, take your positions! *J Health Econ* 19:439–59.
7. Broome J. QALYs. 1993. *J Public Econ* 50:149–63.
8. Birch S, Donaldson C. 2003. Valuing the benefits and costs of health care programmes: Where's the 'extra' in extra–welfarism? *Soc Sci Med* 56:1121–33.
9. Nord E. *Cost-Value Analysis in Health Care.* Cambridge University Press: Cambridge. 1999.
10. McGregor M. 2006. What decision-makers want and what they have been getting. *ViH* 9:181–5.
11. Williams I, Bryan S. 2007. Understanding the limited impact of economic evaluation in health care resource allocation: A conceptual framework. *Health Pol* 80:135–43.
12. McGregor M, Caro JJ. 2006. QALYs: Are They Helpful to Decision Makers? *PharmacoEconomics* 24:947–52.
13. McCabe C, Claxton K, Culyer AJ. 2008. The NICE cost-effectiveness threshold: What it is and what that means. *PharmacoEconomics* 26:733–44.
14. Birch SGA. 2006. Information created to evade reality (ICER). Things we should not look to for answers. *PharmacoEconomics* 24:1121–31.
15. Weinstein MC. 2008. How much are Americans willing to pay for a quality-adjusted life year? *Med Care* 46:343–5.
16. Evans C, Tavakoli M, Crawford B. 2004. Use of quality adjusted life years gained as benchmarks in economic evaluations: A critical appraisal. *Health Care Manage Sci* 7:43–9.
17. Eddy DM. 2006. Accuracy versus transparency in pharmacoeconomic modeling. Finding the right balance. *PharmacoEconomics* 24:837–44.
18. Griffin S, Claxton K, Sculpher M. 2006. Probabilistic analysis and computationally expensive models: Necessary and required. *ViH* 9:244–52.
19. Caro JJ, Getsios D, Moller J. 2007. Regarding probabilistic analysis and computation all expensive models: Necessary and required? *ViH* 10:317–8.
20. L'Ecuyer P. Efficiency improvement and variance reduction. *Proceedings of the 26th conference on winter simulation,* Orlando, FL, 1994: Society for Computer Simulation International, 122–132.
21. Getsios D, Migliaccio-Walle K, Caro JJ. 2007. NICE cost-effectiveness appraisal of cholinesterase inhibitors. Was the right question posed? Were the best tools used? *Pharmacoeconomics* 25:997–1006.
22. Gyrd-Hansen D. 2005. Willingness to pay for a QALY: Theoretical and methodological issues. *PharmacoEconomics* 23:423–32.
23. Robinson R. 1999. Limits to rationality: Economics, economists, and priority setting. *Health Pol* 49:13–26.
24. Chong C. 2003. QALYs: The best option so far. *CMAJ* 168:1394–5.
25. Fryback DG, Methodological issues in measuring health status and health-related quality of life for population health measures: A brief overview of the "HALY" family of measures. Appendix C in Field MG, Gold MR, Eds. *Summarizing population health: Directions for the development and application of population metrics.* National Academies Press, 1998. 85 pages.

26. Gafni A, Birch S. 2003. Inclusion of drugs in provincial drug benefit programs: Should "reasonable decisions" lead to uncontrolled growth in expenditures? *Can Med Assoc J* 168:849–51.

27. Institute for Quality and Efficiency in Health Care (IQWiG). Methods for Assessment of the Relation of Benefits to Costs in the German Statutory Health Care System. Available at http://www.iqwig.de/download/08–10–14_Methods_of_the_Relation_of_Benefits_ to_ Costs_v_1_1.pdf. Accessed: January 29, 2009.

28. Eddy DM, Schlessinger L. 2003. Archimides: A trial-validated model of diabetes. *Diabetes Care* 26:3093–101.

29. Palmer AJ, Roze S, Valentine WJ, Minshall ME, Foos V, Lurati FM, Lammert M, Spinas GA. 2004. The CORE Diabetes Model: Projecting long-term clinical outcomes, costs, and cost-effectiveness of interventions in diabetes mellitus (types 1 and 2) to support clinical and reimbursement decision-making. *Curr Med Res Opin* Suppl 1:S5–26.

30. Luce BR, Paramore LC, Parasuraman B, Liljas B, de Lissovoy G. 2008. Can managed care organizations partner with manufacturers for comparative effectiveness research? *Am J Manag Care* 14:149–156.

31. Coffey CS, Kairalla JA. 2008. Adaptive clinical trials: Progress and challenges. *Drugs R D* 9:229–42.

32. Caro JJ. Role of simulation to set up the design and to guide the adaptation process in Issues in Comparative Effectiveness Research: Seeking Efficiency Exploring Bayesian Adaptive Trial Methods. Short Course at 30th Annual Meeting of the Society for Medical Decision Making—Comparative Effectiveness Research: Practice and Policy. Challenges and Opportunities Oct 18 – Oct 22 2008, Philadelphia. Available at: www.smdm.org.

33. Caro JJ. Using Pharmacoeconomic Studies to Guide Drug Development in SPECTRUM—Pharmaceutical Industry Dynamics 1996. 124:1–11. Available at: http://www.decisionresources.com/ stellent/groups/public/documents/wfp/IndustryReports. hcsp?Topic=IndustryDynamics.

34. Wolin J, Ayers PM, Chan EK. 2001. The emerging role of medical affairs within the modern pharmaceutical company. *Drug Inf J* 35:547–5.

Index

A

Absorbing Markov model, 51–54
Actuarial analysis, 202, 207
Administrative claims databases
  description of, 64
  outcomes analyses using, 74–75, 100
Agency for Healthcare Research and Quality, 63, 176, 203
Agent-based simulation, 29–30
Aggregation, 135–136, 140
Analogy, 145
Anchor-based approaches, 158
ARBITER, 218
Argumentation modes, 145
Atherosclerosis Risk in Communities database, 74
Atopic dermatitis, cost-of-illness analysis of, 38–41
Australia
  human papillomavirus vaccine in, 182–183
  pharmacoeconomics in, 176–178, 180–181, 194
Austria, 165
Authority, 145

B

Baltic, 165
Base-case analysis, 167
Bayesian networks, 218–220
Belgium, 165
Bentham, Jeremy, 142
Best-case analysis, 164
Beta distributions, 172
Bias, 76–77
Binary chance nodes, 22, 24
Bivariate sensitivity analysis, 26, 164, 168–169
Branch and node decision tree. See Decision tree
Brazil, 165
Budget impact analysis
  calculations, 116
  comparators, 114–115
  cost-effectiveness analysis model and, 115
  data sources, 115–116
  definition of, 113
  guidelines for, 112–117
  health condition, 113
  model, 115
  outcome of, 113
  reporting of results, 116–117
  target population of, 113–114
  time horizon of, 114
Burden-of-illness, 37

C

Canada
  human papillomavirus vaccine in, 183–184
  pharmacoeconomics in, 165, 178, 180–181
Canadian Agency for Drugs and Technologies in Health, 178
Caregiver-reported outcomes, 6
Centers for Medicare and Medicaid Services, 176
Central limit theorem, 172
Cerner Health Facts, 61, 72
Cervarix, 182–184
Cervical cancer
  claims database application to, 65
  Markov model of, 55–57
China, 165
Claims databases, 64–67, 74
Clinical equivalence, 85, 87–88, 90–92
Clinical trial evidence
  equivalence trial as source of, 87–89
  non-inferiority trial as source of, 88–89
  optimizing of, 85–86
  sources of, 86–89
  superiority trial as source of, 85–87
Clinical trials, market-oriented, 233–234
Clinician-reported outcomes, 6
Clopidogrel, 204
Code of ethics, 3–4
Coin flipping, as stochastic process, 48
Common Drug Review (Canada), 178
Comparative effectiveness, 176, 188–189, 191
Comparative molecular field analysis, 211
Comparative molecular similarity indices analysis, 211
Computers
  decision making uses of, 214–221
  molecular design aided by, 211–214
  pharmaceutical industry uses of, 210
  pharmacokinetic/pharmacodynamic modeling and simulations, 210
  quantitative structure-activity relationships, 210–214
Confounding bias, 77
Construct validity, 155–156
Consultation form, 11–13
Content validity, 155
Convergent validity, 155